A Complete Plain-English Guide to Living with a Spinal Cord Injury

A Complete Plain-English Guide to Living with a Spinal Cord Injury

✦

Valuable Information From a Survivor

Carolyn Boyles

iUniverse, Inc.
New York Lincoln Shanghai

A Complete Plain-English Guide to Living with a Spinal Cord Injury
Valuable Information From a Survivor

iUniverse books may be ordered through booksellers or by contacting:

iUniverse
2021 Pine Lake Road, Suite 100
Lincoln, NE 68512
www.iuniverse.com
1-800-Authors (1-800-288-4677)

ISBN: 978-0-595-45864-6 (pbk)
ISBN: 978-0-595-70590-0 (cloth)
ISBN: 978-0-595-90166-1 (ebk)

Printed in the United States of America

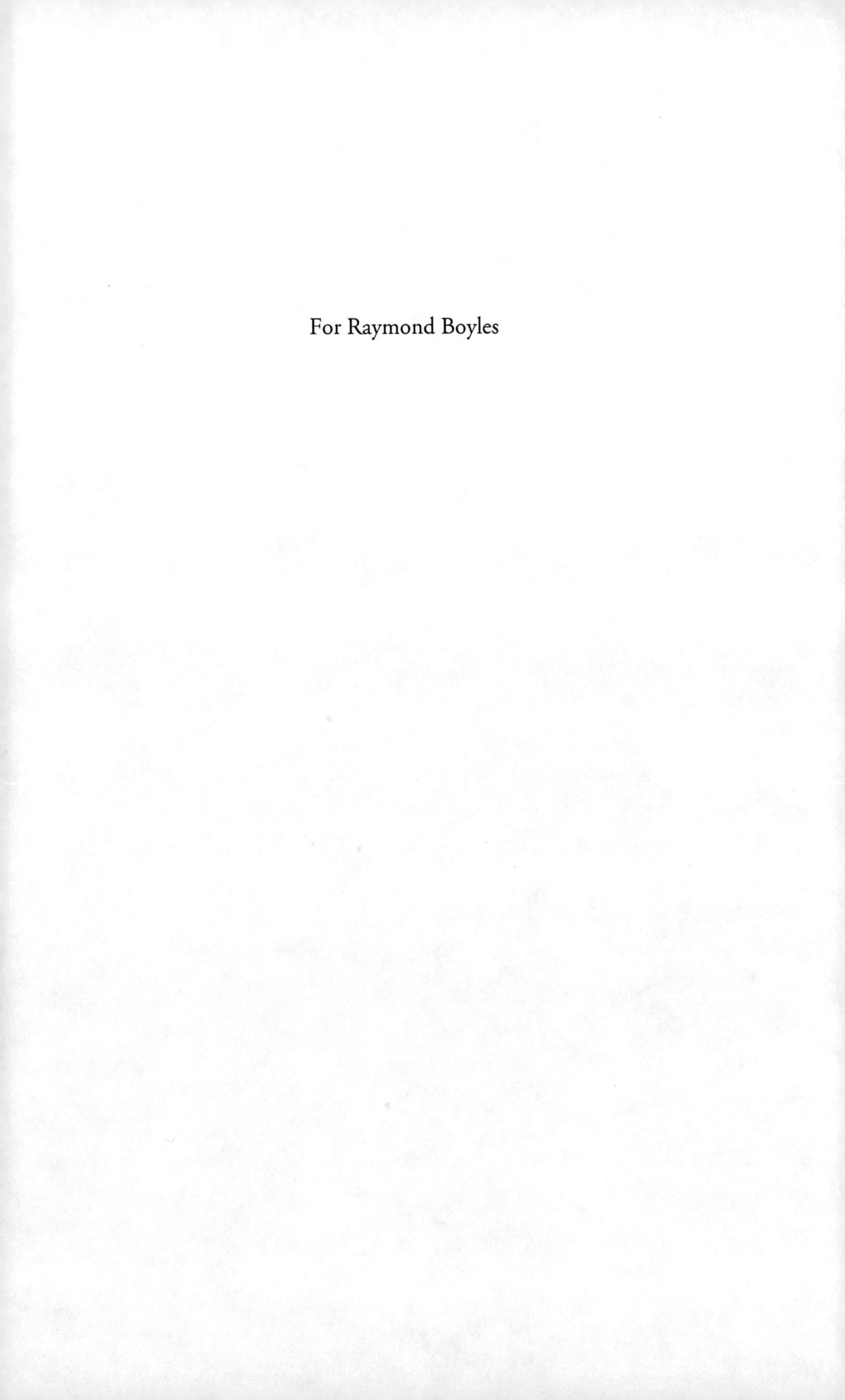

For Raymond Boyles

Contents

Understanding Your Injury

People Don't Treat Me the Same Way After the Accident

The Questions Nobody Wants to Ask After a Spinal Cord Injury

Getting Help and Quality of Life Improvement

Final Thoughts

Acknowledgments

I want to thank my husband, Raymond, for always being there for me every day since my accident in 1994.

I also want to thank Brett Herndon, Terry Lowe, and my family and friends for encouraging me to follow through writing this book after I had the initial idea.

I want to thank Dr. Ramona Bates for her time during the research phase of this book.

I could not have done this without the help of the wonderful people at iUniverse.

I had invaluable help from the staff at the medical school library at the University of Arkansas for Medical Sciences during the research phase of this book.

I want to thank Cheryl Vines, the Executive Director of the Arkansas Spinal Cord Commission, and the Commission staff for their help and encouragement during the research and writing of this book.

Finally, I am grateful for the company of my Maine Coon cats, Max and Brother, for keeping me sane while I sat at the computer for the long hours on end writing this book.

Abbreviations

aka: Also Known As
CDC: Center for Disease Control
CT Scan: Computed or Computerized Tomography Scan
EMT: Emergency Medical Technician
ENT: Ear, Nose and Throat Specialist
MRI: Magnetic Resonance Imaging
NSCIA: National Spinal Cord Injury Association
paraphrase: a statement or remark explained in other words or another way, so as to simplify or clarify its meaning.[1]
PTSD: Post Traumatic Stress Disorder
sic: This indicates that an incorrect or unusual spelling, phrase, punctuation, and/or other preceding quoted material has been produced verbatim from the quoted original and is not a transcription error.[2]
SCI: Spinal Cord Injury
TDD: Telecommunications Device for the Deaf
TTY: Teletypewriter for the Deaf
V: Voice telephone number
verbatim: means an exact reproduction of a sentence, phrase, quote or other sequence of text form one source to another. The same words appear in exactly the same order, with no paraphrasing, substitution, or abbreviation of any kind, not even trivial changes that wouldn't have affected the meaning in any way.[3]

Preface

Humpty Dumpty sat on a wall.
Humpty Dumpty had a great fall.
All the king's horses and all the king's men
Couldn't put Humpty together again.—
Mother Goose Nursery Rhyme

Quadriplegia: caused by damage to the spinal cord at a high level (cervical spine) or the brain. The injury causes the victim to lose use of the arms and legs. The condition is also termed tetraplegia. Both terms mean "paralysis of four limbs."[1]

Quadriplegic: a person who is paralyzed in both arms and both legs, sometimes shortened to "quad" in conversation. Also called Tetraplegic. I have never heard of anyone being called a "tet."

Paraplegia: a condition in which the lower part of a person's body is paralyzed and cannot willfully function. It is usually the result of a spinal cord injury or a congenital condition.... [2]

Paraplegic: a person who is paralyzed in the lower part of the body, sometimes shortened to "para" in conversation.

A spinal cord injury can happen to *anyone*. Most people would not or did not believe this until the late Christopher Reeve was injured in 1995. "A celebrity with a spinal cord injury? Wow, it really can happen to anyone!" was the general public's reaction. A spinal cord injury was certainly the last thing I ever expected to have happen to me.

I am a C3-7 incomplete quadriplegic after an auto accident in 1994, and complications in 2004 and 2006. I was originally a C5-7 incomplete quadriplegic.

A spinal cord injury is an "odd duck" as a medical condition. Each injury is unique. Not all spinal cord injuries follow standard medical protocols. Mine sure didn't. More details on my injury later in the book.

And even years later when I applied for state-level benefits years later, the medical evidence of my spinal cord injury was considered "soft" because again, I did not match "standard" medical protocols.

To learn to adapt to having a spinal cord injury, I sought solace in books written by and about spinal cord injury survivors. But I found I could not relate to their situations. So many of them were more severely paralyzed than I was.

I continued my research years later once the Internet had developed to the point where it was useful. In 1994 the Internet barely existed. When I started my research in 1995 there was, if you will pardon the pun, "virtually" nothing out there. I read medical journal articles and everything else I could find related to spinal cord injury. I was going to say "get my hands on" instead of find, but I realized it was a poor choice of words under the circumstances.

By 2005, I was starting to see people posting on spinal cord injury support forums who were in the same boat I was ten years ago. Desperately looking for others they could relate to, and for information about living with a particular type of incomplete spinal cord injury.

Much has changed between 1994 and 2007. Awareness of spinal cord injury has increased. Surgical techniques have improved above and beyond what they were in 1994. New lighter weight wheelchairs are on the market. Time spent in rehabilitation is shorter; both because of advances in techniques, and as a result of HMO regulations. More is known about how the human body's functions go wrong after a spinal cord injury. The Internet is well established, and full of information on spinal cord injury.

But still "the book" about spinal cord injury I have been looking for all these years had not been written. I found some excellent books that were close to what I was looking for. But they were written by medical professionals, not by actual injurees. I wanted a "blend" of the factual information from a medical perspective, and a guide from someone who has been through a spinal cord injury.

I couldn't find "the book" I wanted, so I decided to write it. Many of the topics covered in this book are the same as in other books about spinal cord injury, such as pressure sores. Others are not, like dealing with survivor guilt.

Understanding a spinal cord injury requires basic information, a framework to put that information in, and an understanding of the emotional aspects of the injury. My original focus in writing this book was to write a book for spinal cord injurees like myself who can walk with the assistance of crutches and/or a walker.

But I wanted to write something more than just "my story." I wanted to give people information they could really use. So I expanded the focus of the book to cover the variety of spinal cord syndromes seen in incomplete spinal cord injuries.

Then I realized that the same information could be useful to those in wheelchairs as well. What about family members and friends of the spinal cord injured? They needed a "handbook" that wouldn't take a lot of time or concentration to read. Something they could pick up and put down as they had a free minute here and there.

Finally, I started thinking about busy medical professionals who might want to learn more about spinal cord injuries, but who didn't have the time (and maybe not the desire) to wade through highly technical medical books or journal articles.

But thinking about writing a book, and actually writing a book are two very different things. The final motivation for me to begin writing was seeing posts on the National Spinal Cord Injury Forum from people who had injuries similar to mine. They were also looking for "the book" on spinal cord injuries which would answer their questions. I had been looking for such a book for more than ten years. I decided if no one had written it by now, I would. And I decided I had better write it before someone else did so.

I asked myself "what are my qualifications to write such a book? I'm not a doctor." My basic experience comes from being a spinal cord injury survivor. I have first hand knowledge of the emotional and physical challenges a spinal cord injury brings with it. I realized I could research the medical information I did not know.

I was injured in an auto accident in 1994. It was a classic "t-bone" wreck, with my car being the stem of the "t." Another car pulled out in front of me. I had no chance to hit the brakes, and broadsided the car at thirty-five miles per hour.

My head hit the roof of the car, despite the fact I was wearing a seatbelt and shoulder harness. My car was a pre-airbag model. In the accident, I suffered a closed head injury, and badly ruptured my C5/6 and C6/7 cervical discs. The accident occurred with such force that the two discs mentioned above were literally liquefied from their original cartilage-like state. The insides of the discs had been pulverized and squeezed out, like a smashed grape. What was left of the discs, now only husks, were pressing on my spinal cord. However, I did not break my neck. I did suffer a closed head injury though.

When all was said and done, I had to recover from three separate spinal cord injuries, not one. The initial accident caused damage to my spinal cord. The stress of the spinal fusion caused the upper adjacent disc, C4/5, to fail. It was also pressing on my spinal cord. I had to be fused at C4/5 in 2004.

I repeated the process in 2006 after the C3/4 disc failed from the stress of the fusion. This situation was more critical than the previous two operations because the C3/4 level of the spinal cord controls involuntary breathing. Too much damage to the spinal cord at this level from either the failed disc or the surgery would have caused me to be on a ventilator for the rest of my life.

To briefly sum up my physical condition, I am an technically an incomplete C3-7 quadriplegic. My neck is fused solidly from the levels of cervical disc 3/4 through cervical disc 6/7. Because I can "walk" with a walker or a crutches, I am would be known in the spinal cord community as a "walking quad." As are others like me. The doctors are trying to keep me out of a wheelchair as long as my condition will allow it.

I have lost fine motor control in my body from the neck down. I have use of my shoulders, arms, hands, and fingers. I do not have neither normal strength or coordination. I have difficulty holding onto things without dropping them. Writing by hand is almost impossible. I don't have the motor control to write. It becomes painful to write by hand after only a few minutes. I can't read my own handwriting most of the time. Thank goodness for the age of computers, or you would not be reading this book.

I have lung problems as a result of the accident. I have bladder and bowel problems. I suffer from spasticity, like many spinal cord injury survivors. This is a condition where the muscles are no longer under proper control from the brain, and contract on their own. This condition, while occasionally useful, can be very painful. I also have difficulty swallowing.

My particular type of spinal cord injury happens to be the most painful of the various types of spinal cord injury. I live my life in constant, searing, chronic nerve pain. Medication eases this pain to a point, but the pain never completely goes away.

I have memory problems because of the closed head injury. I communicate much better in writing than by speaking. This is because the part of my brain that controls speech was damaged in the accident. I have difficulty thinking of the right words to say. My short-term memory is quite impaired. My long-term memory was not as badly damaged from the accident.

Much of my ability to perform higher reasoning functions was damaged in the accident. For someone with an MBA, this was a catastrophic injury. So much of an MBA's function is to make recommendations on business decisions.

I may not be in a wheelchair, but the injuries I experienced were, and still are, devastating. My ability to hold full-time employment has been severely compromised. My ability to even be considered for a position, despite my credentials, has been negatively affected. Being a disabled person, and especially a disabled woman, carries with it a stigma that even my excellent credentials cannot overcome. Pushing fifty does not help either.

In addition to my actual injuries, I have been to several spinal cord injury conferences here in Arkansas. I have also been to a conference on disability in general. I have been regularly attending the monthly support group meetings of the Arkansas Spinal Cord Commission. I have become friends with other spinal cord injury survivors, and have talked with them in detail about their experiences.

In doing the initial research for the article that eventually became this book, I made contacts in the state of Delaware; and was appointed as a consultant to the Traumatic Brain Injury and Spinal Cord Injury Team of the Delaware Coalition for Injury Prevention.

As for actually writing a book, it is something I have always wanted to do. Even as far back as a teenager. I thought it would be a nice family tradition to continue (see the next paragraph). I had no idea what to write a book about. I had heard that you should write about what you know. The only problem was that I didn't know anything about anything. There are a lot of topics in the world I didn't want to know anything about. Spinal cord injury was high on that list.

I had some large shoes to fill in writing a book. My grandfather, Paul H. Vieth (1895-1978), was one of the foremost Christian educators of the early twentieth century. My father, David M. Vieth (1925-2004), was considered by many to be the world's expert on John Wilmot, the Earl of Rochester. Each of them wrote several books in his chosen field of expertise.

The final question I had to ask myself was if I had the writing talent to put such a book together. I did well in English classes in high school and college. Never mind the fact that my parents would never have let me hear the end of it if I didn't do well in English. My father was an English professor, and my mother was a former schoolteacher, after all.

I graduated from college with a bachelor's degree in history from the University of Illinois, Urbana, a school with an excellent academic reputation. I went on to get an MBA in marketing from Southern Illinois University, Carbondale. I completed a year of a master's degree in sociology, and a year of law school at the University of Arkansas, Fayetteville. All my academic studies required a large amount of reading and writing.

I worked in traditional employment roles for many years. I was a Research Assistant at the University of Arkansas, Fayetteville; where I made recommendations on policy decisions. I served a similar function at Southwest Missouri State University (now Missouri State University) in Springfield where I was a member of the President's Staff.

In the corporate world, I have been an Account Executive/Consultant for Sygnis, a marketing research subsidiary of Alltel; the telecommunications company. I have worked for a small privately-owned company called Burgett & Dietrich in

Little Rock. In that position, I made cost reduction recommendations in medical insurance programs for client companies.

My final full-time employment before becoming disabled was as Manager of Marketing and Business Development for Southwestern Bell Wireless (SWBW), and then briefly as SWBW became Cingular Wireless. The company is now known as AT&T Wireless. All of the above positions required extensive research and writing.

I also had written or co-written three professional journal articles during my working years. One was published in *College & University*. One appeared in *Research in Higher Education*, and the third article was in *The Paralegal.*

In addition, I had been a reporter for *The Daily Illini*, the newspaper at the University of Illinois. I wrote a newspaper column many years ago for the *Augusta Advocate/McCrory Leader* newspapers (Augusta/McCrory, Arkansas). So I decided I had enough writing experience to write this book.

To further my newly-found career as a freelance writer, I have joined the American Medical Writers Association, as well as several writing groups in Arkansas.

I stay active, despite my disability. I am a member of the Arkansas Increasing Capabilities Access Network (ICAN) advisory council. This is a federally funded program designed to make technology accessible and available to those who need it.

I am a member of the Illini Media Alumni, having worked for *The Daily Illini.* Finally, I also attend support group meetings related to my injury when the opportunity presents itself, and my schedule and health will allow it.

But back to the book itself. I have done my best to do two things in writing this book: 1) to "translate" technical language into language the average person can understand, and 2) to inject a sense of humor into an otherwise dry and terrible subject.

Don't be intimidated by all the footnotes (technically endnotes). I had to provide the source material for the information in this book. It is mainly there for the medical professionals.

If you are not familiar with research; at the end of material quoted from or which refers another source, there will be a tiny number at the end of the sentence. You would then look in the Endnotes in the back of the book under the corresponding chapter. You will see the same number, and the information for the source material. If you want to look at the actual source material for yourself.

The Bibliography lists the material in the Endnotes in alphabetical order by the author's last name. If there is no author, then alphabetical by title. You would then search the Internet. Or take the information to a reference librarian in a public library, college/university library, or a medical school library. The librarian will explain to you how to find the original source material in the library or by Interlibrary Loan. I certainly don't expect you to look up the source material unless you are a medical professional. You have more important things to deal with right now. Otherwise, you wouldn't be reading this book. But now you know what the Endnotes and Bibliography are there for.

My emphasis is on teenage, young adult, and adult spinal cord injuries. Spinal cord injuries in children follow different patterns than in adults. Because such injuries are often fatal in very young children, I will leave the discussion of these injuries to medical journals and textbooks except for a few selected places in the book.

I have also tried to adopt a worldwide focus in this book. I have included information for countries other than the United States where I could find information. There are also resources for other countries in the Resources chapter. Many spinal cord injury books are specific to the country of the author. Spinal cord injuries happen all over the world.

I decided not to use illustrations because there are already so many good books on the subject of spinal cord injury that contain illustrations. The information is also readily available on the Internet.

I have not specifically discussed causes of spinal cord injury such as Guillaume-Barre Syndrome. The effects are going to be similar to other spinal cord injuries from other causes such as trauma.

I had a more than a few challenges during the writing of this book beyond my physical and mental limitations. I had a large Maine Coon Cat who insisted on jumping into my lap while I was trying to type. He would grab my forearms away from the keyboard, and start licking them. He also had a bad habit of trying to anchor himself by kicking his back legs against my keyboard drawer, which pushed the keyboard back under my computer desk.

I had a death in the family of someone very close to me. My computer corrupted some of the files. My keyboard died, worn out from many years of use. I had to borrow my husband's computer to finish the manuscript, because I no longer trusted mine.

This book may have its critics, claiming there is "nothing new" in the book. Or it is pretty much the same as other "guides" to spinal cord injuries written by medical professionals. I beg to differ. The perspective is different in this book. A spinal cord injury survivor wrote it. Someone who has been through the injury.

Perhaps not a textbook case of spinal cord injury. But a spinal cord injury, nevertheless.

I found books by medical professionals on spinal cord injury often did not touch on the emotional aspects of the injury. Or they were discussed in a clinical, professional third-person viewpoint.

I have discussed other topics in this book often not seen in "typical" spinal cord injury books. These include claw hand deformity, addiction after a spinal cord injury, and the differences between the hangman's fracture historically and in modern medical usage.

In some chapters and the Resources chapter I have mentioned products or services. Just because I have included a company, a company's product, or a company's services does not mean I endorse it. I have discussed some products I have successfully used, but these products may not be suitable for everyone. There are the occasional products or services I highly recommend. These are noted accordingly.

The information in the Resources chapter was current as of the time of my research. Companies go out of business, change locations, and change names. I cannot guarantee the accuracy of the information beyond a reasonable time after my research was performed. If you have any doubts about dealing with a company, check with other people, local or national organizations as applicable (such as the Better Business Bureau in the United States). You might also want to check with your state or regional attorney general's office (or the equivalent in your country) to see if any complaints have been filed against the company. Just because a company is in business to serve the needs of the disabled does not mean the company is legitimate.

I have made every effort not to focus on myself in this book. While "my story" may be interesting, it is not information a spinal cord injury survivor needs. I have included information on "my story" so the reader will have some background about me. And so the reader will be able to understand what I have gone through that makes it possible for me to write this book.

If even one person who reads this book finds something useful in it, then my injury has served a purpose.

Carolyn Vieth Boyles
August 2007

Beginning Thoughts

1

"Thoughts Immediately After a Spinal Cord Injury"

Don't fear change, embrace it.—
Anthony J. D'Angelo

This isn't my body. My body works. It does what I tell it to do. What kind of joke is this? When am I going to wake up and find out it was all a dream. All a joke? This is all temporary, right? It will go away.

How can parts of my body hurt so much, but I cannot move them? Cannot feel them. "No pain, no gain." I must be having plenty of gain then.

I want to scream. I want to start screaming and not stop.

What did I do to deserve this?

Why are the doctors and nurses so serious? Why are my family and friends crying?

It happened in a heartbeat. In the time it takes to blink an eye.

I wish I could have that moment back again. To do it again. Differently. Or not do it at all.

It was a stupid thing to do.

(Or it was a stupid thing for someone else to do).

(Or I was in the wrong place at the wrong time).

I know I am the same person inside. But I don't feel like the same person.

I'm scared. Yesterday I thought I knew exactly how my life would go. Now I don't know what to expect. Neither do the doctors and nurses.

I wish I were dead. This is worse than death.

Nurses and doctors are doing things to my body. All day. All night. Seeing parts of my body they shouldn't see. I'm embarrassed.

People who know me look at me like they don't know me. Like I am a stranger.

I feel like a stranger to myself.

I have started the book with this chapter to explain what sort of thoughts go through your mind right after you have a spinal cord injury.

This isn't my body. My body works. It does what I tell it to do. What kind of joke is this? When am I going to wake up and find out it was all a dream. All a joke? This is all temporary, right? It will go away.

Initially you experience a feeling of "unreality." Your mind and body are both in shock after the injury. Nothing seems real. If you have never been a patient in a hospital before, being in a hospital is a strange and terrifying experience by itself. Even without a terrible injury.

Once you get over the initial reaction that the situation can't be real, then you start to focus on yourself. You realize your body no longer functions the way it did before the accident. You may have lost control of your bladder or bowels, or both. This is very embarrassing. To suddenly have been regressed to the state of an infant before toilet training.

No matter how hard you try to move the affected parts of your body, they don't react properly. They may not move at all. They may move erratically or slowly.

It is human nature to assume the consequences of the injury are only temporary. Once you wake up from this nightmare, everything will be back the way it used to be.

How can parts of my body hurt so much, but I cannot move them?

This is a difficult concept for anyone to understand, with or without a spinal cord injury. It is possible to have lost normal feeling in an area of the body, and yet still feel pain. And the pain experienced with some types of spinal cord injuries is the most intense pain a human being can have.

I want to scream. I want to start screaming and not stop.

The frustration a person feels after a spinal cord injury is indescribable. One of the worst feelings a person can have is to lose control in a situation. We, as human beings, value control. It helps define our self-image, and our feeling of value in society.

Every one of us takes the ability to control our own bodies for granted. We have been doing it for so long we don't have to think about it. We know how much effort it takes to raise a hand six inches. Or to grasp a glass of water. We can sense whether we are standing up or sitting down. We know without looking where each arm and leg is "in space" relative to the rest of our body. We know whether something is hot or cold, smooth or rough, dry or wet. Simply by touching it.

When we are in the hospital immediately after a spinal cord injury, we have not only lost the ability to control our own bodies, we have lost control over our situation. Who wouldn't rather be home watching television, reading a book, or out on the lake water skiing? But we no longer have that choice. We are stuck in a hospital. And not only can we not watch television at home, read a book (and turn the pages on our own), or be water skiing at this very moment.

There is doubt if we will ever be able to perform these abilities again. At all or even with assistance.

What did I do to deserve this?

This is a very normal thought for anyone who has been seriously injured. I believe it relates in some way back to the desire to maintain control in a situation. "I" must have done something. "I" must have taken some action. The action was wrong. Therefore, "I" deserved to be punished. It still preserves control in an odd sort of way.

Why are the doctors and nurses so serious? Why are my family and friends crying?

We are in a strange place, a hospital. We are in a situation that we are neither emotionally or physically prepared to handle. Therefore, much of our reaction must be based on others we come in contact with.

Immediately after a spinal cord injury it can be difficult for doctors to provide an accurate prognosis. What appears to be a complete injury may turn out to be an incomplete injury. What appears to be a permanent injury may heal given time. Sometimes there is no visible sign of injury to the spinal cord, and yet a person is completely paralyzed.

We are looking for some form of stability. Some form of hope after this type of injury. And we look to the doctors' and nurses' facial expressions, along with the facial expressions and reactions of our family and friends.

It happened in a heartbeat. In the time it takes to blink an eye.

It is almost inconceivable that such a devastating injury can happen so fast. Misjudging the depth of water on a dive. Losing control of a car. Getting shot in the spinal cord from out of nowhere.

I wish I could have that moment back again. To do it again. Differently. Or not do it at all.

It would be so easy to repeat the moment, and make the accident not happen. If we would only be given the chance.

It was a stupid thing to do.

Sometimes accidents just happen. Sometimes people use poor judgment in situations. It would be great if we could realize in advance that doing something is a stupid thing to do. And it is going to cause a spinal cord injury. But the best we can do is realize it in hindsight. This emotion also leads into the very difficult area of survivor guilt. Depending upon what the spinal cord injury survivor's situation was to cause the accident; there may be guilt and other negative emotions to confront during recovery, rehabilitation, and the rest of a person's life. These emotions can be as dangerous as the spinal cord injury itself, if left unresolved.

(Or it was a stupid thing for someone else to do).

This is again dealing with the problem of survivor guilt. What if you were hurt as a result of something stupid someone else did? How do you deal with this emotion?

(Or I was in the wrong place at the wrong time).

This is again trying to exert some form of control over the situation. Let me go back in time. Let me be someplace other than where I was when the accident happened.

I know I am the same person inside. But I don't feel like the same person.

You cannot be the same person emotionally after a spinal cord injury. At least not immediately after the injury. You may be the same person again emotionally after time. Such devastating injuries have an emotional effect on a person for the rest of a person's life. A spinal cord injury changes the way you see yourself. It changes the way family, friends, and co-workers see you. Some people will see the disability before they see the person. This is a troubling fact of life. Sometimes even we, as the spinal cord injury survivors, see our own disability before we see our own self image.

I'm scared. Yesterday I thought I knew exactly how my life would go. Now I don't know what to expect. Neither do the doctors and nurses.

This goes back to the lack of control we feel in the situation. And also addresses the uncertainty that goes hand in hand with the prognosis for recovery.

I wish I were dead. This is worse than death.

This is all too common an emotion after a spinal cord injury. It is difficult to envision how life can ever be "the same" after such an injury. Immediately after a spinal cord injury, a person will be at their maximum degree of disability; except in rare instances. Then, depending upon the injury, the rehabilitation received, and the length of time since the injury; function may begin to return. With the physical and emotional challenges that lie ahead, a person may feel death would be a simpler solution.

Nurses and doctors are doing things to my body. All day. All night. Seeing parts of my body they shouldn't see. I'm embarrassed.

This goes back to the lack of control, and just the general indignity of the situation. Most people don't want to be seen naked by total strangers. Let alone the terrible feeling of losing control of your bladder and/or your bowels. Infants and the elderly lack control of their bladders and their bowels. This is not something normal children, young adults, adolescents, or adults should experience.

People who know me look at me like they don't know me. Like I am a stranger.

Not only does the person injured have to adjust physically and emotionally to the situation, so do the person's family and friends. They may see the disability before they see the person. They feel a lack of control in the situation, the same way the injured person does. Their expectations for the future have been changed as well. They are unsure of what their roles and responsibilities will be. Will they have to take care of the injured person for the rest of the injured person's life? Will the injured person be able to earn a living? Will they and their injured family member or friend be able to enjoy the activities they shared before the accident again?

A family member or friend of the injured person may feel responsible in some way for the accident. Even if the guilt is not justified. "I should have told him not to go out so late," for example. The family member may look at the injured person differently because of his or her own guilt in the situation.

I feel like a stranger to myself.

This describes the utter alienation you feel after a spinal cord injury. You can no longer relate to "normal" people who can move their limbs properly. Or who have normal bladder and bowel control. But neither can you relate to people in wheelchairs you see in the hallways of hospitals and rehabilitation centers.

Again, these are all perfectly normal thoughts. Part of the journey toward recovery from a spinal cord injury. I will discuss both the physical and emotional recovery throughout the course of the book.

“My Story”

2

"A Little About Me"

One good anecdote is worth a volume of biography.—
William Ellery Channing

I led an uneventful and pretty boring life growing up. Nothing special. Being that my dad was a college professor, we moved whenever dad got promoted. Sort of like being an "army brat." I was an only child. I was very shy and self-conscious growing up. I was picked on in school. I was the clumsy kid who could trip over the pattern in the linoleum. I had thick hair that curlers would simply not stay in, causing many tears in junior high and high school trying to get ready for school. I had a space between my two front teeth, and my complexion could have been the subject of a horror movie.

I liked to read. As far back as I can remember. My parents used to find me on the floor in my father's study reading whatever I could get my hands on. Even if I shouldn't have been able to understand it as a toddler, I tried reading it. I liked dinosaur books, so my parents told me. Reading was an escape for me. I could go places I had never been or never would be able to go. I could do interesting things. I liked Nancy Drew mysteries growing up. I wished I could be more like her.

My high school years were "nothing to write home about." I had the usual crushes on boys. I had a total of three dates in high school. I was very shy. I never went to a high school prom. I never learned how to ballroom dance. I kept telling my parents I would never need to know how. I never had the occasion before my accident. Since my accident I no longer have the ability. There are times I hate being right.

Being an only child, I wanted to get away from home when I went to college. Despite having excellent grades in high school, colleges weren't interested in me because I had an average ACT score. I chose the University of Illinois, because it had a good reputation as a school. And it was a reasonable distance away from home. Far enough to be away but close enough to get home conveniently for the holidays. I was too nervous to get too far away from home.

My college years were pretty much a disaster. I also didn't know at the time that I couldn't see worth a darn. My parents blamed my bad grades on spending too much time partying, and not enough time studying. They didn't believe me when I told them I wasn't partying. I had spent my entire life needing glasses, despite regular eye exams. Nobody believed me when I told them "I couldn't see."

After changing majors, I finally managed to get a bachelor's degree in history. It was the vogue in those days to have a liberal arts undergraduate degree and an MBA. So I got an MBA from Southern Illinois University in Carbondale. I lived at home while I went to school.

I wasn't emotionally ready for the working world. Is anybody ever emotionally ready for the working world? I took a business law class during my bachelor's degree and loved it. I decided to go to law school after finishing most of my MBA work. One class short of graduation with my MBA, I packed up and went to Fayetteville, Arkansas to start law school. I would have liked to finish my MBA at the time, but I couldn't start law school in a spring semester because it wasn't allowed.

My law school days were a disaster. This is when I found out I really couldn't see. I am farsighted (can't see close) and have astigmatism. This made the long hours or reading impossible without proper correction. The only good thing about law school was that I met my husband to be. It was love at first sight, literally. Shame he was so blurry (just kidding). Don't worry. I still loved him even when I could finally see him properly.

I dropped out of law school to go to work. If Wal-Mart had been the corporate monster it is now, I would have had no trouble getting a job in Northwest Arkansas. Either with Wal-Mart or one of the companies with a branch office there to deal with Wal-mart. But it wasn't. The only job I could find put me into a career track I would spend the next twenty years trying to get out of. I was now a "statistician." A "great" career track for someone with an MBA in marketing.

I worked various professional jobs over the years. Whatever would pay the rent. But almost always underpaid. Sometimes overworked.

I spent two years trying to "recover from the accident." I was determined to be functional again. My neuropsychologist had said I would only be able to function as a housewife. He said my working days were over because of the closed head injury. I had seen an acquaintance after a closed head injury. I didn't want to spend the rest of my life like that.

I started as a receptionist in a temporary job. When my brain had rewired itself enough to where I was comfortable with that, I looked for a slightly more challenging job. I became a legal secretary. When my brain had rewired itself enough to where I was comfortable with that, I became a loan processor. I tried being a financial advisor. I didn't like that. At that point my mom became seriously ill and died.

I had to put my dad in a nursing home and take care of him. By 1997 I got his situation stable. My brain had recovered all it was going to recover. It would never be the same again, but I was at least functional at this point.

I saw an ad in the local newspaper for an MBA-level position. I applied for it and got it. I stayed in that position from mid-1997 until early 2001 when I got laid off. But by that time my physical condition had started to deteriorate.

I will continue the story in the chapter "My Complications One."

3

"My Accident"

You better believe there will be times in your life when
you'll be feeling like a stumbling fool. So take it from me:
you'll learn more from your accident than anything
that you could ever learn in school.—
"You're Only Human"—Billy Joel

I don't remember much about the weather on November 14, 1994. Other than the fact that it wasn't raining. It was a chilly day, as November days are often in Arkansas. I remember it was chilly because I had on my raincoat with the lining in it. I always felt like *Columbo* wearing that raincoat.

I was on my way home from work. I was working on assignment for a temporary service while I looked for permanent work requiring an MBA degree and paying accordingly. It was a little bit after five in the evening, but it was still light outside. Dusk had not quite started.

I was driving a 1987 Dodge Colt. It was a light metallic blue. Dodge Colts were great little cars. Comfortable, and with good gas mileage. I was sorry when Dodge decided to replace them with the Neon. I think Dodge Colts are one of the best cars ever produced in America.

Even though it was not dusk yet, I had my lights on. I preferred to maximize my visibility and increase the chances of being seen by other drivers. Today I drive with my lights on even during the day even in my bright candy apple red Subaru.

I was driving from Little Rock, Arkansas through North Little Rock, Arkansas to my home in Sherwood. Several suburbs share boundaries north of Little Rock along the state highway 67/167 corridor, with North Little Rock coming first, then Sherwood, then Jacksonville, and finally Cabot, and Beebe further northeast.

On each side of highway 67/167 there is a two-lane access road that parallels the highway. The access road that parallels highway 67/167 south is called Warden Road. The access road that parallels highway 67/167 north is called Landers Road. Each access road has businesses with parking lots that open onto the access road.

Today, in 2007, each access road only has traffic flowing one way. The access road on each side of the highway parallels the traffic on the highway itself. This was changed because of the number of accidents on the access roads. My accident could not have happened today because of the one-way traffic flow. For all I know, my accident may have contributed to the decision to make the access roads one way.

I was on my way home from work driving on Landers Road doing the speed limit of thirty-five mph. I am and always have been meticulous about following the speed limit. It is just one of my "oddities."

Traffic on Landers Road at rush hour has been bad for years. An increasing number of families moved out of Little Rock as desegregation issues began hitting the public school system. "White flight" became very common, with families moving either southwest of Little Rock to Alexander, Benton, and Bryant. Or northeast of the city to Cabot and Beebe.

A new shopping mall had been built in the area, just off Warden Road in the 1970s. I wasn't living in the area at that time so my reports of what it was like come from friends who are lifelong residents. I understand that this new mall, called McCain Mall, because it is located on McCain Boulevard, caused frantic residential and business expansion in the area as well, fueling the increase in traffic.

A growing number of businesses began building along the two access roads as the population in the suburbs and outlying communities northeast of Little Rock increased. Strip shopping centers were built. Big name chain restaurants such as The Outback Steakhouse went up along with big name retailers such as Wal-Mart (which is headquartered in Northwest Arkansas for anyone not familiar with the state), Best Buy, and Circuit City.

Landers Road itself in 1994 was a paved two-lane asphalt road with well-defined road markings. Landers Road was known as "car row" because there were so many car dealers located on it. Today Warden Road has just as many if not more car dealers, but at the time more of them were located on Landers Road.

In the early 1990s a section of Landers Road became a well known area for Little Rock metro area residents. A Wal-Mart store was built, perpendicular to the road, with its large parking lot opening onto Landers Road. Sharing that parking lot was Best Buy, directly across from Wal-Mart. Parallel to the road a grocery store was built at the back of the parking lot.

Arkansans are passionate about Wal-Mart. There is "no other place to shop" for many of them. Despite the fact that we had K-Mart stores competing effectively with Sam Walton's "offspring" in price and location, there was just no convincing Arkansans to buy any place else. As a result, the parking lot of the Wal-Mart store on Landers Road was almost always filled with cars and a wide variety of pickup trucks (Arkansans are also passionate about their trucks).

Dusk was nearing, and I was on my way home from work. I don't remember my day at work being anything atypical. The drive home, however, was one I was never going to forget.

I was driving northeast, away from Little Rock. We bought this car at the salvage auction, and my father-in-law restored it. In those days my father-in-law would buy vehicles from the salvage auction and restore them. Something of a hobby for him.

One thing we did not do in restoring the car was to replace the seatbelts. They had no obvious defects. We will never be able to confirm if having the original seatbelts in the car contributed to the accident.

Traffic was typical rush hour traffic for the metro area. While driving conditions weren't optimal, they weren't bad either. Visibility was good. It can be difficult driving at dusk in heavy traffic.

I was driving on Landers Road heading northeast to Sherwood. There were several different routes I could have chosen to get home. But for some reason that day I chose that one.

My speed was thirty-five mph. I am a cautious driver, and I do not exceed the speed limit. The posted limit on Landers Road was thirty-five mph. Traffic was bumper to bumper, but it was moving. I had just passed the first part of "car row," with the new and used car dealers. I was approaching the section of Landers Road with Best Buy, Wal-Mart, National Home Center, and Sam's, before "car row" resumed again.

I saw a car stopped at the first stop sign in the Wal-Mart/Best Buy parking lot on my right. I got an odd feeling that something bad was about to happen. Then I saw the car move forward to make a left turn onto Landers Road. I took my right foot from the accelerator and had enough time to move it over above the brake pedal. Before I could put my foot to apply pressure to the brake pedal I heard the awful sound of metal on metal. Then I blacked out.

When I woke up I was several car lengths down the road from where the initial impact had taken place. I knew that I had blacked out. I knew I shouldn't move around too much, but I didn't have the slightest idea why. I realized I was very confused as well.

There happened to be an ambulance a few cars behind me in traffic when the accident happened. So there was no wait for an ambulance to be on the scene.

I remember once my car came to a stop after the impact I put the automatic transmission in park. Then I leaned back in the seat. One of the paramedics came to my driver's window. He asked me to roll the window down. He asked me if I was ok. I said no. He asked me what hurt and I replied, my neck and my back.

At some point in time someone must have taken my glasses off me because I realized I did not have them on. I don't know to this day whatever happened to that pair of glasses.

The paramedics put me on a backboard. They put a hard neck collar around my neck. Then they asked me which hospital I wanted to go to. I kept changing my mind back and forth as to what hospital. I finally settled on St. Vincent Infirmary/Medical Center in Little Rock. I realized I was still unusually confused. I didn't know why I was so confused.

During the ambulance ride I was in and out of consciousness. I don't think the paramedics ever noticed. Nobody ever asked me about blacking out.

When I reached the emergency room at St. Vincent's I was taken into an examination room, still on the backboard and in the neck collar. Dr. Lloyd Warford was the doctor on duty. I will never forget that name. I will always wonder what damage might have been prevented if he had done his job properly. Since I could not prove what damage I would not have suffered if Dr. Warford had done his job properly, I had no case for malpractice. Now if I had become paralyzed from the neck down as a result of him not doing his job, then I would have had a malpractice case. I'll take the no malpractice case option.

In the mid 1990s the awareness of spinal cord injury that exists today did not exist. Among the general public or the health care industry. Unless you couldn't move from the waist down or the neck down, you weren't considered to have a spinal cord injury.

Dr. Warford took the neck collar off me, and loosened me from the backboard. He asked me where I hurt. I gave him the same response I had given the paramedics. "In the neck and in the back." This wasn't mild pain. I had been in auto accidents before. I was a bit banged up and sore after those accidents. This pain in my neck and my back was *different.* It was a burning, searing pain.

Dr. Warford had me walk around the examination room. He had me move my arms in various positions. I soon learned that I could not physically raise my arms above my shoulders. I told this to Dr. Warford. He did not even order a simple x-ray. He wrote me out a couple of prescriptions for muscle relaxants and discharged me.

I asked repeatedly to call Raymond, and let him know where I was. My request was repeatedly denied. I wasn't coherent, so I wasn't in any shape to deal with this unusual situation that had suddenly been thrust upon me.

The accident had taken place shortly after five at night. It was now close to eight. I was finally able to call Raymond, and ask him to come get me. He was, of course, worried sick because he didn't know where I had been for the last three hours.

He arrived about twenty minutes later. I explained everything to him. It was too late at night to get the prescriptions filled, and he had to wait until morning. This was also before pharmacies stayed open as late as they do now. We both agreed it was pretty stupid that the emergency room doctor couldn't give me actual pills instead of just handing me two written prescriptions.

I also don't remember if we stopped and got some fast food on the way home, if we found something to eat at home, or if Raymond dropped me off at home and then went out and got us something to eat.

All I remember about that night is that I was very sore, in a lot of pain, very confused, and scared. It would become even more obvious to both of us in the days to come that I was far from alright.

The next day wasn't any better. I didn't know where anything was in the house. I knew the room layout. I was the one who had organized (if you can use that word in our household) things in that house. I didn't know where I had put anything. I was having trouble remembering phone numbers (I was always a whiz with phone numbers and friends' and relatives' birthdays).

Not only was I still very confused, my left arm had started to hurt above the elbow. The pain was so bad I wanted to gnaw my arm off. Between the confusion and the pain it was no wonder I couldn't think straight.

I had a sharp pain in my right forehead, at the hairline. I didn't know where it came from. I also had terrible fits of rage if I anything touched that spot.

The bruises on my body were beginning to come out. I had deep bruises where the seat belt and shoulder belt held my body back. I would also have bruises on my knees and thighs. The bruises would take months to disappear.

An odd symptom I developed overnight was severe diarrhea. Every time I would eat I would have to run to the bathroom. This was a nuisance, but it was the least of my problems.

My speech was slurred, and I did not know why. I sounded like I had been out partying for days. I could not think of the words I wanted to say. And I could not read properly. I had to sound out the words on the page. Some words would just not register. Pinecone, for example. I kept interpreting it as "pin-e-cone."

I remember Raymond talking about closed head injury. He had been to a seminar not long before on the effects of closed head injury. He told me I was showing the symptoms, and we needed to keep an eye on me over the next few weeks. We both hoped in the next few weeks my mental processes would clear up.

Unfortunately, I was the one who would have to deal with the after accident details such as dealing with insurance adjusters. This was going to prove challenging, since I could not think straight. Raymond was tied up with work.

A few days later I got the idea into my head that I should go to one of the other hospitals that my insurance covered, and have myself checked out. I was in no shape to drive, and I did not have a functioning car. I did not want to disturb Raymond at work. I also realized I had no money on me to pay for a cab ride. The nearest ATM machine was about an eight-block walk from the house. So I walked to the ATM machine, and got the cash for the cab ride. Not the most logical thing to do. But it gives you some idea of just how confused I was.

I had the cab driver take me to the University of Arkansas Medical School emergency room. I gave them my insurance information, and they put me in an examination room. Ten different people must have come in to see me. I repeated the same story to each person about the auto accident.

After head to toe x-rays, the doctors determined I had no broken bones. They could not explain why I was in so much pain or why I was so confused. So I went home just as frustrated and confused as I had gone to the emergency room.

I also had the issue of my missing glasses. Fortunately I was farsighted so I could drive without glasses if I had Raymond's car. But I was getting a headache from not wearing glasses. I went to my eye doctor's office in Little Rock, and I explained my glasses had been lost in an auto accident.

I could not get the technician to understand that they would not have to wait for the accident settlement to get paid. I was going to pay for the glasses out of my own pocket, and then be reimbursed by my insurance. I finally got her to understand. But I would still have to wait close to another week before my glasses would be ready because the prescription lenses could not be obtained locally.

It was now the end of November. I had met with the family attorney, Dennis James, for him to handle my lawsuit. He suggested I should see my family doctor in the attempt to determine what was causing my medical problems.

I made an appointment with my family doctor at the time, Dr. Joe Schotts, in Jacksonville. Jacksonville was a short trip from where we lived at the time. I explained what had happened with the auto accident. I also told him what doctors I'd been to see.

He examined me, and decided a visit to a neurologist would be in order. The clinic had a neurologist come in periodically so its patients would not have to drive into Little Rock. The neurologist, Dr. Alonzo "Lon" Burba, was scheduled to come in either later that week or early the following week.

I met with Dr. Burba in offices in the same shopping center as the family practice clinic. He used office space normally occupied by a physical therapist's office. We spoke at length before he examined me. I expressed to him my concern about being unable to lift my arms over my head (no higher than straight out from the shoulders).

Dr. Burba had an EEG (brainwave pattern test) performed. He told me that he did not think anything was seriously wrong with me, but he was going to order an MRI (Magnetic Resonance Imaging) test of my neck. He said he expected it to be normal. The EEG was normal. The only thing it showed was that I had fallen asleep during the test.

I was scheduled to have the MRI performed a few days later at a mobile MRI facility at Rebsamen Regional Medical Center in Jacksonville. I figured Dr. Burba was just trying to humor me since I was female. Obviously I wasn't seriously hurt as far as he was concerned.

Dr. Burba telephoned me early the following week. He was audibly shaken and upset. I could hear the "*oh sh—*" in his voice even though he never said it. What he did say was that he had to get me to a neurosurgeon as soon as possible. The C5/6 and C6/7 cervical discs in my neck were badly herniated, and were compressing my spinal cord.

I told him "I kept telling you I wasn't ok."

4

"My First Surgery"

The practice of medicine is a thinker's art
the practice of surgery a plumber's—
Martin H. Fischer

It was now early January 1995. Raymond and I were sitting in the waiting room of Dr. Scott Schlesinger. Dr. Schlesinger was a neurosurgeon. He was the doctor that Dr. Burba, the neurologist, wanted me to see. Dr. Ron Williams was supposed to the best neurosurgeon in town at that time, according to many people. I had a co-worker who had a disc in her back fixed by Dr. Williams and was very pleased. Dr. Williams and Dr. Schlesinger were partners. Dr. Schlesinger was Dr. Williams' protégé. Dr. Schlesinger took my insurance. Dr. Williams did not.

The waiting room was packed. I had no idea that so many people had so many things wrong with them that they needed to see a neurosurgeon. We must have waited two or three hours before my name was called. I had already picked up the MRI films from the hospital, and given them to Dr. Schlesinger's nurse.

Raymond was quite willing to go into the examination room. I don't remember if the doctor's office wouldn't allow him in, or if I was of the opinion I wanted to do it alone. I only remember I was in the examination room alone.

The examination was very detailed. It took more than an hour. Dr. Schlesinger did some very strange tests I had never had any doctor do. After he tested my knee reflexes, he ran the sharp tapered point of the rubber hammer across the bottom of my foot. He also scraped a fingernail across the fingernail of the middle finger on my right hand. He also had me walk up and down the hall while he watched.

I remember him taking me into the hallway, and showing me what was wrong on the MRI films. In those days they still used film for MRI. Now everything is transferred onto a CD-ROM drive.

Dr. Schlesinger told me I had two options. I could either do nothing, or I could have surgery. He did not think physical therapy, which is prescribed for so many cervical disc problems, would do me any good.

If I chose not to have surgery, then any fall I took would run the risk of severing my spinal cord, he told me. This would result in permanent total paralysis from the neck down.

If I chose to have surgery, Dr. Schlesinger would remove the herniated discs from my neck, and fuse the discs with bone taken from the arch of my hip. This was state of the art surgery in 1995. If I chose to have surgery, the risk of permanent paralysis from the neck down from a fall would be eliminated.

I told them I would have to think about my decision, and I would get back to them in a few days.

5

"My Complications One"

This is more significant....
it's a very big complication.—
John Silvia

Obviously I chose to have the double disc fusion at C5/6 and C6/7 or I wouldn't be writing this chapter.

I had the surgery and it went fine without complications. I spent the first month after the surgery in a soft neck collar except when bathing. After the first month, I had to wear the neck collar while driving for the next three months. My recovery went without complications.... initially.

I was very sore from muscle spasms after the first surgery. I had been holding my body in an unnatural position because of the spinal cord injury. Now my body was back in a normal position. My muscles weren't used to it. The only thing Dr. Schlesinger gave me for pain was Motrin. I had no restrictions of any kind, except not to try to look up or down. I had no lifting restrictions.

It is now summer 2003. Raymond and I have been living in our house since 1997. For the last two years I have been very physically active in the yard as an amateur landscaper.

During the previous summers I had been trying to build up landscaping beds. Our soil was rock with a little dirt thrown in. It could "technically" be described as "soil." I had built up beds along the sides of the back yard, and had started along the back border. "Little Rock" didn't describe our soil adequately. We had rocks the size of footballs in our yard.

But something this year was different. I was getting terrible pain in my wrists. I also didn't have the stamina I had had the previous years.

My family doctor, Dr. Rob Barrow, repeatedly wanted to refer me to an orthopedic surgeon for carpal tunnel release surgery. I told him that I did not want the surgery. I had heard of too many cases where the surgery had been unsuccessful.

I had spent all of my working career chained behind a computer writing business cases, building spreadsheets, doing computer programming, that sort of thing. The perfect career to generate carpal tunnel syndrome.

Raymond and I had "met" James Thompson, a retired Air Force sergeant, when we all played *Everquest*. For those of you not familiar with *Everquest*, it is an online computer game set in a fantasy world where players interact with each other and with creatures that are supposed to be killed to gain experience, money, and loot.

James and I had gotten to know each other well in the game. Raymond and James and I had the opportunity to meet in person when James was on a business trip to Little Rock for training. We kept in touch regularly via the game, and talked several times a week.

James and I talked frequently about my wrist problems. He was a knowledgeable fellow about medicine, as he repaired medical equipment in his VA hospital. He repeatedly asked me if anyone had looked at my neck recently to see what its current state was after the fusion in 1995. No one had.

Finally I relented, and insisted that "Dr. Rob" as his patients know him, send me for an MRI of my neck. Dr. Rob didn't think it would show anything, but he humored me and authorized the procedure.

A few days later his nurse called. I had ruptured the cervical disc between C4/C5, one level *above* the fusion at C5-C6/C6-C7. Dr. Rob wanted to refer me to Dr. Scott Schlesinger, who had performed the previous fusion. I declined.

The previous fusion had gone well, but I had heard of other patients of Dr. Schlesinger's who hadn't had such good luck. I decided not to risk it. Instead, I asked for a referral to Dr. Steven Cathey, a neurosurgeon who had been featured in the *People* section of the Little Rock newspaper. The appointment was scheduled.

I don't remember how long I had to wait until my appointment with Dr. Cathey, but I don't think it was more than a couple of weeks. I had a long wait in the waiting room and then a longer wait in the exam room. Raymond had gone with me, fearing the worst.

Through the paper-thin walls we overheard conversations between Dr. Cathey and other patients. The other patients were all people in chronic pain, pleading with Dr. Cathey to operate, to do *something* to stop the pain. In every case Dr. Cathey discussed their x-rays and told them there was nothing he could do to help. He said as much as he would like to operate because he made money when he operated, he could do nothing for them.

I liked the sound of what I heard. The last thing you want in a surgeon is a scalpel-happy doctor who will operate on everybody, especially when your spinal cord is involved.

Finally we heard the door open and Dr. Cathey walked in. He had a bouncy walk; longish sun bleached reddish hair, and from my perspective looked just too young to be a neurosurgeon. Yet he was supposed to be one of the best. I also found myself thinking "*oh no, not again.*"

Dr. Cathey must have spent an hour, hour and half with us very carefully perusing my past medical records and my MRIs (the films themselves, not just the radiologist's report).

He finally said that he didn't see any alternative *but surgery* for me. He described in detail, however, that surgical technical for spinal fusion had changed drastically in the ten years since I had had my last fusion done. Options and materials were available now that weren't available ten years before.

He described to us how he was going to remove the ruptured C4/5 disc. He was going to insert cadaver bone to replace the ruptured disc and plate the new fusion to the existing fusion. Fortunately, the existing fusion was good and solid.

He said he truly hated to perform a triple fusion, because I had lost enough neck movement already; but there was no choice in this case.

If I'd known then what I'd knew now, I would have made a few decisions differently. The last thing in the world I expected was that things would get worse. I didn't know in 2003 they were going to get even worse.

6

"My Complications Two"

Oh no, not again—
Douglas Adams in *The Hitchhiker's Guide to the Galaxy*

This is a difficult chapter to write because I don't remember many of the details.

I remember during the summer of 2005 I was not feeling well. I started having terrible pain in my neck and in my back between my shoulder blades. I went back to my family doctor, Dr. Barrow, and he examined me. When he touched the spot in my upper back between my shoulder blades that hurt, I screamed. I remember him telling me I was having muscle spasms, and he prescribed physical therapy for me.

I was dubious about the physical therapy because the person Dr. Rob referred me to was his office mate. He sent me next door to a sports medicine clinic. I met with the fellow running the clinic. He had enough credentials to his name in sports medicine. He was not a doctor. He did physical therapy. He suggested that I undergo some nerve conductivity testing. The fellow he referred me to was a friend of his.

So I had the nerve testing done. I knew during the testing that this friend of his did not know what he was doing. Anyone who has ever had nerve conductivity testing done knows that it hurts. And it hurts with a capital "h." This testing did not hurt.

The results of my nerve conductivity came back saying there was nothing wrong with me except for some nerve conductivity loss in my wrists, which would be typical of mild carpal tunnel syndrome. I had been working with computers since 1984. Tell me something I didn't know.

I continued with the physical therapy. At first it helped some. It reached the point where it was making the pain worse. And the pain was bad enough on its own. I told the therapist and Dr. Rob I would not undergo more physical therapy.

Dr. Rob decided to send me to a chiropractor. I was dubious again, but I went. The physical therapy room was impressive. It was huge. It must have had every type of exercise equipment known to man. I felt like I was in Richard Simmons' house. The walls were all glass to show a wonderful view. There were people there of all races and ages working very hard on the exercise equipment. They all seemed to be very happy with the results they were getting.

I found out early on, that like most of the doctors I was being sent to; that this chiropractor had no experience with spinal cord injury. I decided there was going to be a limit to what I was going to let him do in the way of neck manipulation. I didn't want to end up a complete quadriplegic.

I did get some relief in the way of increased range of motion in my neck. I had little enough range of motion with three fused discs, so I was happy to get any range of motion back. But when the chiropractor increased the degree of manipulation and the pain got worse, I said "no more."

I may be wrong in the order these events occurred, but you get the general idea. Dr. Rob decided to send me to a pain management specialist.

By this point in time, I was losing additional fine coordination of my arms, hands, and fingers. I was having enough trouble walking that I was using forearm crutches (also called Canadian crutches). I knew something was very wrong. I had an awful feeling I knew exactly what it was.

So I went to see the pain management doctor, Dr. Lawrence Ault. He decided that my cervical discs were compressed. He wanted to stretch my spinal cord to get the pressure off it. He also wanted me to ice down my neck for twenty minutes each day with a special ice bag that his office happily sold me for about thirty dollars.

I iced my neck down, and that did feel better. I decided I would give the stretch machine a try, and see what happened.

I did ok on the first two or three visits. The pain wasn't getting any worse. Each visit the technicians increased the "pull" on my spinal cord. By about the fourth visit I told the technicians to stop the machine and get me out of it. You had to be strapped onto the machine in a harness like a pilot in an airplane.

I was in absolute agony. The doctor's assistant tried to convince me that pain was a necessary part of the healing process. He tried comparing it to physical therapy done on his knee after knee surgery. I informed him that this kind of pain was not normal, and I was not going to continue.

I decided to request to have a look at my medical records from the pain management doctor. This took some doing. His office was quite unwilling to let me look at my own medical records. They finally gave in. I could not believe what the doctor had recorded during my initial examination. Despite the fact I had come into his office on forearm crutches, and the crutches were next to me on the examination table; and I complained I was having trouble walking, my medical records indicated I had no trouble with ambulation.

Another symptom I had started noticing that I was becoming concerned about was that breathing was becoming more difficult. I noticed that I had to concentrate to breathe when normally breathing required no thought whatsoever. I kept telling this to all the doctors, and they kept ignoring me.

Sometimes I would lose the ability to control everything below the waist, typically when I was lying on the bed. Other times my legs would just collapse under me with just a few seconds of warning.

By this point the pain in my neck and my back was becoming absolutely agonizing. I was spending my days and nights in bed on the strongest pain pills I had, which were nothing. They weren't even coming close to touching the pain. I was getting no sleep. This was pain unlike anything I had ever experienced, and I had been through spinal cord pain.

I happened to speak with our friend, James Thompson, the former Air Force Sergeant, in Texas and told him what was happening. He said it sounded like I had another ruptured disc in my neck, and I should insist my family doctor order an MRI.

So I went back to Dr. Barrow. And I insisted he perform an MRI on my neck. He did. We got the results. Back to Dr. Steven Cathey, the neurosurgeon. The MRI showed I was badly ruptured at C3.

By this time it was February 2006. On March 15, 2006, I had surgery to fuse my C3/4 disc to the existing fusion. This would mean I was fused at four levels. Dr. Cathey told me that they do C5/6 fusions all day long without thinking about them; as it were, because they are so commonplace. He explained that C3/4 is the level of the spinal cord that controls breathing. He further explained if they nicked the cord, I'm on a ventilator. He said they would proceed very slowly and cautiously during the surgery. It was expected to take about an hour and a half.

During the operation Dr. Cathey discovered that my C3 disc was so badly herniated, there was nothing left of it. It was a husk. And that husk was sitting directly on my spinal cord. Since there was nothing left of the disc, the vertebrae on either side of the disc were grating against each other. No wonder I was having trouble breathing, and was in agonizing pain.

Dr. Cathey and I both knew that it would take months to determine what function would return and/or pain reduction would occur, if any, after the surgery. We waited.

I had been having severe pain in both elbows, the left worse than the right. After about a year, the pain in the right elbow vanished. The pain in my left elbow slowly improved.

But none of the coordination in my arms, wrists, and hands came back. The disc had been on my spinal cord too long.

7

"Good Days, Bad Days, Even Still"

If anybody can have 3 of out 2 medical conditions, it's you.—
My husband to me many years ago

One inescapable fact after a spinal cord injury is that you (or your family member) are going to have good days and bad days. Immediately after the initial injury, the days are all going to be bad for a long time. Then gradually you start having a slightly less bad day here and there. Then you have neutral days. Then a good day here and there.

Good days and bad days are going to continue for the rest of your life. Depending on how your health was before the accident will determine how you react to having good days and bad days.

If you were a healthy person before the accident, you may find it difficult adjusting to the ups and downs of your health. On the other hand, if you were a person with health problems before the accident, you may find the adjustment a little easier.

There are so many factors that can go into whether you feel good or not on any given day. Pressure sores, urinary tract infections, constipation, diarrhea, pain, the weather, how well you slept the night before, what particular stresses you are under, what you have to do that day, can all contribute to how you feel.

I have never enjoyed great health, so the adjustment for me was not as difficult. But it was difficult to get used to the idea that my body no longer works the way it is supposed to.

I hate the days with pain. Pain, screaming, stabbing into my consciousness. I cannot completely escape.

I miss having the stamina I used to. Like many people, I could really drop a few pounds.

I miss being able to tolerate the heat. Arkansas is hot. And humid. In the summer the temperature hovers around one-hundred degrees, and the humidity hovers near one-hundred percent. I have to be very careful now about going outside, because the heat can make me sick very quickly.

But I remind myself I am alive. And I go on.

8

"What If....?"

It is not every question
which deserves an answer.—
Publilius Syrus

In the years since the accident I have gone over the scenario of the accident in my mind many times. I have done this voluntarily. This is different from Post Traumatic Stress Disorder where the scenario plays in your mind over and over again involuntarily.

A little on Post Traumatic Stress Disorder (PTSD) before I continue the "what if" discussion. According to the National Center for PTSD:

> People with PTSD experience three difference kinds of symptoms. The first set of symptoms involves reliving the trauma in some way such as becoming upset when confronted with a traumatic reminder or thinking about the trauma when you are trying to do something else. The second set of symptoms involves either staying away from places or people that remind you of the trauma, isolating from other people, or feeling numb. The third set of symptoms includes things such as feeling on guard, irritable, or startling easily.[1]

I will admit that, sometimes, when I am passing the location of the accident I get unnerved. Also if I see a car wreck on TV in the same scenario as mine, it can bother me. But this does not happen all the time.

As I discussed on the chapter about my accident, it was a t-bone wreck. For the reader who does not know what a t-bone wreck is, I will explain. The Urban Dictionary defines a t-bone as: "When a car crashes into another car forming the shape of a T."[2] My car was the stem of the t.

The first "what if" thought, is, of course, what if the accident hadn't happened at all. The effects of this "what if" thought are far too broad to imagine and impossible to know. It is not a realistic "what if."

The second "what if" thought is what if I had had time to hit the brakes. This would have slowed the speed of the impact.

The third "what if" thought is "what if I had had a car with air bags?" I do have an answer to this question. I saw an episode of *Crash Test Human* on The National Geographic Channel. The episode was titled "Cars." In this show they demonstrated a t-bone collision in a car with air bags. The car they were running into looked like an old Ford Escort. This would have been slightly smaller than the actual car I ran into, which was a Dodge Intrepid. The car they were driving looked like a Chevrolet Cavalier or similar sized car; which would have been slightly larger than the car I was driving, which was a Dodge Colt.[3]

The other difference between the re-enacted collision, and my accident is that the other car was moving in my accident. In their re-enacted collision, the car was stationary. The effective speed of their wreck would have been slightly less than the actual effective speed of my accident. In the accident re-enaction, the speed was not sufficient to set off the air bags.

I have also wondered about "what if my head had not hit the roof of the car?" I might not have suffered the closed head injury, but I can't be certain of this because the suddenness of the change of momentum was so great. I might still have suffered a closed head injury from the suddenness of changing from a forward direction to being slowed down by hitting the other car.

The other "what if?" question I have always had is "what if the paramedics/ER doctor had realized I had a spinal cord injury, and had treated me with Prednisone. Prednisone is a commonly used drug to prevent progressive damage to the spinal cord.[4] It has been standard treatment for spinal cord injuries since about 1998, three years after my accident.[5] In my research I found an author who cited several articles worldwide that discussed the lack of evidence Prednisone is an effective treatment to prevent damage in acutely injured spinal cord patients.

So it appears that having airbags and not having been given Prednisone did not make any difference.

I realized something while writing this book that has not occurred to me in the previous twelve, almost thirteen years. I was driving northeast. The suns rises in the east and sets in the west. The other driver would have been looking west, into the sun. It was also getting close to dusk. I was driving a sky blue metallic car. The other driver may never have seen me.

I will never know.

9

"Carolyn, What Syndrome and Symptoms Do You Have?"

It's a tough question and it requires introspection—
Jonathan Smith

This chapter may seem out of place here because I don't discuss the different incomplete spinal cord syndromes and symptoms that spinal cord injury survivors can have until later in the book. It will make more sense after you have read some of the later chapters.

I'm not going to go into extreme detail on how my body does and doesn't work. I know many spinal cord injury survivors in their books have done so, On some things, I will share the specifics. I reserve the right to keep intimate details to myself, but I will share the generalities where I feel comfortable doing so.

I'd like to start with the question of what spinal cord syndrome I have. I've never been told specifically by a doctor which one, so my conclusions are my own.

Since I have feeling and movement below the level of injury, although abnormal, I obviously don't have a complete injury. That's a no-brainer.

I wrote in my posts on the National Spinal Cord Injury Discussion Forum that I have Central Cord Syndrome (see the Central Cord Syndrome chapter). I came to that conclusion before I wrote this book.

I had come to the conclusion I had Central Cord Syndrome because of the way my injury happened. I had a hyperextension injury of the spinal cord in the neck at the C5/6 and C6/7 levels. From my research I had found that hyperextension injuries cause Central Cord Syndrome without neck breakage. I did not break my neck according to any of the x-rays or MRI scans that were done.

I had also found in my research that Central Cord Syndrome affects the upper body more than the lower body, In Central Cord Syndrome, the legs recover function, as do the bladder and bowels,

My legs are weak, requiring me to use forearm crutches or a walker. My legs collapse out from under me. At times I can feel my legs, but I cannot move them. My bladder and bowel function are far from normal.

I found an excellent comparison of the different spinal cord syndromes in *The first 48 hours* [*sic*] by Paul Harrison.[1] This resource gives good information on the initial management and evaluation of spinal cord injuries. It also has drawings of how the most common spinal cord injuries happen.

After reading the discussion of Anterior Cord Syndrome being not only the common form of incomplete injury, but also typically being induced by a high speed accident, I began to wonder if I had Anterior Cord Syndrome. As I mentioned in the Preface, with a t-bone accident I certainly had the high-velocity impact for an Anterior Cord Syndrome injury. I was restrained, but my head hit the roof of the car where the windshield and car roof meet.

Anterior Cord Syndrome also results in weakness below the level of injury with reduced pain and temperature below the level of the lesion. The senses of crude touch, position (proprioception) and vibrations are usually well preserved below the level of injury."[1]

Central Cord Syndrome can come from trauma also, It costs strength in the arms but the strength in the legs is usually normal. There are negative effects on the ability to sense pain and temperature below the level of injury. [1]

I have arm function below the shoulders, but my arms are very weak. I have lost the fine coordination in my hands and fingers. My abdominal muscles are weak. I can still sense position in my entire body, And of course, the crazy thing about my condition is that my spinal cord "shorts out" as my neurosurgeon puts it. Sometimes signals get through. Sometimes they don't.

My neurosurgeon has also diagnosed me with the equivalent of post-polio syndrome from a spinal cord injury. I am continuing to lose function. One of the articles I read discussed how people with Central Cord Syndrome can lose function over time, instead of gaining it as in other types of spinal cord syndromes.

Incomplete spinal cord injuries can be so different from each other. It can be very difficult to force them to fall into categories. And who ever heard of a spinal cord that works sometimes, but not others? This is not covered in any of the spinal cord injury syndromes I found in my research.

Things You Need To Know Right After a Spinal Cord Injury

10

Ways The Spinal Cord Can Be Injured

"He who joyfully marches to music in rank and file has already earned my contempt. He has been given a large brain by mistake, since for him the spinal cord would surely suffice."—
Albert Einstein

What can I say? For all its importance in the body, there just aren't many quotations on the spinal cord. It's not something most people talk about.... until after they have injured it.

But how exactly does the spinal cord come to be injured? We hear almost daily of automobile accidents damaging the spinal cord, diving accidents damaging the spinal cord, or gunshot injuries to the spinal cord.

An understanding of how the spinal cord is damaged requires a quick discussion of the two types of spinal cord injuries: complete and incomplete. A person who has no function or sensation below the level of injury to the spinal cord is considered to have a complete injury. A person who has any function or sensation below the level of injury to the spinal cord is considered to have an incomplete injury.

Comparing one person's spinal cord injury to another person's spinal cord injury is like comparing apples and oranges. So doctors needed to come up with a more universal way to "measure" the degree of spinal cord injury.

The method they chose was to figure out if any part of the body universally lacked sensation in a complete injury. And, yes as it turns out, there is. If a person has no motor or sensory function in the lowest level of the spinal cord, at S4/S5; then that person is considered to have a complete injury.

What this means in real life terms, is if a person cannot feel or cannot control the area around his or her anus ("asshole," "butt hole," "bunghole," or whatever other common term you are familiar with), he or she has a complete injury.

Incomplete spinal cord injuries are as varied as there are spinal cord injurees. But more on that in the next chapter. A person can initially be classified as having a complete spinal cord injury only to be reclassified as an incomplete injury days, weeks, months, or years after the initial injury. This was true for Christopher Reeve, perhaps the most well-known spinal cord injuree in recent years.

I suppose it is theoretically possible for a person to be initially diagnosed as having an incomplete injury, and then later losing function to be reclassified as a complete injury.

Back to how the spinal cord can be injured. Let me clear up a common misconception first. Most people assume that when a person has suffered a complete spinal cord injury that the spinal cord has actually been torn in two, with two separate pieces. Like cutting a spaghetti strand in two. This is not necessarily true.

Although the spinal cord can be literally cut in two by damage from a bullet or bone fragments, this happens less frequently. What happens more often is the spinal cord is so badly damaged that it cannot transmit a signal from the part of the spinal cord above the level of injury to the level of the spinal cord below the level of injury.

In incomplete injuries there are two common ways the spinal cord can be injured. The first is when a bone fragment from a broken vertebra or broken vertebrae press on the cord. A bullet puts pressure on the cord in the same way bone from broken vertebra or vertebrae could. The second is when one or more of the soft cervical discs press on the spinal cord.

A group of doctors presented a new theory on how the spinal cord is injured in 2002. They proposed the cause of the damage in a spinal cord injury is the same as the cause of damage in a closed head injury. They theorized that it is not the initial injury that causes the damage. Instead it is the lack of oxygen, and lack of blood flow to the damaged location. The blood carries oxygen and nutrients to the area.

In addition cell membranes are damaged or destroyed. When the cell membranes are those of nerve cells, this disrupts the flow of vital information from the brain to the body and vice versa.[1]

For more information on closed head injury see the appropriate chapter.

11

The Neck Bone Is Connected To The Hip Bone....?

Unsolved Mysteries Of Anatomy

Where can a man buy a cap for his knee
or the key to a lock of his hair?
Can his eyes be called an academy
because there are pupils there?

Is the crown of your head where jewels are found?
Who travels the bridge of your nose?
If you want to shingle the roof of your mouth,
would you use the nails on your toes?

Can you sit on the drum of your ear?
Can the calf in your leg eat the corn off your toe?
Then why not grow corn on the ear?
Can the crook in your elbow be sent to jail?
If so, just what did he do?

How can you sharpen your shoulder blades?
I don't know, do you?—
Author unknown

Let's get the anatomy lesson out of the way first. You need to understand how your body is built to comprehend what has happened to you, your friend or family member. I am going to try and do this in plain English. You're under enough stress as it is. You don't need to go to medical school as well right now.

For those of you who are determined to have a nice, formal discussion of human anatomy with pictures, read *Still Lives: Narratives of Spinal Cord Injury* by Jonathan Cole (see Additional Reading and Movies chapter for the full citation).

Let's talk about your neck. We've all heard the expression "pain in the neck." Necks *hurt* when they are injured, even slightly. And they can hurt a lot. It's a difficult type of pain to ignore. And that's how the expression came about.

But why do necks hurt when they are injured? There is a limited amount of stretching the human neck is designed to take. If you were a cat, it would be different. Cats are designed to take a lot of stretching, and not get hurt. But we're not cats.

Some body parts must be rigid to support you. Others are more flexible and softer. Your neck is a combination of rigid parts and flexible parts. Remember as a child playing with a toy that was a wire with different types of large beads on it? They were different colors and different shapes? Your neck is somewhat like that wire with the beads on it. You have a wire in the middle (your spinal cord), except it is more like a strand of spaghetti instead of a wire. It is the same texture and hardness as a strand of spaghetti. Your spinal cord carries the message from your brain to lift your left arm or lower your right leg and by exactly how much.

The "hard beads" on your body's "wire toy" are there to make it possible for you to stand upright. Doctors felt this urge a long, long time ago to name everything in the body in Latin. They call each "hard bead" a vertebra, and they call more than one vertebra vertebrae. Vertebrae are made of bones; the same as in your arm, leg, hands, feet, fingers, and toes.

The "soft beads" on your body's "wire toy" are there to serve as a cushion between the "hard beads" so the "hard beads" don't rub against each other. The "soft beads" also make it possible for you to stretch and turn. Those doctors who named everything in those funny Latin words call these discs. But wait! Isn't disc an English word? Yes disc is. But it comes from the Latin word discus. For those of you who are sports-minded, this is the same word discus as the flat plate-like object that is thrown in competition.

Are the discs disc-shaped? Nothing in the world is easy, is it? Well, most of them are. The very top two in your neck are not. They are more square and smaller.

So, assuming you have been constructed as a "normally," you have eight vertebrae in your neck (the "hard beads"). Then you have the "soft beads" between them. The discs are referred to by their relative location to each pair of vertebrae. Thus, if you (or your family member or your friend) have injured the disc between the fifth vertebra and the sixth vertebra; you have injured C5/6 (alternatively referred to as C5-6).

I guess all those years ago, doctors decided to be very specific. So they divided the discs in your neck and your back into subsections. The vertebrae in your neck are called cervical vertebrae. The Latin word for neck is cervix. The discs in-between are referred to as C1-C8.

The next twelve vertebrae connect the bottom of your neck to the bottom of your rib cage, more or less. These are larger than the vertebrae in your neck. As you go down the spinal cord, each one is larger than the one above it. These are called thoracic vertebrae.

Thoracic comes from the word thorax. Thorax is a little more complicated in its origin. It comes from both Latin and Greek. It meant breastplate or chest. The word is commonly used today to refer to the area of the body between the head and the abdomen (belly). Not all creatures that have a thorax have a neck, so that's why it's between the head and abdomen. The discs in-between are referred to as T1-T12.

Let's go down further into your back. Next you've got five vertebrae in your low back. These are called lumbar vertebrae. Lumbus in Latin means loin. These five vertebrae (L1-L5) are even larger than the previous twelve thoracic vertebrae. They support most of the weight of your body.

Finally, you've got what doctors call a sacrum. Here I've got to get a little more complicated on you. The sacrum in an adult human is a single triangular-shaped bone. In a child the sacrum consists of five vertebrae. They fuse together as the child grows. They are *supposed* to fuse together, anyway. They don't always. Mine didn't. So I've got an extra vertebra.

Think of your sacrum as a fancy hinge that connects the vertebrae in your low back with your pelvis (your hip bones). The discs are referred to as S1-S5.

And last, but not least, is your coccyx. This is what people in the real world call a tailbone. Most of us have fallen on our tailbones at some point in our lives, and that really hurts. Especially if you've ever broken your tailbone. If you were a cat, you would have more bones past your tailbone. But you're not so you don't. Your coccyx is like your sacrum. It is made of three to five fused bones in an adult. The bones are not fused in a child.

That covers the bones that make up the spinal column. But there's still a little more to the spinal cord. There's a section at the bottom of the spinal cord doctors call the cauda equina. This is (you guessed it) Latin for horse's tail. If you were to see this section of the spinal cord, it looks like a horse's tail. Where a horse has hair in its tail, we have the spinal nerve roots. The cauda equina lines up roughly with the L2 vertebra and on down through the S5 vertebra.[1]

You might be wondering about the name of this chapter. In the earlier days of spinal fusion surgery, it was common to take a piece of bone from the crest of the hip bone, and use it to replace either a soft disc or broken vertebra(e) or both. This procedure is still performed in some situations. Today it is more common to use cadaver (dead person) bone and titanium hardware in many situations.

12

"You Are Not Alone"

I know SCI is about the biggest curve ball as life can give us....—
Richard Hollicky in *Roll Models*

One of the first feelings I experienced upon having a spinal cord injury is that I was suddenly *alone.* I was no longer the person I used to be. I no longer knew my body. I felt there was no one else like me. I didn't fit among "normal" people anymore. I didn't fit among most spinal cord injury survivors either because I wasn't in a wheelchair. I couldn't find much on the Internet in 1994 about what I was going through.

You (or your family member) are not alone.

You have become part of a group of people who know exactly how you feel. And they are willing to help. You have friends you have never met.

During one of the first spinal cord injury support group meetings I went to, one of the spinal cord injury survivors made a comment I want to share with you. This particular gentleman is an incomplete quadriplegic in a power wheelchair. He told the group how important it was to him to be present at every meeting. He said he would come back from vacation just to attend the support group meeting. It was that important to him. He went on to say, "in here we are all normal." That thought really stuck with me.

And he's right. When you are with other people with a similar disability, you lose the feelings of alienation from non-disabled people.

I will continue this discussion in the chapter on Peer Support.

13

A Brief History of Spinal Cord Injury and Treatment

History is the sum total of things that could have been avoided.—
Konrad Adenauer

Oh no. History. Boring….!

Don't fret. This is a short history. There is no pop quiz at the end of the chapter.

I attended a wonderful presentation during one of the Arkansas Spinal Cord Commission support group meetings. It was on the history of spinal cord injury and treatment given by Ben Hollis from the local Little Rock Veterans' Administration office. I'm trying to re-create what I can from his presentation.[1]

Possibly the earliest medical quotation regarding spinal cord injury dates from around 3000-2500 B.C. in the Edwin Smith Surgical Papyrus, a 17th century B.C. manuscript which copied the earlier manuscript. Until the mid part of the 20th century the following statement was true regarding doctors' attitudes toward treatment of spinal cord injury, "One having a dislocation in a vertebra of his neck, while he is unconscious of his two legs and his two arms, and his urine dribbles—an ailment not to be treated."[2]

You've probably heard of King Tut. Maybe through the exhibit that toured the U.S. If you're old enough, maybe through Steve Martin's hilarious song. But did you know that King Tut may have been the earliest recorded celebrity with a spinal cord injury according to some sources?

Maybe you've heard of General Douglas MacArthur? He was a famous American army general in World War II. He suffered a spinal cord injury in a jeep accident.

A man responsible for advances in military aviation during the early twentieth century, Frank "Spig" Wead, was also a spinal cord injury survivor. He was injured in a fall. The 1957 John Wayne movie "The Wings of Eagles" was based on his life story.

American musicians Teddy Pendergrass and Vic Chesnutt were both rendered paraplegics after accidents from driving drunk.[2] [3] Missouri state senator Chuck Graham is also a paraplegic.[5]

I found an article that provides a very detailed discussion of the history of treatment of spinal cord injury in the nineteenth and early twentieth century for wounds sustained in military conflicts.[6]

Many of the advances in treatment of spinal cord injuries were the result of World Wars I and II. Spinal cord injuries were common because of jeep accidents. Jeeps had a tendency to flip over, injuring the occupants. Lee Goldstein provides one of the best summaries of the history of spinal cord injury I have seen in his book, *So Far So Good.*[7]

As Goldstein quite succinctly states, "Up until World War II, almost all spinal injured patients died." Goldstein goes on to relate that Nancy Reagan's stepfather was a doctor named Loyal Davis who pioneered treatment of spinal cord injuries.

Goldstein also discusses two advances that made recovery from spinal cord injuries a possibility. In the 1930s two men whose names are now synonymous with wheelchairs, Everest and Jennings, invented the folding wheelchair. The second event was the invention of automatic transmissions in cars. Goldstein mentions one more event that meant increased freedom for spinal cord injury survivors: the advances in incontinence equipment over time that made being away from home for long periods of time possible.

14

Why You Need a Sense of Humor After a Spinal Cord Injury

I think the next best thing to solving a problem is finding some humor in it.—
Frank A. Clark

After a spinal cord injury, people are going to be telling you (or your family member) how important it is to have a sense of humor. For anyone who isn't exactly sure what a sense of humor is, Wikipedia defines humor as "the ability or quality of people, objects, or situations to evoke feelings of amusement in other people." A sense of humor is defined as "the ability to experience humor, a quality which all people share...."[1]

A spinal cord injury isn't exactly the type of situation that people find funny right off the bat. We as human beings don't like change. We don't generally find humor in things we are uncomfortable with.

Richard Hollicky states in *Roll Models*: "We move at our own speed and in our own ways, and some of us take awhile before we can begin to question how SCI is affecting our lives and what we should be doing about it."[2]

Don't worry if you don't have a sense of humor. If you didn't have a sense of humor before your accident, it may take time for you to develop one. If you did have a sense of humor before your injury, it may take time for it to come back. It's possible you may never develop one after the accident.

Getting on with your life will be a lot easier if you have a sense of humor.

15

Know Your Surgeon and Anesthesiologist

Knowledge is Power.—
Sir Francis Bacon

If you have already had spinal surgery after your accident, then this chapter will be of no use to you. If you are considering surgery, the information in this chapter may be useful.

You want to find a good neurosurgeon or a good orthopedic surgeon, but how?

If you have to have emergency spinal cord surgery, asking around to find a good surgeon (either a neurosurgeon or an orthopedic surgeon) is not an option. A neurosurgeon specializes in surgery on the nervous system. Often a neurosurgeon will specialize in either spinal cord surgery or brain surgery. An orthopedic surgeon specializes in surgery on bones and connecting tissues, such as tendons, ligaments, and muscles.

If you are not in an emergency situation, ask around your community. Try in your church, synagogue, or place of worship if you attend regularly. Some forms of spinal cord surgery have become routine these days. You can probably find someone who has had a disc fused. Talk to that person. Find out who his or her surgeon was, and if the person is happy with the results.

If you are having a spinal cord operation, you are having an operation to restore function. You may be having the operation to restore stability in your spinal column as well. Many doctors do not perform spinal cord operations only for pain without a loss of function because the surgery is risky.

You may find some return of function and/or lessening of pain when you wake up in the recovery room after surgery. It may take months or years after the operation for you to experience your maximum recovery. You may require more than one operation in a short period of time or over a period of time.

You are, of course, limited in your choice of surgeon to the doctors that are covered on your health insurance, Medicare, or Medicaid. But you can take steps to insure that your surgical results are as successful as possible.

If your situation is not an emergency, your family doctor has probably given you a referral to either a neurosurgeon or an orthopedic surgeon. I will discuss the different types of spinal surgery in the next chapter. Ideally, you want your surgery to be performed by the person your family doctor would have the surgery performed by if it were him or her in your position.

Ask around your community to find out who is the "best" doctor for your operation. Doctors develop reputations. People are happy to talk about a good experience with a surgeon. You may also find out which doctors to avoid.

You also need to be comfortable with your anesthesiologist. You do have choices on your anesthesiologist. If you wish to request as specific anesthesiologist, you must make arrangements in advance.

Be sure to communicate to your surgeon and anesthesiologist any medical conditions you have which might affect the outcome of your surgery. Do you have high blood pressure? How about asthma? Do you smoke or drink regularly? Have you had surgery before and if so, when and why? Did you have a bad reaction to the anesthesia in a previous surgery? Have any of your family members had a bad reaction to anesthesia in a previous surgery? Are you allergic to any medications? Be sure to tell this information to your surgeon and anesthesiologist.[1]

If you are a family member or friend of the injured person, and the injured person is unable to communicate medical history; make sure the doctors and nurses know the person's medical history, allergies, and prescription medications being taken.

16

Surgery for Spinal Cord Injuries

Picking up the pieces, they don't fit
Looking for the good life, what became of it
Looking for some answers, find that I have none
Feel like I'm stranded a long way from the sun
Look into the future and know that I'm not scared
Long as I'm breathing I can be repaired
"Right To The Top"—The Kings

Surgery for a spinal cord injury is very important. If you have suffered broken vertebrae, the longer those pieces of bone are pressing on your spinal cord, the lower chance of recovery you have.

Most spinal cord injury patients are operated on within a few days of their injury. Their injury is diagnosed promptly in the emergency room, making a quick response by either a neurosurgeon or orthopedic surgeon possible.

There are several different schools of thought in the medical community on how to repair a spinal cord injury. Spinal cord surgery also changes as advances are made in medicine. The surgery that was performed on me in 1995 is very different from most spinal cord operations today.

Today you can have a disc fusion, a bone cage, or an artificial disc. In a disc fusion, the broken vertebrae are repaired with either donated cadaver bone or bone taken from your own hip (see below). The damaged soft disc is removed and replaced with bone. Titanium screws and plates are used to hold the whole thing together. The fusion takes up to a year to fully heal.

Depending on the injury, the surgeon may operate on the neck from the front (anterior), the back (posterior), or both.[1]

In a bone cage, the surgeon builds a titanium cage and seeds it with bone fragments from the broken vertebrae. If the vertebrae were not broken, then the surgeon uses donor bone or bone harvested from the hip.

With artificial discs, the damaged disc is removed and replaced with an artificial one. This provides more freedom of movement than a fusion or a bone cage. It also has the advantage that a person does not have to wait for the fusion to heal or have plates and screws inserted. Another advantage of an artificial disc is that it maintains motion and lessens the chances of transition syndrome (see Transitional Syndrome chapter).[2]

An article in the June 2005 *Managed Care* magazine discusses an artificial disc made of cobalt chromium, the Charité Artificial Disc. It is very expensive ($11,500). The article goes on to discuss that not just anybody with a spinal cord injury can have an artificial disc used in his or her surgery. The FDA (Food and Drug Administration) has very strict requirements about the type of injury in which the artificial devices are used.[3] The FDA's rules only cover the United States.

There is another artificial disc approved by the FDA. It comes in two versions, one for the neck and one for the back. The neck version is called PRODISC-C®. The back version is called PRODISC-L®. The first is called "C" for cervical (neck). The second is called "L" for lumbar (back). Both discs are made of a cobalt-chrome alloy and plastic.[4] [5]

Depending on the procedure, the surgeon may use bone grafts. There are three different sources of bone that may be used: 1) a man made bone graft substitute 2) a sterilized cadaver bone from a bone bank or 3) a bone graft taken from the patient's own body.[6]

Bone is normally taken from the hip if a bone graft is taken from the patient's own body. The bone can be taken from the front of the hip or the back of the hip. Pain after bone donation has been reported in surveys, and varies lasting more than three months in between approximately three to thirty-nine percent of patients. Pain lasting up to two years was reports in fifteen to thirty-nine percent of patients.[7]

If the surgery is being performed on the front of the neck, the surgeon will usually try to conceal the incision in one of the folds of the neck. I have found a great product for minimizing the scarring from the surgical incision. It is called ScarMassage. See the Resources chapter for more information.

If you are still self-conscious about your surgical scar, even after using ScarMassage, then there is another product that can also be used by both males and females. It is called Dermablend. It is a concealing cream that a professional at a makeup counter matches to your skin tone. Its purpose is to minimize the appearance of the scar. It is commonly used by people with scars or other skin discolorations. It is available online, and is also sold in department stores.

I can comment on the pain from a bone hip graft from personal experience. Oddly enough, I ended up talking with a man who had had the surgery done with a bone graft from his hip while I was in the hospital being prepared for my first surgery. He told me he had more pain from his hip than he did from his neck. He said it took five years for the pain to stop. It also took five years for the pain to stop for me. And it still hurts from time to time. Fortunately on my second and third operations my hipbone was not used.

There are several factors that influence the amount of pain produced in the bone graft from the hip:

1. The sensory nerves that exit in this region may be cut, bruised, or stretched.
2. Blood vessel injury can cause significant blood loss and blood clot formation.
3. If the bone is taken from the back of the hip, the join where the pelvis attaches to the spine can be damaged.
4. The hip can be broken if the bone graft is taken too close to the anterior iliac spine [this is the edge of the hip you can feel most prominently if you feel your hip].[8 9]

As with any surgery there are risks. Infection of the surgical site occurs in approximately one to five percent of patients. The risk of infection is higher if hardware is used in the surgery. If a patient is diabetic or overweight the risk of infection is higher.[10]

There are so many advances being made in materials science that I think eventually almost every person with a spinal cord injury needing surgery will receive an artificial disc.

17

Communicating With Your Doctor

Every accomplishment starts with the decision to try.—
Anonymous

One of the unfortunate realities of having a spinal cord injury is that many different doctors are now going to be part of your life on a regular basis. You will have regular checkups by certain specialists. You may have emergency situations take place as well. Effective communication with your doctor(s) is essential to your recovery and continued good health.

To be able to communicate with your doctor, you need to understand what the communication process is. Communication is the process of passing information and understanding from one person to another. In the communication process there must be a sender, which is you. There must be a receiver, which is your doctor. There must be a message, which is what you have to say to your doctor. There must be understanding, which means your doctor must receive and comprehend your message. There must be feedback from your doctor to you, which indicates your doctor understands what you said.[1]

I found some guides on the Internet to make communicating with your doctor easier. There are two basic scenarios when you will be communicating with your doctor(s): 1) immediately after your injury (while you are in the hospital/rehab and during follow-up care) and 2) months and years later.

Here is a list of useful suggestions:

Basic Advice

1. You (or your family member) should make a list of any medications you are taking and bring it with you to every doctor visit.
2. Make sure your doctor knows about any previous operations you have had.

3. Make sure your doctor knows about any allergies you have, whether to prescription medications, or everyday items (such as latex), or foods.
4. Make sure your doctor knows about any medical conditions you have such as autonomic dysreflexia, diabetes, high blood pressure, etc.
5. Make sure your doctor knows about your family medical history where appropriate.
6. Don't be afraid to do (or have a family member do) independent research such as on the Internet about your condition.
7. Ask plenty of questions and make sure you understand the answers.
8. Follow through on the agreed-upon treatment and if it is not working, don't be afraid to contact your doctor's office as soon as possible.
9. If you think of a question after you leave your doctor's office, don't be afraid to contact your doctor's office and ask the question.
10. Be sure to take all your medication. Not finishing your medication as prescribed may cause your condition to worsen.[2]

Questions
1. Ask your doctor "what do you think is causing my problem?"
2. Ask your doctor "is there more than one condition (disease) that could be causing my problem?"
3. Ask your doctor "what tests will you do to diagnose my problem and which of the conditions is present?"
4. Ask your doctor "how accurate are the tests for diagnosing the problem and the conditions?"
5. Ask your doctor "how safe are the tests?"
6. Ask your doctor "what is the likely course of this condition? What is the long-term outcome with and without treatment?"
7. Ask your doctor "what my treatment options? How effective is each treatment option? What are the benefits versus the risks of each treatment option?"
8. Ask your doctor "if my symptoms worsen, what should I do on my own? "When should I contact you?"
9. Ask your doctor "are you aware of the medications I am taking? Can they adversely interact with the medications you are prescribing for me?" (if your doctor is prescribing medication).
10. Ask your doctor "should we monitor for side effects of the medications that you are prescribing or for their interactions with other medications I am taking?" (if your doctor is prescribing medication).[3]

Don't be afraid to communicate with your doctor. Your recovery depends on it.

18

The Importance of Peer Support After a Spinal Cord Injury

Really great people make you feel that you too,
can become great—
Mark Twain

I have been accused of not staying up with current events. It only took me some eleven years after my spinal cord injury to discover support groups exist for spinal cord injury survivors. I only found out about a local support group while doing research for this book.

I became curious about peer support for people recovering from a spinal cord injury. I knew how it fit in with my own situation, but I was curious if there was anything universal about peer support related to a spinal cord injury.

The first thing I noticed in my quest about peer support is that *everybody* who has experienced a spinal cord injury seems to be writing a book about it these days. *Their story*. The number of "my story" books on the market is ever increasing. Whether this is to satisfy a desire to provide peer support to other SCI survivors or a means of increasing one's income, I can't say for any individual book. Maybe a little bit of both.

Richard Hollicky in *Roll Models* has interviewed many people with a spinal cord injury in his book. He indicates that these individuals were successful in having happy and productive lives after their injuries because they relied on peer support. They listened to other people who had been in wheelchairs for longer periods of time. The "old-timers" as Hollicky calls them, were more than happy to help.

Hollicky comments that peer support may become more necessary as the time increases after the initial injury. He points out that hospital and rehabilitation stays are becoming more limited, so people must find their support through other means. Those means include peers, the Internet, and their own communities.[1]

There are many ways to mentor others with a spinal cord injury. You can do so with another person in a rehabilitation hospital. Other ways of doing so are in community or rehabilitation support groups, volunteering at a rehabilitation hospital, or in chat groups.[2] You can even write a book like I did.

The existence of the many forums on the Internet for people who are looking for information about spinal cord injury also supports the theory that spinal cord injury survivors feel a need to help their fellow survivors. I know that I have felt a strong need to help other spinal cord injury survivors since my accident.

I have a theory about spinal cord injury survivors, and their need to help others in similar circumstances. Some were, of course, the caring sort before their injuries. Others were not. Not all spinal cord injury survivors become involved in the effort to help other survivors. Some never recover from the injury emotionally, and stay in a self-pity mode.

Steve Fiffer in his book about his own spinal cord injury and recovery, *Three Quarters, Two Dimes, and A Nickel*, describes that he may not be a dollar bill, but he's still "three quarters, two dimes, and a nickel."[3] In other words, you are not exactly like you were before a spinal cord injury, but you are basically the same person.

I think people who have overcome a spinal cord injury feel the need to help others in similar circumstances because it provides a *reason* for their injury. I discuss the problem of survivor guilt in later chapters. People asking "Why me?" Being able to help another spinal cord injury survivor answers that question.

Don't be afraid to seek out help from others. Or offer it to someone who needs it.

19

Family and Friends Adjustment to a Spinal Cord Injury

All biologic phenomena act to adjust;
there are no biologic actions other than adjustments.
Adjustment is another name for Equilibrium.
Equilibrium is the Universal, or that
which has nothing external to derange it.—
Charles Fort

The phone rings. You listen in disbelief. The phone call every person dreads has just come in. Your family member or friend has just been in a terrible accident. He or she has a spinal cord injury.

What now?

You feel shaken and numb. You experience disbelief, shock, anger and terror.[1]

The world as you know it has just been ripped apart. Your mind starts to race with questions:

Did the emergency medical people get to my family member or friend as soon as possible? Did they do everything they could for him or her? Is he or she getting the best medical care at X Hospital where they took him or her? Will he or she walk again? Will he or she live?

Your sense of "normal" and "routine" have just gone out the window. And why shouldn't they? Nobody has ever prepared you for this situation. You don't know what to do, how to act, how to help.

You may experience denial about your family member or friend's condition. You may feel grief. You may feel a sense of unfairness about the accident and injury. You may feel like something about the situation was your fault.[2]

Family roles are going to change. The injured person is going to need the help of friends and family. Not only during hospitalization and rehabilitation, but also after returning home. Other people are going to have to take over the responsibilities of the injured person until the injured person can either resume those responsibilities or another person takes over them.

The first thing you need to do is get answers to the endless list of questions you have. Ask the doctors. Ask the nurses. Ask the professional staff. Research on the Internet. Find a local support group and ask members of it.[1]

People react differently to stress. Some people feel like they have to take control of the situation. They want to make lists. They feel like they have to be constantly busy. Others prefer to put the situation out of their minds. They keep their minds occupied doing other things.

You need to prioritize your tasks. Decide what is really important to do in the situation. Put everything else on hold. Yes, you need to visit the injured person in the hospital or rehabilitation if they are local. But you also need to take care of yourself. Don't forget to eat, even if you don't feel hungry. Rest even if you don't sleep. At least lie down. Exercise to reduce stress. Find someone who is a good listener and talk about what is on your mind.[3]

A few general guidelines on the situation are:

1. Try to be a good listener.
2. Do not try to talk the injured person out of negative feelings.
3. Express your feelings too. Keeping up a "brave front" is not always a good idea.
4. Express your support and reassurance.
5. Hold on to hope.[4]

You may never have dealt with a disabled person before. It may cause you to feel awkward when you are with your family member or friend. Here is some general advice:

1. People with disabilities are people. Your family member or friend is the same person he or she was before the accident.
2. People with disabilities know they are disabled. Don't avoid the subject of the person's disability.
3. A person with a disability does not have a contagious disease. You won't get sick by coming in contact with him or her.
4. Don't be condescending.
5. Don't hold a person with a disability in awe or treat him or her like a hero.
6. Adults with disabilities are adults. Don't treat them like children.
7. People with disabilities can respond on their own. Don't talk to a third person as if the disabled person is not in the room with you.

8. It may take longer for a person with a disability to get dressed or catch a bus. Be considerate.
9. People with disabilities can have—and enjoy—sex.[5]

If you are the spinal cord injury survivor, you need to remember to be patient with your family and friends. They are having to adjust to the new situation. They may keep trying to deny the injury is permanent. Don't lose patience with them if they do. They need time to accept the permanent change of circumstances.

If you are the family or friend(s) of the spinal cord injury survivor, do your best to be patient as well. Adjustment to the new circumstances will take time for everyone. Life will never be the same. It's possible it could be better than before.

Life can take unusual twists.

20

Trauma Centers

Getting out of the hospital is a lot like resigning from a book club. You're not out of it until the computer says you're out of it.—
Erma Bombeck

Many factors go into recovering from a spinal cord injury. The injured person has control over some. Not others. The chances of surviving a spinal cord injury are much better now than in the middle of the twentieth century. Many advances in medical care have been made, and more will be made in the future.

One of the factors the injured person does not have control over is where the accident takes place. Accidents happen everywhere. Major urban areas. Suburbs. State parks. Remote areas. Backyards. Bathtubs.

The sooner a person can receive medical care and a spinal cord injury is diagnosed, the sooner corrective measures can be taken.

In this chapter I want to briefly discuss the concept of trauma centers. As you are probably aware, some communities don't even have a hospital. Large metropolitan areas have several hospitals. Depending upon its facilities, type of staff and hours dedicated to handling emergencies, each hospital in the United States has a level rating.

A trauma center is formally defined as a hospital equipped to perform as a casualty receiving station for the emergency medical services by providing the best possible medical care for traumatic injuries twenty-four hours a day, three hundred sixty-five days a year. Trauma centers were established as the medical establishment realized that such injuries often require immediate and complex surgery to save the patient.[1]

There are four levels of trauma facilities. The number of patients admitted yearly also contributes to the level grading of a facility. The level ranking of a facility may change periodically as each facility is periodically reviewed. [1]

A Level I trauma center has a full range of specialists and equipment available twenty-four hours a day. It admits a minimum required annual volume of severely injured patients. Additionally, a Level I center has a program of research, is a leader in trauma education and injury prevention. It is a referral resource for communities in nearby regions.

A Level II trauma center works in collaboration with a Level I center. It provides comprehensive trauma care, and supplements the clinical expertise of a Level I institution. It provides twenty-four hour availability of all essential specialties, personnel and equipment. Minimum volume requirements may depend on local conditions. These institutions are not required to have an ongoing program of research or a surgical residency program.

A Level III trauma center does not have the full availability of specialists; but does have the resources for the emergency resuscitation, surgery and intensive care of most trauma patients. A Level III center has transfer agreements with Level I and/or Level II trauma centers that provide back-up resources for the care of exceptionally severe injuries.

A Level IV trauma center provides the stabilization and treatment of severely injured patients in remote areas where no alternative care is available. [1]

A complete list of verified trauma centers is available from the American College of Surgeons Trauma Programs website.[2] I am not going to reproduce the listing because it changes over time.

21

How an Incomplete Spinal Cord Injury is Diagnosed

Bedside manners are no substitute
for the right diagnosis.—
Alfred P. Sloan

I'm going to start this chapter with a simple explanation of how a spinal cord injury is diagnosed. Then I will explain in more detail how a spinal cord injury is diagnosed. The more detailed explanation is for medical professionals and anyone else who is interested in the subject beyond a brief explanation.

If you have already had a spinal cord injury, you will be quite familiar with the diagnostic process already. Your family members and friends may not be familiar with the process.

Diagnosis of a complete spinal cord injury is much less complicated than the diagnosis of an incomplete spinal cord injury. The person with a complete spinal cord injury, if conscious, will usually complain of the inability to feel anything or the inability to move anything below a certain level of his or her body. For example, this person would complain of being unable to move anything below, say, the shoulders.

Diagnosis of an incomplete spinal cord injury is more complicated. The person may still have feeling below the level of injury. The person may still have the ability to move below the level of injury. The person may complain of feeling weaker below the level of injury. The person may complain of pain below the level of injury. The person may complain of loss of control of the bladder and/or bowels. The person may start out as if he or she has a complete injury, but may recover function and/or feeling over time.

Emergency medical professionals on the scene of your accident will ask if your neck or back hurts. If you have answered "yes" to either of these, it should raise the suspicion of the emergency medical professionals that you may have a spinal cord injury.[1]

You may be asked if you can feel and move your arms and legs. You may be asked if you are under the influence of alcohol or drugs to see if either or both of these might be masking any symptoms. You may be asked if you have any other pain that might be drawing your attention.[2]

If the emergency medical professionals suspect you have a spinal cord injury, they will immobilize your spinal column. This is ideally done with your entire spinal column in what is called a neutral position (not bent) on a flat surface. You may be placed on a flat backboard (or suitable substitute), in a cervical (neck) collar, and/or in side head supports, and/or in strapping (usually tape). You should be strapped about the shoulders and pelvis and head.[3]

Once you reach the hospital, the emergency room staff will likely perform what is called a "log roll" on you. It is the standard procedure to allow examination of the back and transfer on and off of backboards. It takes four people to perform (not including the patient). One person holds the patient's head and directs the roll. One person holds the patient's chest. One person holds the patient's pelvis and one person holds the patient's arms and legs. The patient should only have a "log roll" performed as few times as possible to avoid further injury.[4]

Once you get to the hospital, you can expect to have a series of tests to check for spinal cord injury. The first are standard x-rays to check for broken bones. The next set is CT scans (computed or computerized tomography). The final tests are MRI scans (Magnetic Resonance Imaging).[5] You may not have all three series of tests performed.

CT scans have become standard diagnostic procedures. MRI scans are much more expensive and are reserved for situations where more detailed results are necessary. CT scans are non-invasive (the doctors don't have to cut you open!) tests. They function by creating a three-dimensional image from a series of two-dimensional images.[6] To clarify the difference between two-dimensional and three-dimensional images, a piece of paper is two-dimensional and an apple is three-dimensional. CT scans are used for examination of body components where there are many different densities of body components involved.

MRI scans are also non-invasive. MRI scans also use a series of two-dimensional pictures to create three-dimensional images. MRI scans are better than CT scans because they show the difference between different body structures with more detail.[7] For example, an MRI scan is better than a CT scan at showing ruptured discs in the spinal column. While a broken vertebra may show on a standard x-ray and will likely show on a CT scan, the soft tissue of a ruptured disc does not show as well.

Now let's look at a spinal cord injury from the perspective of a medical professional, beginning with a/an First Responder/Paramedic/Emergency Medical Technician [EMT] to a doctor.

One author in his book on spinal cord injury discusses "safe assumptions" to when initially encountering a trauma victim in order to avoid missing the diagnosis or worsening the injury. This is the list he presents:

1. Every patient with a head injury and every unconscious patient have an SCI.
2. Every patient with multiple traumas has an SCI.
3. Every motor-vehicle accident victim has an SCI.
4. Every victim of a sports or recreational accident has an SCI.
5. Every severely injured worker has an SCI.
6. Every victim of a fall at home has an SCI.
7. Every SCI has an unstable spinal column and any movement of the spinal column after trauma will cause further damage to the spinal cord.[8]

A doctor may check to see if you can determine the difference between the feel of sharp objects and dull objects. If you have sudden shooting sensations like electric shocks that spread down your body or into your limbs when your neck is flexed, this is another indication of a spinal cord injury in the neck.[9]

There are two medical signs, Hoffman's Sign and Babinski's Sign, that the doctors may test for. More on these in the next chapter.

The author listed above also provides a list of "spinal clues" which can be obtained from a combination of a physical exam and vital signs. I will "translate" the medical terminology into plain English. The plain English in brackets is mine. The list is as follows:

1. Hypotension [low blood pressure] and bradycardia [a resting adult heart rate of less than 60 [*sic*] beats per minute] occur in spinal shock
2. Paradoxical respiration [deflation of the lung while breathing in and inflation while breathing out (this "translation" took a translation of its own because the definition was in medical terms)].
3. Low body temperature and high skin temperature
4. Priapism [persistent erection of the penis in men, often painful, and not related to sexual arousal]
5. Bilateral paralysis of arms and legs, especially flaccid [paralysis on both arms and both legs especially if lacking in normal muscle tone (This author may be

the only doctor I know of who uses "erect" and "flaccid" in two adjacent sentences in a non sexual context.)]
6. Bilateral paralysis of legs, especially flaccid [see above for flaccid definition, Isn't he repeating himself here? He's already talked about paralysis of the legs, But what do I know? I'm not a doctor.]
7. Lack of response to painful stimuli [I've had many visits to an OB/GYN where this would have been welcome. I'll bet most men would welcome this on a rectal exam.]
8. Detection of an anatomic level in response to painful stimuli [I'm not really sure on this one what he is trying to say, I'm guessing that this is the ability to detect something painful only above a certain area in the body and below that level a person cannot detect the pain.]
9. Painful stimulation produces only head movement or facial grimacing [I've got to guess on this one also, I think he's trying to say that a normal reaction to something painful would be to try and jerk away from the pain, If a person is not trying to jerk away from the pain, it would indicate an inability to move the areas of the body where the pain is being felt.]
10. Sweating level [Again I've got to guess but I'm more certain on this one, I think he's trying to say if a person is not sweating below a certain area on the body but is sweating above that area.]
11. Horner's syndrome [This seems to cover just about everything from my research, Some of the symptoms listed were inappropriate reaction to light by the pupils of the eyes, the eyes sinking into the face, lack of sweating on the face, eyelids drooping, facial sweating, rapid eye movements in which the eyes are moving up and down or back and forth.]
12. Brown-Sequard syndrome [As above, the ability to move one side of the body but not the other] [10]

On the subject of symptom four above, priapism, I have a story. (No, you're not going to get any "juicy" details of my sex life here). Raymond and I are long-time friends with a married couple in Arkansas. Both of them are volunteer fire-fighters in their community. The man's wife is an EMT/paramedic. They were doing emergency preparedness drills for a large scale accident. A female friend of theirs was also participating in the drills. The man was down on the ground, "obviously injured." During the initial exam of the man by the female friend, the man's wife shouted "*No Checking For Priapism!*"

Doctors, always wanting standardization, devised a scale to measure and grade spinal cord injury beyond that of level in the body, The original scale was devised before World War II at Stokes-Mandeville hospital in the United Kingdom, A Dr. Frankel popularized the scale in the 1970's, but it was not without its flaws. The original test was later modified and called the ASIA Impairment Scale, categorized spinal cord injuries into one of five letter classifications:

> A. Complete: No motor or sensory function is preserved in the sacral segments S4-S5 [In plain English, you can't feel or control your rectum, This is probably the only test in the world a person doesn't want to score an "A" on, If I had been devising the scale, I would have reversed the lettering, but that's just me.]
> B. Incomplete: Sensory but not motor function is preserved below the neurological level and includes the sacral segments S4-S5, [In plain English, you can feel everything below the level of injury, including the rectum, but you can't move or control anything.]
> C. Incomplete: Motor function is preserved below the neurological level, and more than half of key muscles below the neurotically level has a muscle grade less than 3 [*sic*].
> D. Incomplete: Motor function is preserved below the neurological level, and at least half of key muscles below the neurological level has a muscle grade of 3 [*sic*] or more.
> E. Normal: Motor and sensory function are normal.

I don't want to get into a long discussion of the differences between the Stokes-Mandeville/Frankel test and the ASIA test beyond saying that the original Stokes-Mandeville/Frankel test left more description up to the examining physicians while the ASIA scale is more specific about the requirements for each category and added categories D and E.[11]

The main difference between the two tests is the original test simply said nothing below the level of injury could be felt or moved, After years of observation and experience with spinal cord injuries, doctors had more quantifiable experience on which to base a scale, The ASIA test specifies that the difference between having a complete and an incomplete injury is whether or not a person has movement and feeling in their rectum.

And for those who are curious about where I fall on the ASIA scale, no one has ever told me. I know I'm not a category A and I know I'm not a category E so I must be some place in-between, My guess is a C or a D.

22

Hoffmann's and Babinski's Signs

Gratitude is the sign of noble souls.—
Aesop

As unthinkable as it is, there are people who try to fake a spinal cord injury after an accident. They do this because they want to draw state and federal government benefits for being disabled. Not having a disability and trying to claim one is fraud. However, doctors have two different tests to diagnose a spinal cord injury. These tests are impossible to fake.

Let's do another anatomy lesson real quick. Don't worry. This lesson is pretty basic. As you already know, inside the human body are the brain and the spinal cord. The brain and the spinal cord together form the central nervous system.[1] The brain sends signals to the spinal cord. The spinal cord must then send the signals to the appropriate part of the body. This is done through the peripheral nervous system. It consists of nerves and nerve cells (neurons) that run between the spinal cord to the parts of the body. Neuron can also be spelled neurone.[2 3]

Then we have what are called motor neurons (neurones). There are different types of neurons, but for our purposes motor neurons are the only type we are concerned with. Motorneurons are also called motoneurons. Motor neurons, as you might expect, directly or indirectly control muscles.[4]

Are you with me so far? If you are, then let's go on. If you're not, then reread the previous two paragraphs until you are comfortable with the concepts.

There are two types of motor neurons relevant to this discussion. There are upper motor neurons, and lower motor neurons (upper motoneurons and lower motoneurons). Upper motor neurons are in the brain and spinal cord. Lower motor neurons run from the upper motor neurons to the muscles in the peripheral nervous system.[5 6]

Symptoms of upper motor neuron damage are spasticity, exaggerated reflexes, and loss of voluntary muscle control. Symptoms of lower motor neuron damage are involuntary twitching of muscles, paralysis, weakening of muscles, and muscle atrophy (wasting).[5 6]

Got that? Ready to talk about the tests now? The first test is called Hoffmann's Sign. It is also known as Hoffmann's Reflex or the Finger Flexor Reflex. It is used to test for hyperactive reflexes in the upper extremities. Hyperactive or exaggerated reflexes are a symptom of upper motor neuron damage. Upper motor neuron damage occurs with a spinal cord injury (or brain injury).

If you hold a person's middle finger loosely and flick the fingernail downward, the finger will rebound slightly into extension. The thumb may also flex and draw toward the body. This is a positive Hoffmann's Sign.[7] The test may also be done on the second, third, or fourth finger.[8]

Every doctor that has performed it on me has done it with the middle finger. It is always positive on me, and has been since my accident. In a person without spinal cord injury, the fingers would not react the way they do, and show a positive Hoffmann's Sign. Disease could also cause a positive sign.

There is a second test that doctors perform to test for spinal cord injury. It is called the Plantar Reflex test. It is a similar test to Hoffmann's Sign. It is performed on the foot. It can also identify damage to the brain. It is also called the Babinski Reflex or Babinski's Sign.

There are two situations in adults where the Babinski's Sign will be normal on an adult without spinal cord or brain injury: while asleep and after long periods of walking, such as soldiers marching. Young babies also show a positive Babinski's Sign because the pathways for walking that run from the brain to the feet have not developed yet. Around twelve to eighteen months of age the proper adult response is present.[9] In other words, once a baby has learned to walk, he or she will show a negative Babinski's Sign or no response. Again, disease could cause a positive sign.

The test is performed on the sole of a person's bare foot. A blunt instrument is rubbed across the bottom of the foot in the arch of the foot on the side of the big toe in a curving motion. There are three responses possible: 1) The toes curve inward and the foot turns outward. This is the normal response. 2) There is no response. 3) The large toe extends upward and the other toes fan out. This is a positive Babinski's Sign.[1] My Babinski's Sign is also positive.

So you've got two different tests that test for basically the same thing. A trained medical professional should only perform these tests. Don't try performing them on yourself, even if you have the capability of doing so. Don't try having a family member or friend perform them on you either. And certainly don't try committing fraud to obtain government benefits.

23

"What Does Paralysis After a Spinal Cord Injury Feel Like?"

The ability to move is something you do not notice
until you can no longer do it.—
Carolyn Boyles

I am including this chapter for the friends and family members of spinal cord injured individuals as well as for medical professionals.

Paralysis is defined as "the complete loss of muscle function for one or more muscle groups." Paralysis may be localized, or generalized, or it may follow a certain pattern. Most paralyses caused by nervous system damage are constant in nature. Paralysis often includes loss of feeling in the affected area.[1] Those are the fancy words.

"*But what does it feel like*?" family and friends may ask you. Different from anything an uninjured person feels or can imagine.

I have asked people with complete injuries to describe how it feels. Some people have said they have absolutely no feeling below the level of injury, and do not experience pain. The sensation just *stops.* Others have no feeling below the level of injury, but do experience pain. Imagine trying to describe *that* to an uninjured person.

I have the problem that my spinal cord "shorts out" at times and sometimes I can feel everything below my waist, but I cannot move anything below my waist for brief periods of time. I believe twenty minutes is the longest amount of time this has happened. This would be called intermittent paralysis.

"How does it feel when you can't move something?" you may also be asked. The feeling of starting to move something is the same. It is still there. But the parts of the body you have told to move *don't.* Or they move in ways different from what you have instructed. They may experience sudden jerky movements. Or they may move very slowly.

Again, each injury is unique and each person's loss of motion and sensation is different.

Understanding Your Injury

24

An Introduction to Spinal Cord Injuries and Syndromes

Sobering stuff, this spinal cord injury—
Richard Hollicky in *Roll Models*

Spinal cord injuries fall into one of two categories: complete or incomplete. Complete injuries are injuries in which the damage to the spinal cord is beyond recovery, and the patient has fewer rehabilitation options.

Incomplete injuries are injuries in which a person regains neurological function and/or feeling hours to years after the original injury. Spinal cord injuries can also be temporary or permanent. The combinations of injury that exist are: 1) complete and permanent 2) complete and temporary 3) incomplete and permanent and 4) incomplete and temporary.

For my list of incomplete spinal cord syndromes, I am using a list found in one of the medical textbooks on spinal cord injury. The list is as follows:

1. Anterior Cord Syndrome
2. Brown-Sequard Syndrome
3. Central Cord Syndrome
4. Posterior Cord Syndrome
5. Cauda Equina Syndrome
6. Arachnoiditis [this is mentioned in the literature related to Cauda Equina Syndrome so I'm adding it to the list]
7. Conus Medullaris Syndrome
8. Cervicomedullary Syndrome
9. Anterior Spinal Artery Syndrome [I have added this one because it is so closely related to Anterior Cord Syndrome although it may occur by itself]
10. Spinal Cord Concussion
11. SCIWORA
12. SCIWORET
13. Burning Hands Syndrome

14. Contusio Cervicalis
15. Hysterical Paralysis[1]

The article has an oddity that I'm surprised no one caught in the proofreading. The table of the syndromes lists Contusio Cervicalis and Hysterical Paralysis, but the article does not discuss them. The article discusses SCIWORA and SCIWORET, which the authors may have intended to cover Contusion Cervicalis. But the authors never discuss hysterical paralysis.

For you to get a better understanding of all these medical terms, I'm going to simplify things as best I can. The spinal cord has sections to it in addition to having levels as discussed previously. Depending on which section has been damaged determines what neurological losses the patient suffers.

Let's pretend we are looking down on a person from above. Their spinal cord looks like circle from this position. Anterior means front. This is the part of the spinal cord closest to the front of the body. Posterior means back. This is the part of the spinal cord closest to the back of the body. Central is the middle of the spinal cord. It is like a round core of the spinal cord. Unilateral hemisection is a fancy way of saying one side or the other, like the right side or the left side of the spinal cord. Make more sense now?

An article I found by two athletic trainers has this observation on the cervical spine:

> The cervical spine anatomy makes little sense; considering that it is one of the most delicate structures of the body and yet has little protection. This leaves the area susceptible to injury, especially in high-risk contact sports. The cervical spine has 4 [*sic*] protective factors, which include curvature (lordosis) that acts as a shock absorber, musculature to provide strength, ligaments to resist excessive motion and bones to protect the spinal cord. The cervical spine can be injured in the following ways: hyperflexion injury (forcing the neck forward), hyperextension (forcing the neck backward), lateral flexion (forcing the neck to the side), axial loading (compression of the neck from a hit on top of the head, and rotational forces (twisting of the neck).[2]

You should have a context for the discussion of the syndrome by knowing the categories spinal cord injuries fall into, complete or incomplete and temporary or permanent. You also need to know what types of incomplete syndromes exist to have a full understanding of incomplete injuries.

I want to insert a quick note on complications of spinal cord injuries. There is no real good place to put it in the book, so I am inserting it here. The list is as follows:

1. Skin breakdown [see the appropriate chapter]
2. Osteoporosis (bones losing calcium and breaking easily) and fractures
3. Pneumonia, Atelectasis [full or partial lung collapse], and inhaling liquid or solid objects into the lungs (if the level of injury is above T4)
4. Heterotopic Ossification [body joints that normally aren't bony becoming so]
5. Spasticity [see the appropriate chapter]
6. Autonomic dysreflexia [see the appropriate chapter]
7. Deep vein thrombosis or pulmonary embolism [blood clots, some of which may travel to the lungs] [see the chapter on Blood Flow Problems]
8. Cardiovascular Disease
9. Syringomyelia [enlargement of the central canal of the spinal cord]
10. Neuropathic/Spinal Cord Pain [see the Pain After a Spinal Cord Injury chapter]
11. Respiratory Dysfunction [see the Breathing Problems After a Spinal Cord Injury chapter]
12. Involuntary control of bladder and bowel [see the Kidney and Bladder Problems chapter]
13. Urinary tract infection [see the Kidney and Bladder Problems chapter]
14. Kidney and bladder stones [see the Kidney and Bladder Problems chapter]
15. Slow healing of any injury to the paralyzed limb.[3]

Now I have learned something. I wondered why I keep inhaling things while I'm drinking or eating. I figured it was the closed head injury or my asthma. Now I know because of number three above.

As for number fifteen above, I can personally attest to this one. I sprained my right foot and ankle badly in May 2007. When the injury had not healed in the expected period of time, Dr. Rob (my family doctor I mentioned previously) sent me to an orthopedic specialist. The specialist said it would take longer to heal because of my spinal cord injury. He expects it to take at least six months to heal from the time of the original injury. You may have heard or read about pressure sores after a spinal cord injury taking a long time to heal.

I have not covered Syringomyelia in the book. If you need additional information, I recommend going to a library, medical school library, or searching the Internet.

25

Anterior Cord Syndrome

Don't approach a goat from the front, a horse from the back, or a fool from any side.—
Yiddish Proverb

Anterior Cord Syndrome is the worst of all the spinal cord syndromes. It has the worst prognosis of any of the spinal cord syndromes.[1] It is the syndrome closest to having a complete spinal cord injury. As a reminder, the anterior part of the cord is the front.

You would think that damage to the front of the spinal cord and damage to the back of the spinal cord would have opposite effects. Spinal cord injuries are strange, though. In Anterior Cord Syndrome the legs are affected more than the upper body.[2] Central Cord Syndrome has the opposite effect in that the upper body is affected more than the lower body (see the chapter on Central Cord Syndrome).

With Anterior Cord Syndrome, unless the patient shows improvement in the first twenty-four hours, there will be no improvement. Only ten to fifteen percent of patients with this syndrome show improvement.[3] Most patients with Anterior Cord Syndrome usually have complete loss of strength below the level of injury.[4]

Now for the anatomy details. The anterior part of the spinal cord carries the sense of light touch and the muscle control for the upper extremities and the neck. The posterior (back) part of the spinal cord carries sensory impulses from the sacral, lumbar, upper thoracic, lower thoracic areas of the body and the upper extremities. In English, from the very low back, the low back, and the upper and lower chest.

Damage to this part of the spinal cord causes an absence or decrease of the sense of position and movement, a loss of the ability to tell the difference between being touched in two different places (two-point discrimination), a loss of the ability to sense vibration, and a loss of the ability to sense deep touch and pressure; although the latter is questionable in some studies. Damage to this part of the spinal cord also interrupts impulses for voluntary motion and pain and temperature sensation.

Anterior Cord Syndrome is not as complicated [as some other syndromes], one article stated. It is characterized by an immediate, complete paralysis with hyperesthesia [increased or altered sensitivity to neural stimuli] and hypalgesia [diminished sensitivity to pain] below the level of the lesion, together with preservation of touch, motion, position, two-point discrimination, and vibration sense. It is usually associated with flexion injuries of the cervical spine, producing a fracture dislocation commonly referred to as a "tear-drop fracture."

Two main factors are present with Anterior Cord Syndrome 1) direct damage to the anterior part of the spinal cord by a dislocated bone fragment or herniated disk, and 2) disruption of the blood supply to the anterior spinal artery. [5] For more information on Anterior Spinal Artery Syndrome, see the chapter on this subject.

26

Brown-Sequard Syndrome

All emotions are pure which gather you and lift you up; that emotion is impure which seizes only one side of your being and so distorts you.—
Rainer Maria Rilke

Damage to the hemisection of the spinal cord (one side or the other) is also known as Brown-Sequard Syndrome (sometimes called Brown Sequard). Brown-Sequard Syndrome is rare. There is little information in medical literature about it, despite the fact the syndrome dates back to the 1840's in medical literature.[1]

PeaceHealth.org has a nice description of Brown-Sequard:

> Characteristically, the affected person loses the sense of touch, vibrations and/or position in three dimensions below the level of the injury.... The sensory loss is particularly strong on the same side as the injury to the spine. These sensations are accompanied by a loss of the sense of pain [*sic*] and of temperature on the side of the body opposite to the side at which the injury was sustained.[2]

A list of causes for Brown-Sequard is as follows:

1. Spinal cord tumor
2. Penetrating or blunt trauma (including injection of illicit substance)
3. Degenerative disease such as disk herniation
4. Loss of blood flow
5. Infection or inflammation (meningitis, empyema, herpes, myelitis, tuberculosis, syphilis, multiple sclerosis)
6. Hemorrhage
7. Chiropractic manipulation (more on chiropractic treatment in a later chapter)[3]

Brown-Sequard can be complete or incomplete. Complete Brown-Sequard is rarer than incomplete Brown-Sequard.[4]

I went out on the Internet to the National Spinal Cord Injury Association Discussion Forum to see what messages people had posted about Brown-Sequard Syndrome. There weren't many, but there were enough for me to get a better understanding of what people with the syndrome are experiencing.[5 6 7]

One person, who I will refer to as "Poster1," an incomplete C1/C2 quad, reports that he/she has Brown-Sequard Syndrome and has impaired movement on the right side but somewhat normal sensation. His/her left side has normal movement but no sense of temperature or pain. This person reports that he/she was completely paralyzed initially but has recovered to the point of being able to walk, which is unusual.

A guest to the forum reported the case of a forty-year-old male patient in broken English. I will do my best to interpret the case into better English. The patient apparently experienced a rupture at C6/7. He deteriorated post operatively (after surgery) because of Brown-Sequard. His left lower limbs were weak but sensations were intact. His right side was stronger than his left, but still weaker than normal. He initially had poor sphincter control. He started walking three months after surgery, and strength improved to normal on both sides. However, the right side of his body experienced reduced sensation. He has spasticity (more on this in the chapter on spasticity) and tightness around his chest.

Another person, who I will call "Poster2," reported having Brown-Sequard from a C4-C7 rupture three years before his/her posting on the website. Poster1 answered the post discussing his/her abilities and limitations further beyond the original posting on the forum, such as walking with a cane, left side has full movement with no temperature or sharp dull sensation, right side has impaired movement with hypersensitivity to temperature and touch. The person's right hand is "like a quad hand." He/she cannot "do ponytails or zippers," but can do just about everything else. His/her sense of proprioception [sensory awareness of part of the body] is "messed up," so he/she cannot walk in the dark. He/she also mentions the lack of temperature regulation like other quads.

A third person, who I will call "Poster3," posted in the thread that he/she is a C3/4 incomplete with Brown-Sequard with a hypersensitive left side and limited movement. On the right side this individual has no temperature sensation but good motion. Five years post injury this individual is experiencing deterioration of his/her condition. He/she is now having "tremendous difficulty walking." His/her legs are "numb from mid-thigh to just below the knee." His/her arms are "so painful" that he/she "can barely move them." This person also says that he/she is going to end up in a wheelchair if no medical personnel can find a way to help him/her.

'Poster1" posts that he/she has gained weight from a low of eighty-four pounds to his/her current weight of ninety-six pounds. He/she discusses the sensitivity/burning problems and difficulty with showering because the water hitting his/her skin "feels like pins and needles." He/she says the shower "water has to be warm and not hot." He/she says he always sleeps on the side that "isn't burning" and the burning keeps him/her awake. He/she says that he/she wears a glove on his/her right hand because "it gets cold easier." He/she also says with the glove on he/she "can touch things" because of the sensitivity of fingertips.

A fourth person, who I will call "Poster4," responds that he/she has Brown-Sequard also as a result of a tumor on the spinal cord root at C3-5. He/she says the nerve roots were cut during the surgery. He/she has no feeling in the left leg, foot, or right arm and his/her right hand "burns when under pressure or tired." He/she says his leg feels like it is five times its normal size if he/she does not take medication, and his/her foot aches. He says that Brown-Sequard people can't feel pain or temperature but aching is present. He/she says that he/she can walk and use his/her arm and hand now and also has a very small amount of sensation in the left foot. He/she is working.

Another person, who I will call "Poster5," from the UK joined the discussion because her daughter has Brown-Sequard. She said that no one mentioned Brown-Sequard Syndrome to her but only "cervical disc mylopathy" [myelopathy] but fortunately the condition was discovered before damage was permanent otherwise her daughter would have ended up in a wheelchair. She says her daughter has trouble falling down a lot and dropping things but her daughter does manage to work. She indicates her daughter has problems with pins and needles sensations, general numbness and difficulty telling hot and cold and extreme tiredness. Her daughter had been injured fourteen years previously in a car accident where her spinal cord was "just crushed completely flat."

Another person, who I will call "Poster6," posted to ask the others if they had ever felt like they were the only one with Brown-Sequard Syndrome. She says that people looked at her like she had three heads when she mentioned the name of the syndrome and she is glad to have found the site where she can talk to people who really understand what she is going through. She says that if she tells people that she can't feel temperature and her foot is on fire but her leg is cold they don't understand. She posted that she had C5/6 surgery. She was paralyzed for a time but has regained movement since. She says she has weakness on the right side and "the temperature pain sensation thing on the left."

A man posted that he has recently been injured, and has Brown-Sequard; but is still in the hospital and not in rehabilitation yet.

Douglass John Mack in his book, *The Walking Quadriplegic: Defeating Paralysis*, relates his incredible recovery from an incomplete C5-7 Brown-Sequard syndrome injury. While in college, Mack was injured in a fall. After many months in the hospital, Mack regained the ability to walk. He was able to return to college. Today Mack is leading a normal life, and is able to pursue many of the outdoor activities he enjoyed prior to his injury.

27

Central Cord Syndrome

Every beloved object is the center of a paradise.—
Anonymous

By far the most common incomplete injury to the spinal cord is Central Cord Syndrome. In one study, seventy percent of the patients in the study had this type of injury. Because it is the most common of the syndrome-type injuries, more is known about this type of spinal cord injury.

Here is a quotation on the physical findings of Central Cord Syndrome:

> It is characterized by disproportionately more motor impairment of the upper than the lower extremities, bladder dysfunction, usually urinary retention, and varying degrees of sensory loss below the level of the lesion. The amount of recovery depends on the degree of edema [swelling] present compared to the extent of hematomyelia [hemorrhage of the gray matter of the spinal cord]. The lower extremities tend to recover motor power first, bladder function returns next, and finally strength in the upper extremities reappears, with the finger movements coming back last. The varying degrees of sensory impairment do not follow any set pattern of recovery.

The authors of the previous quotation go on to discuss that the usual cause of Central Cord Syndrome is a hyperextension injury of the cervical spine where bone spurs are present in the spinal column. This may occur with or without fracture.[1]

An excellent illustration of the different types of spinal cord syndromes with illustrations comes from Jim Pointer, MD, FACEP, Medical Director of the Alameda County EMS. He clarifies the cause of the damage to the spinal cord in a Central Cord Syndrome injury by explaining that the bony spurs on the discs pinch the spinal cord between them when the neck is hyperextended.[2]

Central Cord Syndrome was first mentioned in "modern" medical literature in 1954. This article is one of the best at explaining the mechanism of Central Cord Syndrome even today. The article explains that in Central Cord Syndrome, the spinal cord is compressed from both the front and the back (anterior and posterior to you medical professionals).[3] Dislocation does not have to occur in Central Cord Syndrome.[4] Fracture of the spinal column does not have to occur in Central Cord Syndrome.[5] Hyperextension of the neck has to be severe for Central Cord Syndrome to occur.[6] The article mentions some case studies on the syndrome as early as 1887.[7]

Let me give you some everyday examples of how Central Cord Syndrome would work if it happened to something else other than your spinal cord. Imagine a round balloon. Hold the round balloon between your hands. Now squeeze it together. This is the way the initial damage is done to the spinal cord.

Now imagine a piece of paper. If you crumple the paper in your hands, this is the same way Central Cord Syndrome does the initial damage to the spinal cord. The same as the balloon example above. Now take the same piece of paper. Expand it back out to full size. Twist it and rip it into two pieces. This is how the secondary damage takes place in Central Cord Syndrome. It is a graphic example, but it does get the point across.

Central Cord Syndrome happens most often in the mid to lower cervical cord.[8] It is easy to confuse Central Cord Syndrome with other syndromes, such as Brown-Sequard. Some of the characteristics are shared. Central Cord Syndrome is rare in athletes.[9]

I found a thread on the National Spinal Cord Injury Association Forum on Central Cord Syndrome. I have left in misspellings where the authors of the posts put them.

First, a bit of clarification. I am going to use the same naming conventions for people who have written on Internet spinal cord injury forums in this chapter as I used in the chapter on Brown-Sequard. The person I labeled "Poster1" in the chapter on Brown-Sequard is not the same person as "Poster1" in this chapter.

A man ("Poster1") started a thread on the NSCIA forum looking for others with Central Cord Syndrome. He was especially interested in the C4/5 levels. He stated that he could "walk, run, snow ski, play golf, yet half of his upper extremities were atrophied." He said he "experienced incredible amounts of pain, arthritis, join pain," and was wanting to know if anyone could relate.[10]

A woman ("Poster2") responded that she was what was called a "walking quad," and was a C2-7 injuree. She indicated that she did not have the function that the man has, but that the upper half of her body was "weaker or worse than the lower." She said she "can only stand and move a bit at a time," but that *she could* [italics hers]. She continued that she felt "extremely lucky" and especially when she was first hurt felt guilty about the amount of function she had.

I threw my two cents into the thread. I will call myself "Poster3." My first post in August 2005 was as follows:

> Hi. I am also a 'walking quad' fused at C4/5, C5/6, and C6/7 with central cord syndrome [*sic*]. I am going on 11 [*sic*] years post injury. I am also in the "shouldn't be" category but unfortunately my condition is worsening as literature indicates about ¼ [*sic*] of central cord syndrome patients experience. I have the incredible amounts of pain, arthritis, joint pain, etc. I have lost much motor control in the upper extremities including fine coordination in the hands. I can 'walk' with a walker or crutches but sometimes my legs will collapse out from under me.

A man, ("Poster4,") was the next person to post in the thread. He stated he was "an incomplete C4-5? central cord injury" but that he had more problems with his left later lower leg/foot and left arm. He wanted to know if that made him a Hemi [Brown-Sequard Syndrome]. He said this was his second post and he needed to learn more [don't we all?]. He said he had more atrophy of the left arm than the right and that he was very active. He indicated he uses his physical therapy sessions as "his private weight room" and "amazes everyone with their simple cervical fusions without neurological injury." He said he needs a left arm brace which he would be getting on his next occupational therapy appointment and he thought he also needed an ankle-foot orthosis [a custom fitted brace to hold the foot and ankle in their correct position]. He says he feels that a person can push him- or herself "farther than some of the people think if you are able."

He says he was a Navy SEAL and "still doesn't let obstacles get in his way." He says "the pain is a bummer though and it is getting worst [sp]" in his left foot and arm/hand. He refuses to take narcotics, and had surgery in December and started having symptoms by his own memory in August although his ex-wife says he started having symptoms a year earlier. He says he has watched his Rolex [watch] get loose on his left arm as he atrophied and thought "'oh how very interesting'" over the past several years." He says he has depression but in reading some of the posts in this thread he realized how lucky he was.

A man, who I will call "Poster5," added his thoughts:

> I've gone through two surgical procedures this summer to stabilize a failing cervical spine—and have cord injury at C3, C4 and 5 as well as some periph-

> eral nerve damage. I walk—using forearm crutches, having serious problems with prioproception (balance and gait) have about 50% strength loss on left side from the shoulder down along with lots of spasticity, and all sorts of wild sensory stuff on the right, including intense neuropathic pain.
>
> All this came on quite suddenly in May or June—thought I've probably ignored small signs for years....
>
> I count myself luck to have a good neurologist, a great surgeon, and a really solid rehab Doc.... but counting myself lukcy is not something I do very often these days.... though I understand "Poster2's" sense of guilt over being functional.... I've actually had "friends" suggest that I should look worse than I do....

A woman, who I will call "Poster6," was the next poster under the topic. I have left her typing and spelling errors in the text.

> HI EVERYONE,
> I'M SO GLAD SOMEONE MADE A RECENT POST IN THIS TOPIC. I DIDN'T KNOW YOOU COULD DO THAT. THANKS Poster5
> AND THANKS TO Poster1 FOR OPENING THE TOPIC ALTOGETHER.
> I RELATEE TO ALL OF YOU ALITTLE, EXCEPT ON ONE ISSUE: I AM A COMPLETEE C-6 SO I'M NOT A "WALKING QUAD". I ACUALLY HAVE NO MOVEMENT BELOW THELEVEL OF MY INJURY, SOME MOVEMENT IN MY ARMS BUT NO USE OF MY HANDS I'M COMPLETELY PARALYZED FROM THE NIPPLE DOWN.THE FACYT THAT I HAVE A GOOD DEAL OF SENSATION BELOOW MY INJURY IS DOUBLE EDGED SWORD. I HAVE EXTREME PAIN THERE AND SOMEWHAT LESS IN MY HANDS. I ALSO MUST USE A SPECIAL TOOL TO TYPE, SO PLEASE FORGIVE MY TYPOS.
> MY PAIN RANGES FOM AHELLFIRE BURNING TO IT FEELS AS THOUGH SOMEONE IS BEATING ME WITH A MEAT TENDERERIZER [A METAL ONE].
>
> THE REASON I USE ALL CAPS, THE AUTO ACCIDENT RENDERED MY LEFT EYE SERIOUSLY INJURED THATT REQUIRES SURGERY[NEXT MONTH].
>
> I'M ON A TON OF MEDS ALL SUPPOSED TO ADDRESS TYHE DIFFERENT TYPES OF PAIN, INCLUDING A TON OF OF MORPHINE, NEURONTIN, AND BACLOFEN. NONE OF WHYICH BARELY TOUCH THE PAIN. MOST RESEARCHERS SAY THERE IS NO CURE

FOR SPINAL CORD/CENTRAL PAIN. LETS PRAY THHEY'RE WRONG.
I ALSO RELATE TO THE MUSCLE WASTING SOME OF YOU'VE TALKED ABOUT A ND YES IT IS VERY DEPRESWSING, KEEPING BUSY IS WHAT WORKS BEST FOR ME. FOR THE MUSCCLES I TAKE EXTRA PROTIENN,[IN PILLO, POWDER, OR LIQUID FORM. FOR ARTHRITIS GLUCSOMINE AND CHONDROITIN FOR JOINT HEATH.

I ALSO TAKE A GREEN SOURCE AND EXTRA E AND C FOR SKIN. MILLK THISLE TO PROTECT MY LIVER AND GINGER CAPSULESS TO HELP WITH NAUSEA IMPROVE DIGESTION.
AND FOR THHOSE WHO FEEL GUILTY FFOR BEING HEALTHIER THAN YOU OR YOUR FRIENDS THINK YOU SHOULD BE—LET IT GO. IF YOU CAN'T TALK TO SOMEONE ABOUT "SURVIVERS GUILT" THAT'S WHAT IT'S CALLED.

ONE LAST THING, AFTER DESCRIBING MY PAIN TO MY SCI DOC, HE ACTUALLY HAD THE NERVE TO SAY HE WASN'T EVEN SURE MY PAIN WAS REAL.

TALK TO EACH OTHER
AND ME TOO

I added the next post:

Hi. Me again.

I wanted to pass along something that has helped me with the fatigue from the spinal cord injury. I've talked to other SCI people and everybody mentions fatigue as a problem.
I've started taking digestive enzymes (Garden of Life makes a really good one) and have found a dramatic increase in my energy levels. As normal people age, they lose their ability to break down fat. So do we but since we can't exercise normally we have the increased risk of weight gain.
Yes, I can speak for the pain as wel [sp]. Nothing touches it. My doctors wont' give me anything stronger than ultram because they dont want to get me addicted to anything "at such a young age." I've got a TENS unit and that helps some. I have found that the Nikken elastomag wraps do help as well.

"Poster6" responded to my post:

> HI "Poster3,"
> MY NAME IS "Poster6" AND AS I MENTIONED BBEFORE I'M GLAD THIS TOPIC WAS OPENEDE AGAIN FOR DEISCUSSION.
> YES, I ALSO HAVE FOUND DIGESTIVE ENZYMES HELPFUL IN ALOT OF WAYS. ALONG WITH THE BENEFITS YOU DESCIBE, I ALSO TAKE THEM TO FEND OFF FREQUENT NAUSEA AND TO HELP WITH MY BOWE3L PROGRAM.
>
> SINCE I DON'T HAVE CONTRROLL OF MY BLADDER OR BOWELLS, I MUST SUPPLIMENT MY REGULAR MEDSW WITH HEALTHY6, NATURAL SUPPLIMENTS.
>
> I TAKE ALOT OF VITAMINS, MINERALS, HERBS, AND NATURELL REMEDIES AS YOU CAN SEE FROM MY LAST POST.
> I HAVE ONEE MORE I'D LIKE TO SHARE WITH EVERYONE—MSM-IT IS HELPFUL FOR ALL TYPES OF PAIN AS WELL AS HELPING KEEP JOINTS, LIGAMENTS AND MUSCLES HEATHIER. FOR PAIN YOU SHOULD TAKE IT IN INCREASING DOSES STARTING AT BETWEEN 750MGS AND 1000MGS AND NGOING UP TO BETWEEN 2000 ANND 3000MGS A DAY IN DIVIDED
> DOSES. IT MAY CAUSE LOOSE STOOLS IN SOME, THIS IS LESSENEDD OR ELIMINATED IFR TAKEN THIS WAY.
>
> THIS IS TRULY A GREA6T SUPPLIMENT FOR PAIN! PLEASE TRY IT EVERYONE AND LET ME KNOW IF AND/OR HOW IT'S WORKING FOR YOU.
>
> WELL, THANKS FOR YOUR POST, Poster3
>
> I HOPE TO HEAR FROM EVERYONE SOON, AS WWELL,
> SINCERELY,
> Poster6
>
> P.S. Poster3, I'M CURIOUSB TO KNOW HOW OLD YOU ARE AND WHY AFTER 11 YEA4RS THE DOC THINK YOU ARE STILL TOO YOUNG FOR NARCOTIC MEDS IF THEY THINK IT WOULD HELP?

To which I responded:

> I'm 46 [*sic*] now. I was 35 [*sic*] at the time of the accident. I have tried the MSM and it also does help.

> Doctors in Arkansas for whatever reason don't want to give painkillers to women, especially those with spinal cord injury, from what I've seen. I think they are so controlled by HMOs, medical boards, etc. that they are more concerned with covering their own butts than with taking care of the patients.
>
> I think if I were in a chair they might take me more seriously but since I can still walk with crutches and/or a walker, they still don't consider me really a spinal cord injury survivor.

"Poster5" added his opinion following my post:

> Maybe it's a gender thing—but I too have had problems with Doctors, pain control and neuropathy (I have the molten lava thing going from the shoulder down on the right side—day time it fades to a mere warming oven). My physiatrist has been helpful, and my neurologist really good. My internist and surgeon pretty awful when it comes to treating pain. I'm also lucky enough to have a health plan that requires no preapprovals.
> For me—no response to narcotics, or neurontin, partial relief from zonegran, but so much nausea that I couldn't stay on it. I went off everything a few week prior to my second surgery and will start another med next week.
>
> A neurologist pointed out to me that any given anti-neuropathy drug is at best likely to work for only 1 in 2.5 [*sic*] patients treated. There are lots of meds out there that may work, so I'm still optimisitic.

"Poster6" continued:

dear "Poster3" and "Poster5,"

> i nforgot to tell you i sufffer from a severe panic disordeer, i've had anxiety since before my injury, in my twenties. my injury is 8 moonths old. and i'm almost 42 [nov 6th]
>
> sometimes i'm in such a panic at bedtime all massive amts. of drugs i'm on [including 2 for anxiety] i still can sleep. and since i can't roll myself in bed, i have to wake up my fiancee to roll me. this entails propping me various ways and positions with different sized and shaped pillows. this can't be easy on him,being awakened at leastt once a night to do all this, especially with my pain and trying to find the best position i never really knew what love was 'til this man i've livved with for 12 years promised in icu to take care of me, AND ACTUALLY HAS!

> anyway, my neurologist must be bent on turning his patients into drug addicts because he actually prescribed 200mgs twice a day for my pain [i'm only taking 250 to 300 per day. my tolerance is really high,i've had chronic neck pain and migraine headaches for 4 years before my sci. but i still think these are lethal amt. of morphine, another reason i'm afraid to slleep at niight. i'm having alot of breathing problems,i know some is from the injury itself, alot of the muscles and my diaphram are weaker or paralyzed and i can't cough like i used to. i quit smoking for over 3 months after the accident. but have been at it again since. i'm trying the best i can to stop, the best i've been able to do is cut down. which means i'm still hufff'n down almost a pack a day. it's really twisted "cuz i use a nebulizer and an albuteral rescue enhaler too.
>
> if anyone knows a way to help me quitb smoking PLEASE letme know.
> i know i'm jumping around but back to the docs and meds. i'm ready to quit my sci doctor because h won't even deal with my pain and for the nerve pain, his theory is just keep throwing more and more neurontin at it [up to 900mgs 4 x a day] and 100 mgs a day of baclofen a day for spasms. none of w3hich really don't work. what's that? a sane person may ask,try different meds perhaps not covered? because the doc might have to make one phone call to the ins. co. to get it approved.
> the type of spasms i get are band spasms. i get them around my chest and stomach and it feels as thoug someone has wrapped a steel band around me and is tightening it with a vice. [really really tight]
> can anyone relate to this??
>
> as always, thanks for listening and hearing from you also a pleasure,

My buddy,"Poster7," who I have chatted with extensively through the NSCIA website, and who has been greatly supportive to me, chimed in at this point:

> Back in May of 2005 I had a deer get out in front of me while motorcycling through Pennsylvania. I went down at about 70mph and was thrown over the bars, landing on my head and becoming entangled in a bunch of 1-2 inch saplings. Fortunately I wear a full helmet, leathers, etc. The helmet was totaled but ended up saving my life.
> I spent two weeks at the level one trauma center in central PA and underwent a laminectomy and fusion from C2-T1. I also suffered dislocation in both shoulders. Immediately after the accident I experienced EXTREME hypersensitivity from fingertip to fingertip. Simply blowing on my skin caused me to fade in and out of consciousness. I was transferred back to my home state of Connecticut where I spent the next two months at a rehabilitation hospital called Gaylord. This place proved to be one of the finest facilities I've encountered in my lifetime.

> I had to learn everything all over again; walking, eating, etc. Because of the central cord injury and the dislocation of both shoulders I was unable to use my arms for the first 30 days after the accident. My wife, great friends and lots of determination kept me going in a time when I thought my life was over.
>
> Fast forward to today: I still suffer from severe spasticity/increased tone, weakness in my upper extremities, curling pinkie and ring fingers, residual nerve pain, etc. However, I walk fine, drive to work and lead a pretty normal life. I've got use of both arms but my shoulders are still weak and external rotation still causes me some trouble. Things aren't the same but I've got no room to bitch knowing how lucky I am to be able to get around without a chair.
>
> I had been on huge dosages of Neurontin (Gabapentin), Flexoril (Cyclobenzaprine) and Ultram (Tramadol) but I've managed to wean myself off these medicines without severe complications. Currently I'm taking Baclofen (30mg three times daily) and it seems to be helping to reduce tone and spasticity although I still have plenty of room for improvement.
>
> Anyway, I just wanted to stop in and say hello and spill my story. If I can offer advice or help to anyone out there with SCI (patient or family), please don't hesitate to send a message.
>
> My name is Poster7 and I'm just a dork who fell on his head.
>
> I'm just another dork who fell on his head
> I'm just a dork who fell on his head

"Poster7" always "signs" his posts to the website with a drawing of a skeleton on a motorcycle with the caption "shut up and ride." You can see this on the website if you have access to a computer.

"Poster8" added her opinion next:

> "Poster1," I have central cord syndrome too and have the atrophied shoulders which are clicking away uncomfortably. I have no deltoid in my left shoulder but my right is functional. Both are functional. Do you have full mobility in your upper extremeties. How long is your injury. I am just wondering does the bone clicking get worse. I am 3 [*sic*] years post.
>
> I need to add an explanation at this point or my next post in the thread will not make any sense. Poster7 posted a photograph of the x-ray of his neck after his accident in his previous message in the thread. You can see it on the Internet. If you don't have access to the internet, the x-ray shows him with rods

and screws from the base of his skull to the base of his neck where it joins the shoulders. It's frightening!

My post was next:

"Poster7," that is quite an x-ray!

"Poster6" I know several people who quit smoking through hypnosis. Find yourself a good hypnotist. Sorry to hear of your discomfort. I also went to my hypnotist for pain relief and it did help a bit.
I realized after "Poster7" posted I never went into the details of my car accident. I had a "T-Bone" wreck at 35 [*sic*] mph with no chance to hit the brakes. I was the stem of the "T." I had my shoulder belt on but my head hit the windshield anyway.

About six weeks after the accident the doctors finally figured out I had two herniated discs (C5/6 and C6/7) which were on the spinal cord. I had those removed and fused in early 1995 [*sic*].

In early 2004 I had C4/5 fused. Two weeks ago I had C3/4 fused. For the first time since 1994 I don't have any bulging discs in my neck. I've been trying to tell the doctors I was having trouble breathing for a couple of years now and nobody would put the pieces together even though C3/4 was bulged.

"Poster7" responded with the final post in the thread to date as of the writing of this chapter:

Poster3:
How'd you manage to smack the windshield with the shoulder belt in place? Did the seat belt malfunction? Man that really sucks. I pretty much know how it goes though. I had a full helmet, leathers … full protective gear. Dumb luck 'eh?

Poster6:
You can quit smoking I just know it. My wife used to smoke when we first met and she told me that she was going to quit when she turned 35 [*sic*]. I asked her why 35 [*sic*] was so important and she told me that the increased risks of taking the pill and smoking after 35 (stroke, heart disease, etc) wouldn't be worth it. Since she would be turning 35 [*sic*] in less than a year I asked her why she didn't go ahead and quit now. She knew smoking was bad for her. She said "yeah, you're right." and stopped. She stopped because she wanted to stop.

> I agree with "Poster3" that a hypnotist is a great avenue to explore. If you want to stop and know you shouldn't smoke then you are more than half way there. Keep the faith, stay strong and look to friends and family for support.
>
> I'm just a dork who fell on his head

To show what a small world it can be, in the "Sci Life" column of the December 2006 issue of *New Mobility* magazine, a man submitted an article that he has "backwards quadriplegia." The article went on to explain that this man's lower body is nearly normal, but the upper part of his body is severely atrophied and weak. He is also in a lot of pain daily from nerve damage and muscle pain.

I contacted this man by e-mail to learn more about this "backwards quadriplegia" for this book. It turns out that this man is Poster1 from the NSCIA forum. We have spoken at length by phone and via e-mail about Central Cord Syndrome since.

Central Cord Syndrome is also called "inverse paraplegia" or "backwards paraplegia," even though it is technically quadriplegia (tetraplegia).

28

Posterior Cord Syndrome

Even a mosquito doesn't get a slap on the back
until it starts to work.—
Anonymous

Next we have Posterior Cord Syndrome. Posterior means back. This is the least common of the four syndromes. Some authors doubt its existence.[1]

There is a nice summary of the four syndromes, and their effects with illustrations on Apparelyzed.com (see the Resources chapter). Its discussion of Posterior Cord Syndrome says the person injured may have good muscle power, pain, and temperature sensation; but the person may have difficulty in coordinating the movement of their limbs.[2]

I mentioned the presentation by Jim Pointer in the chapter on Central Cord Syndrome. In his presentation, Dr. Pointer discusses the type of injury that typically causes Posterior Cord Syndrome. It is a fall where the person lands with force to the face and chin.[3]

29

Cauda Equina Syndrome

The horse may run quickly, but it can't escape its own tail.—
Russian Proverb

There are some other common spinal cord syndromes I want to discuss. The first of these is Cauda Equina Syndrome. As I have said previously, the cauda equina is the very base of the spinal cord in your lower back (it looks like a horse's tail). Cauda Equina Syndrome can occur as either a complete or an incomplete injury.[1]

The Cauda Equina Syndrome Support Group (CESSG) maintains a website to help those with Cauda Equina Syndrome that offers a complete discussion of the causes and symptoms of cauda equina.[1] I'm going to summarize the findings on their website briefly. In the discussion of Cauda Equina Syndrome below, any text in parentheses is from the support group. Text that appears in brackets is my insertion.

Cauda Equina Syndrome (CES) is a neurological (nerve) condition. It may be regarded as a form of spinal cord injury. CES is seen more commonly as a medical emergency but it may occur as a chronic condition. CES is a descriptive diagnosis that pertains to a pattern of symptoms and signs, but can have various causes.

> If you have the following specific pattern of symptoms, the support group warns, seek medical attention immediately to avoid permanent nerve damage:
>
> - Severe pain in the back, buttocks, perineum [the "saddle area"—the part of your body that comes in contact with a saddle when you ride a horse], genitalia, thighs, legs.
> - Loss of sensation: often tingling or numbness in the saddle area.
> - Weakness: in legs, often asymmetric [not the same on both sides].

- Bladder/bowel/sexual dysfunction: incontinence/retention of urine; incontinence of feces; impotence/loss of ejaculation or orgasm.
- Loss of reflexes: knee/ankle reflexes may be diminished, as may analy an bulbocavernosus (a muscle of the perineum, the area between the anus and the genitals).

If you have chronic Cauda Equina Syndrome, it may be as a result of belated treatment of the acute syndrome or part of an ongoing illness such as Multiple Sclerosis. *If you develop urinary retention (inability to pass urine), seek medical attention immediately.*

Nerve roots in the cauda equina may be damaged through a variety of mechanisms:

1. Compression—by a herniated disc most commonly but also by spinal fracture or chronic compression in a condition called arachnoiditis.
2. Stretching—by slippage of one vertebra on another.
3. Inflammation—in conditions such as arachnoiditis.
4. Demyelination—loss of the myelin sheath [vital for nerve signal transmission] in conditions such as Multiple Sclerosis
5. Toxic damage to the spinal cord—as a result of spinal anesthetics [this is rare]

Cauda Equina Syndrome can be extremely disruptive of a person's life. Sometimes the individual is unable to work because of the levels of pain, the loss of muscle power, or as a result of incontinence. A person may suffer all three of the above problems.

It is easy to understand why loss of bladder and/or bowel control would affect a person's life and certainly his or her self-esteem. The sufferer may also experience frequent urinary tract infections.

The loss of sexual function can also be devastating to a person. Loss of sexual function is not a problem experienced only by men. Women also experience loss of sexual function. It is equally devastating to both sexes.

After surgery, a person may not be one hundred percent recovered from the condition. Residual problems may exist such as continued urinary or bowel incontinence. Fortunately, therapy can be used to retrain the bowel and/or bladder.

Chronic Cauda Equina Syndrome is more difficult to treat. The levels of pain require strong painkillers. Depending on how the bladder is malfunctioning will determine the treatment necessary.

The bladder may develop one of two conditions. The first is where the bladder is unable to empty. In this situation medication can be used to manage the problem. If medication is ineffective, the individual may need to rely on intermittent catheterization.

The other situation is where the bladder control is lost, and the person leaks urine. The options that exist for this situation is to wear appropriate pads or underwear to absorb the leakage or use of a catheter with or without a leg bag (more on this in the chapter on Kidney and Bladder Problems).

The bowel experiences the same extremes as the bladder. A person may inappropriately pass feces or "gas." More commonly a person may be unable to empty his or her bowels. This is because of loss of sensation in the rectum, and loss of muscle control to effectively move the stool out of the body. More on this in the chapter on digestive system function after a spinal cord injury.

Weakness can also be a problem. Exercise may or may not be effective, depending upon whether or not a person also has Arachnoiditis. If a person does not have Arachnoiditis, then exercise may be helpful in strengthening weakened muscles. If a person has Arachnoiditis, then exercise may cause the Arachnoiditis to get worse.

Sexual dysfunction is another problem that can be experienced by Cauda Equina Syndrome sufferers. A family doctor can help with sexual dysfunction. So can an OB/GYN for women. A urologist can help patients of either sex. More on this in the chapters on Sexuality and Sex.

Sensory loss may also be present. Sore feet and foot drop are other symptoms that can occur. Some individuals wear braces to correct foot drop.

Poor circulation is another common symptom. It is advisable to keep feet warm with heavy socks or through the use of massage with warm oil. Very hot baths after the feet have been cold may cause chilblains (swelling).

Depression is also a result of Cauda Equina Syndrome. It is quite understandable for a person with this condition to be depressed as he or she has a debilitating condition. More on depression in the chapter on Depression.

30

Arachnoiditis

The bird a nest, the spider a web,
man friendship.—
William Blake

I'm also going to talk briefly about Arachnoiditis because it is mentioned in the discussion of Cauda Equina Syndrome above. The *arachnoid mater* is a membrane that covers a nerve.[1] "Itis" means inflammation. An organization exists for sufferers of Arachnoiditis, the Circle of Friends with Arachnoiditis (COFWA). Their website, http://www.cofwa.org, offers information about the condition, and the opportunity to discuss the condition with others who have it.

According to the COFWA website:

> Adhesive Arachnoiditis is a disorder which causes severe, chronic, intractable [difficult to manage] pain. It is the inflammation of one of the spinal cord coverings (meninges), the middle meninges, the arachnoid and nerve roots that causes Adhesive Arachnoiditis. This inflammation causes the covering to become "sticky," adhering it to the spinal cord and the nerve roots as they exit the spinal canal....
> .... Adhesive Arachnoiditis can be progressive in some cases. It can also cause loss of motor function, numbness, tingling, loss of bladder and bowel function, the sensation of walking on rocks or glass, burning, groin pain, and can, in some rare instances, cause paralysis. There is currently NO CURE and NO TREATMENT [*sic*] for Adhesive Arachnoiditis other than pain management.[2]

Another article I found discusses that the predominant symptom of Arachnoiditis is chronic and persistent pain in the lower back, lower limbs, or the entire body. Additional symptoms can include:

1. Tingling, numbness, or weakness in the legs

2. Bizarre sensations such as insects crawling on the skin or water trickling down the leg
3. Severe shooting pain (which some liken to an electric shock sensation)
4. Muscle cramps, spasms, and uncontrollable twitching
5. Bladder, bowel, and/or sexual dysfunction

The author of the article goes on to discuss that symptoms may become more severe or even permanent. He explains that the disease can be very debilitating because the pain is constant and difficult to manage. Most people with Arachnoiditis are unable to work, and have significant disability.

The causes of Arachnoiditis are:

1. Trauma/surgery induced
2. Chemically induced through myelograms
3. Infection induced (meningitis or tuberculosis)[3]

The National Institute of Neurological Disorders and Stroke indicates that Arachnoiditis "is a difficult condition to treat, and long-term outcomes are unpredictable."[4]

The term arachnoid can also refer to a spider[5], which I why I chose the quotation I did at the beginning of the chapter.

31

Conus Medullaris

Passion holds up the bottom of the world,
while genius paints its roof—
Anonymous

There is another more spinal cord syndrome I want to mention, Conus Medullaris. I didn't find a lot of information on this syndrome. The Conus Medullaris is a section of the spinal cord near the bottom end of the spinal cord. It is near the lumbar (lower back) nerves L1 and L2. It is located higher than the Cauda Equina.[1]

Differentiating between Conus Medullaris Syndrome and Cauda Equina Syndrome can be difficult from the medical articles I read. If I understand the literature correctly, Conus Medullaris Syndrome often occurs on one side only. It can also be caused by disease such as cancer or sickle cell anemia or by trauma. Cauda Equina Syndrome seems to be caused more by trauma. Cauda Equina Syndrome symptoms involve the nerve roots, whereas Conus Medullaris Syndrome symptoms involve the spinal cord itself.

Cancer, sickle cell anemia, or trauma can also cause Conus Medullaris Syndrome. Trauma seems to be the most frequent cause.

For anyone who wants to read in more detail how to diagnose the differences between the two, I recommend reading "Cauda Equina and Conus Medullaris Syndromes" on http://www.emedicine.com.[2] The article is more technical than I want to reproduce here.

32

Cervicomedullary Syndrome

Cruelty and fear shake hands together.—
Honore de Balzac

This is actually a head injury that is often referred to as a spinal cord injury. It is also called hyperacute encephalopathy. The common name for it is "Shaken Baby Syndrome."

This syndrome accounts for six percent of all inflicted brain injury on babies. The syndrome is almost always fatal. The survival rate after the injury is in the ballpark of one day. The injury comes from a whiplash of the neck.[1]

From time to time on the news, you will see a local news broadcast of a baby having died because he or she was shaken by a babysitter, an irate or drugged biological mother or father of the baby, or by some other family member.

As most of us know, young babies' necks are very floppy and must be supported. Babies are born with neck muscles that adjust during birth so the baby's head can fit through the birth canal. Later the neck muscles strengthen to be able to hold the head in the proper position.

If a person shakes a baby, the lack of strength in the baby's neck muscles causes a whiplash injury. This typically breaks the brain stem, but can also break the baby's neck.

33

Anterior Spinal Artery Syndrome

We all experience many freakish and unexpected events....—
Viggo Mortensen

I want to begin this chapter with a brief clarification. This chapter is about Anterior Spinal Artery Syndrome. This is not to be confused with Anterior Cord Syndrome, which was discussed in a previous chapter. They are two different conditions that cause spinal cord damage.

Anterior Spinal Artery Syndrome is a rare condition which happens under a wide variety of situations. It can happen when a person sustains trauma to another part of the body other than the spinal cord (such as in an accident or gunshot wound). It can happen with several different medical conditions. It can happen during surgery on a part of the body other than the spinal cord.

This condition can cause quadriplegia or paraplegia. It was first reported in medical literature in 1909. The syndrome consists of pain at the level of injury on the spinal cord, partial or complete paralysis below the level of injury, disturbance of pain and temperature sensation, and urinary incontinence.[1]

In simple English, "the cause [of this syndrome] is found in interference with the blood supply of the spinal cord...." There are three to ten arteries that control blood supply to the spinal cord.[2] Something happens to cut off the blood supply to the spinal cord at a particular level. This results in irrevocable (something that cannot be undone) damage to the spinal cord within a short period regardless of the site of interruption.[3]

The article I quoted above says it takes fifteen minutes without blood for damage to occur to the spinal cord that is reversible. The article then says it takes twenty minutes without blood for there to be permanent damage to the spinal cord.[4] Apparently, fifteen minutes without blood is the longest time for the spinal cord to be deprived of blood without permanent damage. I don't know what happens when the time of blood deprivation to the spinal cord is more than fifteen minutes, but less than twenty. The article didn't say.

The article goes on to say that a reduction in blood pressure might be enough on its own to produce damage to the spinal cord. If there is a reduction in blood pressure and interruption of the blood supply, the potential for damage is increased.[5] It is relatively rare for the blood clot to show during angiography. Angiography is a medical imaging technique in which an x-ray picture is taken to visualize the inner opening of blood filled structures, including arteries, veins, and the heart chambers.[6]

I am now going to discuss the medical conditions that can cause Anterior Spinal Artery Syndrome. The first is arteriosclerosis.[7] This is the classic "hardening of the arteries" from deposits inside the artery walls.[8] What happens is the artery or arteries supplying blood flow to the spinal cord "harden" over time. Eventually blood flow can no longer reach the spinal cord.

The next cause of Anterior Spinal Artery Syndrome is infection.[9] If blood vessels become infected, they become inflamed and swell. This reduces blood flow. They can also bleed, which reduces blood flow to the area the artery or arteries supply with blood.

Another cause of Anterior Spinal Artery Syndrome is vasculitis.[10] Vasculitis is a group of diseases that causes inflammation [swelling] of the wall of the blood vessels including veins, arteries, and capillaries.[11] As above, if the blood vessels swell, they cut off blood flow.

The next cause of Anterior Spinal Artery Syndrome is an embolism ("embolic events" as the article calls them).[12] An embolism is what all of us normal people would call a blood clot. Typically the blood clot is formed elsewhere in the body. In the case of Anterior Spinal Artery Syndrome, that blood clot happens to lodge in one of the arteries that supplies the spinal cord with blood.

The fifth cause of Anterior Spinal Artery Syndrome is sickle cell anemia.[13] Sickle cell anemia (sickle cell disease) is a group of genetic disorders that cause red blood cells to be shaped like bananas instead of their normal round shape. These abnormally shaped red blood cells can become stuck in blood vessels, which blocks the blood flow. [14] As with an embolism above, if they become stuck in the artery or arteries that supply the spinal cord with blood, spinal cord damage occurs.

Another cause of Anterior Spinal Artery Syndrome is cervical [or thoracic or lumbar, I'm assuming] cord herniation.[15] During herniation of the spinal cord discs from whatever cause, the arteries supplying the spinal cord can also be damaged, cutting off blood flow to the spinal cord.

An additional possible cause of Anterior Spinal Artery Syndrome is surgery.[16] In the article I found, interruption of the blood supply to the abdominal aorta during surgery most commonly causes this problem. This article indicated that the length of interruption of blood flow can be as little as ten minutes to cause permanent spinal cord damage. There were only thirteen documented cases as of 1970.[17] The aorta is the largest artery in the body. It starts at the heart, and continues down into the abdomen.[18] The earlier article I quoted on lack of blood flow to the spinal cord said damage would not occur until twenty minutes without blood. I cannot explain the difference of opinion between authors.

A final possible cause of Anterior Spinal Artery Syndrome is trauma.[19] Any trauma to the anterior spinal arteries has the possibility of interrupting the blood flow to the spinal cord.

34

Spinal Cord Concussion aka Spinal Cord Shock aka Spinal Shock

Those who are easily shocked should be shocked more often.—
Mae West

The next spinal cord syndrome I want to discuss is Spinal Cord Concussion/Spinal Cord Shock/Spinal Shock.

Wikipedia defines Spinal Shock as "an initial period of hypotonia [a condition of abnormally low muscle tone (the amount of tension or resistance to movement in a muscle often involving reduced muscle strength[1])] that can result from damage to the motor cortex or other brain regions concerned with the activation of motor neurons.

Wikipedia goes on to say that the cause of Spinal Shock is unknown.[2]

Two neurosurgeons in Canada have stated that there are three criteria for meeting a diagnosis of Spinal Shock:

1. spinal trauma immediately preceded the onset of neurological deficits
2. neurological deficits were consistent with spinal cord involvement at the level of injury
3. complete neurological recovery occurred within 72 hours after injury.[3]

Another author discusses Spinal Shock in these words:

> Spinal shock [*sic*] is a type of neurogenic [originating in the nervous system] shock that occurs in major SCI and can be a source of considerable confusion.... [I think the author means confusion for the doctors, not the patient.]

> The more severe the SCI and the higher the level of injury, the greater the severity and duration of spinal shock [*sic*]. Thus, spinal shock [*sic*] is most severe in complete upper cervical cord injuries, less severe in incomplete thoracic [chest] injuries, and minimal in lumbar [lower back] cord injuries.[4]

My take on Spinal Shock, in plain English, is that if you have a spinal cord injury above the belly button, you are going to have Spinal Shock along with it.

I dislike these chapters where I have to be so technical. I found a discussion of Spinal Shock in much better terms for the average person to understand on http://www.multikulti.org.uk:

> For the first few weeks after a spinal cord injury no one can really tell how severe the injury is going to be. The difficulty is that something called spinal shock develops immediately after a spinal injury. This involves all nervous system communication between the spinal cord and the rest of the body, temporarily shutting off below the level of the injury.
>
> Some patients may recover a lot of sensation and movement when the spinal shock phase ends, others may not. There are no tests that can be done during the spinal shock phase to predict the degree of recovery. So, if you are getting frustrated by the inability of doctors or nurses to give you straight answers to some of your questions, please try to understand that they are genuinely unable to give definite information at this early stage. They don't want to make you too optimistic about the future but, at the same time, they don't want you to give up hope.
>
> Once the Spinal Shock phase is over, the true extent of the injury can be assessed and future abilities can start to be predicted more reliably. Careful assessment of the remaining movement and sensation around the body is needed to determine the likely outcome of SCI in a particular individual.
>
> For high-level SCI, meaning injury to the neck or upper back, the effects are always likely to be more serious than with lower level injuries, regardless of how extensive the actual damage is. It's very likely, for example, that the arms, as well as the legs, will be affected. However, people may regain some sensation or movement in their legs and arms, if their spinal cord has only been partially (incompletely) damaged. Some higher-level injuries will require assistance with breathing.
>
> With lower level injuries, meaning injury to the chest and lower back, the legs but not the arms, will be affected. Again, people may regain some sensation or movement in their legs, depending on the completeness of their injury. Retaining full use of the hands and arms makes it much easier to manage the

> everyday tasks involved in daily life. As such, many of the individuals affected will be able to lead an independent life once they have completed the healing and rehabilitation phases.
>
> Aside from the most obvious effects of SCI—the reduced ability to move and feel things below the level of injury—there are [*sic*] a range of additional complications that a person with SCI can expect to face. Perhaps one of the most difficult to come to terms with is reduced ability to control the bowel and bladder function. During the initial spinal shock phase, this control may be totally lost. Over the next few weeks or months, various degrees of control may return, according to the level and severity of the injury. With the right training and good motivation, new routines for dealing with these essential functions can be learned and put into practice. People with lower level injuries or incomplete injuries may retain enough sensation and mobility to completely manage these routines by themselves, while for those whose hand and arm function remains limited or absent, a carer may have to assist with or carry out these routines.[5]

The Ohio State University Medical Center website has a nice understandable discussion of an acute spinal cord injury (even thought as a University of Illinois graduate I hate citing another Big Ten university's website. Just kidding.):

> Symptoms vary depending on the severity and location of the SCI. At first, the patient may experience spinal shock, which causes loss of feeling, muscle movement, and reflexes below the level of injury. Spinal Shock usually lasts from several hours to several weeks. As the period of shock subsides, other symptoms appear, depending on the location of the injury.[6]

As the previous quotation states, Spinal Shock is a temporary condition, fortunately. It is confined to the spinal cord. There is apparently no structural damage to the cord when it happens.[7]

The condition of Spinal Cord Concussion (same as Spinal Shock) is even mentioned in *Pro Football Athletic Trainer* despite the fact the condition does not happen very often:

> Although extremely rare, this is analogous to a cerebral concussion in that a violent impact to spinal column causes function of the spinal cord to shut down due to the electrochemical imbalances. However, instead of losing consciousness, there is a transient [temporary] loss of all spinal cord functions with no structural damage to the cord itself.[8]

I have a comparison that may make understanding this syndrome a little easier. This was true when I was a child. I don't know if it is still true. Picture a light pole in a city. If the light pole suffers an impact, say from getting hit by a car, the light goes out temporarily. Eventually the light comes back on again. As long as there has been no damage to the light or the pole electronics. The same thing is basically true with a spinal cord concussion. I remember watching kids trying to hit light poles as hard as they could to try and make the light go out.

One article defines Spinal Cord Concussion as: "a disturbance of spinal cord function with objective neurologic deficit following trauma and complete resolution within 48 [*sic*] hours. The neurologic deficit must have occurred at the level of spinal trauma, may have affected ascending and descending tracts, and may or many not have been associated with vertebral injury."[9]

The electrical, chemical, or ultrastructural changes that cause this condition were unknown as of 1989. I do not know if modern medicine is much closer to the answers today or not.

A doctor would say "the key to the cause of this injury is the absorption of kinetic energy over a brief period of time." In English, if your spinal cord gets bounced around inside your spinal column, and something doesn't absorb the movement, you will have a spinal cord injury. A narrow spinal canal means less cushion from the cerebrospinal fluid in the spinal canal. The magnitude and direction of force delivered determines the pattern of neurologic deficit.[10]

In English, The wider your spinal canal the better. A larger spinal canal means there is more spinal fluid to cushion your spinal cord. What kind of nerve damage you take depends on how your injury happened.

35

SCIWORA (Spinal Cord Injury Without Radiographic Abnormality)

The colder the x-ray table the more of your body is required on it.—
Anonymous

I also want to discuss SCIWORA, Spinal Cord Injury Without Radiographic Abnormality. In English, this means a person is suffering symptoms normally associated with a spinal cord injury but that regular x-rays show nothing wrong. Abnormalities may show on an MRI (Magnetic Resonant Imaging) scan, but not always.

Until this point in the book I have only discussed children and spinal cord injury very briefly. SCIWORA is a spinal cord syndrome that occurs in children more often than in adults. Although still not a common occurrence in children. SCIWORA was first defined in medical literature in 1982.[1] It will make more sense if I give you some background on this condition, and why it isn't seen in adults more often.

One article, titled "Pediatric Trauma—Unique Considerations in Evaluating and Treating Children" explains why children are so subject to this syndrome compared to adults. [2] The reason children are more likely to suffer this injury is because their necks are relatively weak compared to those of adults. Combined with having a large head compared to their body size, and more flexible soft tissue in their necks; children have a greater risk of force to be transmitted to the spinal cord.

I found varying statistics on the incidence of SCIWORA in children. This may be because, as one article discusses, there is insufficient evidence to support diagnostic standards of this condition and there is insufficient evidence to support treatment standards.

Basically, there have not been enough cases worldwide for doctors to develop guidelines for diagnosis. Without enough cases to develop guidelines for diagnosis, guidelines for treatment are also impossible to develop.

With the rate of spinal cord injuries increasing worldwide, doctors need to get to work, and develop some consistency in the standards before a child dies as a result.

One study indicated "in some studies only half of children with neurologic injuries show radiographic abnormalities." A study in a Turkish journal reported that SCIWORA made up thirty-three to forty-two percent of all pediatric spinal injuries.[3] One series of pediatric spinal cord injuries reported a sixty-seven percent incidence of SCIWORA.[4]

As for adult injuries, one study followed a group of seventeen adult patients with SCIWORA for seven years. Of the seventeen patients using conservative treatment, fifteen showed neurological improvement, one remained quadriplegic, and one died. [5]

In the Turkish article, the rate for adult SCIWORA was quoted as between three and ten percent of adult injuries. [6] Finally in an article which was a study of reported injuries to emergency departments nationwide, 0.08% of all cervical spinal injury patients were SCIWORA patients. Central Cord Syndrome was specifically described in ten of the twenty-seven cases (thirty-seven percent).[7]

SCIWORA excludes spinal cord injuries associated with degenerative changes of the spinal column.[8]

As for how a SCIWORA injury is treated, I could not find anything that specifically explained treatment options. I have seen a TV program, one of these emergency room reality TV shows, that had an adult with SCIWORA. This patient was treated in exactly the same manner as someone with a spinal cord injury documented on an x-ray, and recovered completely.

36

SCIWORET (Spinal Cord Injury WithOut Radiographic Evidence of Trauma)

I was always shocked when I went to the doctor's office and they did my X-ray and didn't find that I had eight more ribs than I should have or that my blood was the color green.—
Nicholas Cage

This particular type of spinal cord injury is described by the diagnosis based on medical testing. As with SCIWORA, regular x-rays show no indication of injury. A CT scan shows injury. This diagnosis is more common in adults than in children. The existence of CT scans has reduced this diagnosis by about nine percent. Often this type of injury will be spinal cord compression.[1]

SCIWORET is common in situations where the patient has narrowing of the spinal canal and herniation of discs. Other conditions that occur with aging such as fusion of ligaments around the spinal canal, and fusion of the spinal discs also come under the diagnosis of SCIWORET.

SCIWORET does include spinal cord injuries with degenerative changes of the spinal column.[2]

37

"Burning Hands" Syndrome aka "Stingers" or "Burners"

A system is a network of interdependent components that work together to try and accomplish the aim of the system. A system must have an aim. Without the aim, there is no system.—
W. Edwards Deming

There is another type of temporary spinal cord syndrome. This syndrome is most likely to happen to athletes. Fortunately, increased awareness that "Burning Hands" Syndrome ("burners" or "stingers" or "burner syndrome") is a symptom of possible spinal cord injury on the part of coaches, team doctors, and players is helping prevent permanent damage.[1] Especially in football.

This injury can also happen in wrestling, cycling, gymnastics, snow skiing, and martial arts.[2] Another source adds basketball, ice hockey, and some track events.[3] In any sport where players can contact each other or a hard object or surface the risk of this syndrome exists.

Some doctors do not consider this syndrome a spinal cord syndrome because it affects the nerve roots coming out from the spinal cord. I found it in one source that listed it under spinal cord syndromes so I am including it.[4]

Let's talk about the anatomy involved. You may remember I talked earlier in the book about upper motor neurons and lower motor neurons. This injury involves lower motor neurons.

Nerve roots exit the spinal canal in the neck. They join together to form cords of nerves. These nerve cords provide sensation to the arms. The intersection where these cords come together for the arms is called the brachial plexus. This is where the injury occurs when an athlete has this syndrome.[5]

Sixty-five to seventy percent of college football players say they have experienced a burner or stinger during their four-year playing career.[6 7] The vast majority of players (up to seventy percent) said they did not report this injury when it happened.[8]

"Burning Hands" Syndrome is a stretch or compression injury to this network of nerves in the lower neck and shoulder. A blow to the head or shoulder can cause it. The stretch injury is more common than the compression injury.[9]

The symptoms of this injury are a "burning" or "electric shock" sensation in one arm. The injured arm may feel "dead" or "numb" following the impact. It is a one-sided injury only.[10] The player's arm may be paralyzed.[11]

The pain, "burning," "deadness," numbness, or "electric shock" sensation will subside quickly, within hours or days. The weakness that accompanies the injury in the arm should go away within two to three weeks after the injury.[12]

Research has shown that an athlete with a narrowing of the spinal canal (stenosis) is more likely to experience "burners." Another study found that athletes who have repeat episodes are also more likely to have a narrowing of the spinal canal.[13]

Initial treatment of the injury should be: protect the injured body part (use a sling for example), rest the injured shoulder and arm, ice the painful neck and shoulder muscles to relieve pain and control the muscle spasms, if swelling is present then use an elastic bandage, and finally elevate the arm or shoulder to reduce swelling.[14]

An athlete can work out on a limited basis after the injury. He or she can also perform strengthening exercises on the injured areas.[15] An athlete should not play until the symptoms are completely resolved.

38

Bruising of the Spinal Cord (Contusio Cervicalis)

The marks you receive in the school of experience are mostly bruises.— Anonymous

This is another spinal cord syndrome that is reversible.[1]

A bruise of the spinal cord generally causes bleeding in the spinal column. This bleeding puts pressure on nerve cells. The pressure on the nerve cells causes the nerve cells to die. Doctors call a bruise a contusion.[2]

Bruising of the spinal cord may not be reversible if it is accompanied by other damage to the spinal cord.[3]

39

The Hangman's Fracture

Having the critics praise you is like having the hangman say you've got a pretty neck.—
Eli Wallach

This is a commonly used term, both historically and in modern times, so I am devoting a chapter to it.

Historically, hanging was a method of public execution for a criminal. The convicted criminal stood on a platform called a gallows. There was a trap door built into the gallows, which the prisoner stood on. A rope was suspended from a beam overhead. The rope was tied into a specific type of knot, called a hangman's knot. The robe was also typically lubricated. The length of the rope and the length of the drop for the prisoner to fall were specifically calculated. The calculations depend upon the prisoner's weight and height. This has become a very exact science over the years.

When the trap door was opened, the prisoner's weight caused the knot to tighten, killing the prisoner. Death could take place instantly or could take some time; depending upon where the knot in the rope had been positioned relative to the prisoner's neck. What typically happened in a hanging to cause the prisoner's death was a fracture-dislocation of the C2 vertebra relative to the C3 vertebra.[1]

In modern times an accident victim can suffer a hangman's fracture. The most common sources of these accidents are motor vehicle accidents and falls.[2] The typical scenario in a car accident for this type of injury is where the victim strikes the windshield with his or her forehead, and suffers a hyperextension and compression of the cervical spine.[3] The late Christopher Reeve suffered this type of injury in his horse riding accident.[4] I had this same scenario of impact inside a car, but I did not have a hangman's fracture.

There is a difference between the hangman's fracture sustained by the condemned prisoner and the hangman's fracture sustained by the auto accident victim. Often there is no spinal cord injury to the auto accident victim because the vertebrae are not dislocated relative to each other. There is only a fracture.[5] If the dislocation occurs, then the injury is the same and is likely fatal.

For an excellent article on the history of spinal biomechanics that also discusses the history of the science of hanging, see "The History of Spinal Biomechanics."[6]

40

Hysterical Paralysis (Ganser Syndrome)

Madness takes its toll. Please have exact change.—
Anonymous

Madness is rare in individuals, but in groups, parties, nations and ages is it the rule.—
Friedrich Nietzsche

This is a temporary (transient) cause of paralysis that is very different from the other syndromes I have discussed.[1] It is the most controversial of the syndromes. Many sources do not even mention it as a spinal cord syndrome. It is also called Conversion Disorder.[2]

One reason this particular syndrome is so controversial is because it is very rare. There are so few cases available for study that it is difficult for medical professionals to really understand its cause.[3] The condition was originally described in medical literature in 1898.[4]

There are some aspects of this syndrome that are agreed upon: it is reversible, it is short-term, it is rare, symptoms usually resolve spontaneously [on their own without medical treatment]. The patient usually does not remember the events that took place during the course of the syndrome, and the patient has experienced a psychological or physical cause of stress before experiencing the syndrome.[5 6 7]

What is not agreed upon is whether the syndrome is psychological (a mental illness) or physiological (a physical illness). Some authors treat it as a form of mental illness. Others treat it as a physiological illness of unknown cause.

A few scientists have attempted to explain the syndrome through the use of modern non-invasive testing. Results have been inconclusive. This means scientists can draw no clear conclusion from the experiments. One study showed decreased blood flow in parts of the brain of the individual(s) being studied.[8] One study showed decreased electrical activity in parts of the brain of the individual(s) being studied.[9]

Known physiological illnesses must be diagnosed and treated, such as meningitis, encephalitis, closed head injury etc. Once these are excluded, then a diagnosis of hysterical paralysis or Ganser Syndrome can be made.[10]

The incidence of hysterical paralysis in the general population is between five and twenty-two cases per 100,000 persons. [11]

*M*A*S*H* even did an episode on dealing with hysterical paralysis where a young soldier was unable to control his body from the waist down after his unit was attacked by enemy tanks.[12]

41

Closed Head Injury aka Traumatic Brain Injury

We want to look for the blood, guts, and gore. And if her head's broken and there's blood, we're gonna think—we know for a fact. But if it's a closed head injury and you don't notice symptoms right away, we're not too sure what's going on there.—
Karen Wilson

The main emphasis of this book is recovery from a spinal cord injury. However, in certain accidents the same accident mechanism also causes a closed head injury.

I suffered a closed head injury in my accident. I know how devastating they are. But you say, "Carolyn, you are writing this book. You don't seem to have any problems." Remember it has been twelve, almost thirteen years since my accident. I have had time to improve, but I am still impaired.

Immediately after my accident I was very confused, as I mentioned in earlier chapters. I couldn't make logical decisions. I couldn't remember where *anything* in my house was. I had testing performed by a neuropsychologist, which rated my mental functioning ability as that of someone unable to work or perform basic functions.

I had an MBA from Southern Illinois University and a bachelor's degree in history from the University of Illinois. I had several published professional articles. I have worked as an advisor to a University President, been a marketing research consultant, and held various other jobs that required a high level of logical analysis.

And suddenly I had no ability to function outside the home. I could not remember anything I had been told five minutes before. I could no longer speak properly without slurring my speech. My sense of smell had been damaged. I could no longer tell if meat was good or had gone bad. It all smelled bad to me. I don't know how much good beef I threw out in the early days after my accident before my husband figured out I had a problem. I no longer recognized some written words that I knew. I still can't think of the right word to say in a given situation (See Word-Finding #1 below). That gives you some idea of the effect that a closed head injury can have on a person in real terms.

I am including this chapter for the friends and family members of the injured person to make you aware of what a closed head injury is, what its symptoms are, and how it is diagnosed.

This is very important material in this chapter.

Please do not skip this chapter. It might make the difference between you and your family member being able to lead a normal life and not. Some individuals have had to suffer for ten to twenty years with a closed head injury before it was diagnosed. Don't let this happen to you or a family member.

A closed head injury is defined as: "A bouncing motion of the brain that results from a blow to the head or severe shaking that does not penetrate the skull or brain tissue. This bouncing motion can cause tearing, shearing or stretching of the nerves at the base of the brain, blood clots, edema (swelling), and even death."[1]

In plain English, a closed head injury is brain damage where there is no visible wound to the head. A closed head injury is also called traumatic brain injury. Closed head injuries are very common after automobile accidents.

I want to make the following point on closed head injuries. *Just because an x-ray of the head, a CT Scan of the head, or an MRI of the head is normal, do not assume the injured person is fine if they start showing any of the symptoms listed later in this chapter.*

The prognosis for recovery for closed head injury victims is better than the prognosis for stroke victims because closed head injury victims are usually younger and have a healthier vascular (heart, lungs, blood etc.) system.[2]

Be prepared that recovering from a closed head injury can take months or years. It is a devastating injury. In one way a closed head injury is like a spinal cord injury to the brain. It is an *invisible* injury. It is not an injury that someone can look at you, and know you have a closed head injury. It is possible to completely recover from a closed head injury, but it is not likely.

Let's talk some numbers so you have an idea just how common closed head injuries are. In the United States, approximately one million people every year sustain a blow to the head. Out of those people, 50,000 to 100,00 have permanent brain damage that will affect their ability to work and/or affect their daily lives.[3]

For you to understand how a closed head injury happens during an auto accident, I need to explain a little bit of physics to you. Don't be afraid you won't understand. I'll make it simple. The term you need to know is *inertia*. This is the tendency of an object in motion to remain in motion and an object that is still to stay still.

In a car accident, this means if you are traveling faster than zero miles an hour, you cannot stop instantly after you apply your brakes. If your car is moving at all, you cannot stop instantly. It will take some period of time, even if very short, for your car to come to a complete stop.

Let's say you are driving along in your car at a particular speed. The speed doesn't matter for purposes of this illustration. Something happens to cause you to stop unexpectedly. Because of inertia, your car, your body, and your brain inside your skull continue moving forward.

Your brain does a really bad thing in this situation. It hits the front of your skull. And then it does a much worse thing. As the rest of your body bounces backward after the impact, your brain hits the back of your skull. You may black out when this happens as I did, or you may remain conscious and be totally unaware it has happened.

Your brain is very soft. It is slightly firmer than Jell-O. It is not made to be thrown around. Inside your brain for your entire life, your brain has been developing. Every new experience, everything you learn, becomes part of your brain. Your brain builds connections that look something like an octopus. These are very, very small. They are too small to be seen by an x-ray technology doctors currently have. These connections tear when the head is subjected to trauma.[3]

Let's talk about the common symptoms of a closed head injury. If you or your family member have multiple "YES" answers to the following questions, you need to make an appointment with your doctor immediately and discuss the results of this questionnaire. Take the questionnaire with you if you have to.

Headaches

1. Do you have more headaches since the injury or accident?
2. Do you have pain in the temples or forehead?
3. Do you have pain in the back of the head (sometimes the pain will start at the back of the head and extend to the front of the head)?
4. Do you have episodes of very sharp pain (like being stabbed) in the head which last from several seconds to several minutes?

Memory
1. Does your memory seem worse following the accident or injury?
2. Do you seem to forget what people have told you 15 to 30 [*sic*] minutes ago?
3. Do family members or friends say that you have asked the same question over and over?
4. Do you have difficulty remembering what you just read?

Word-Finding
1. Do you have difficulty coming up with the right word (you know the word you that you want to say but can't seem to "spit it out")?

Fatigue
1. Do you get tired more easily (mentally and/or physically)?
2. Does the fatigue get worse the more you think or in very emotional situations?

Changes in Emotion
1. Are you more easily irritated or angered (seems to come on quickly)?
2. Since the injury, do you cry or become depressed more easily?

Changes in Sleep
1. Do you keep waking up throughout the night and early morning?
2. Do you wake up early in the morning (4 or 5 am) [*sic*] and can't get back to sleep?

Environmental Overload
1. Do you find yourself easily overwhelmed in noisy or crowded places (feeling overwhelmed in a busy store or around noisy children)?

Impulsiveness
1. Do you find yourself making poor or impulsive decisions (saying things "without thinking" that may hurt others feelings; increase in impulse buying)?

Concentration
1. Do you have difficulty concentrating (can't seem to stay focused on what you are doing)?

Distraction
1. Are you easily distracted (someone interrupts you while you are doing a task and you lose your place [and you can't regain your train of thought]?
Organization
1. Do you have difficulty getting organized or completing a task (leave out a step in a recipe or started multiple projects but don't complete them)?

If you have five or more "Yes" answers, show the results to your doctor.[4]

An excellent way to document a closed head injury is for the person suspected of having a closed head injury to write a daily diary. If this is not possible, have the injured person dictate how he or she is having trouble thinking or functioning to someone who can take notes. Be sure to date each day's entry. This is especially important if there is to be legal action involving the accident, such as a lawsuit or a workers' compensation hearing.

A neuropsychologist is the type of specialist that tests and diagnoses closed head injuries. By definition, a neuropsychologist is a psychologist who specializes in studying brain behavior relationships.[5] A psychologist is a specialist who can talk with patients and their families about emotional and personal matters, and can help them make decisions.[6] Both fields require a substantial amount of college education and additional training.

I tried to find a listing of neuropsychologists by state, but I could not find one. Check your local phone book. I did find a list of doctors compiled by an individual who requested the names of doctors in each state and Canada who have helped with traumatic brain injury. This list is located at http://www.geocities.com/bjscloset/2.html. Omit the final period. If anyone is curious which neuropsychologist I used, my doctor was Dr. Dale Halfaker in Springfield, Missouri.

On a personal note, how I happened to be diagnosed was a matter of coincidence. My husband, Raymond, is an attorney. He happened to have gone to a continuing education seminar on closed head injury a few months before my auto accident. He recognized the symptoms of a closed head injury, and insisted I be tested.

Once a closed head injury or traumatic brain injury has been diagnosed, you may experience problems with your insurance company refusing to pay for ongoing therapy. You may need a friend or family member to help you with this because of your closed head injury. An article I found in *Neurology Now* addresses this problem with this advice:

> 1. First, request a copy of the Master Insurance Policy or Master Provider Agreement if you do not have one. Read the Definitions, Limitations, Exclusions, and Treatment Guidelines. Don't rely on telephone conversations with clerks. Review the policy carefully and get the reason for denial in writing. Insurance companies may say your treatment was denied for one reason and after getting the documentation from you, they will change their reason for denial. The Letter of Denial from the insurance company prevents this.

2. Make sure you understand all the Definitions in the policy. "Cognitive Therapy" may be denied under the policy. Most policies cover "medically necessary" outpatient speech-pathology treatment, occupational therapy, or neuropyschological services. These are all disciplines of Cognitive Therapy.

3. Get a Baseline of Function. Get neuropsychological testing as soon as possible following a brain injury. Testing can also detect problems that were not obvious at first. If you functioned at a high level before your accident, be sure to document this because the degree of impairment of a highly educated person like a doctor or lawyer is greater than the degree of impairment of a person without such education. [An easy way to understand this is: if you jump from a third-story window, you will be hurt worse than if you jump from a second-story window. The higher a person's IQ (Intelligence Quotient, as measured by standardized testing), the more mental damage it takes to bring their IQ down to an average IQ.]

4. Appeal the Denial of Service. Insurance companies have several levels of appeal. If all levels of internal appeals fail, ask for an external appeal. In an external appeal, members of the community not affiliated with the managed care system give evidence. You must start the appeals process early to have a chance to win. Forty two [*sic*] states have an external appeals process. You may also find an independent case manager to be helpful.

5. Find an Expert. Appeals processes are long and difficult. The insurance companies are hoping you will go away with time. An expert can be an independent case manager or an attorney. They can sometimes be paid by funds to be received later during a settlement.

6. Appoint a Legal Guardian. Most people don't do this and it ends up haunting them. Courts don't have to follow the wishes of spouses, parents, children or other family members without a court decree. Court-appointed guardians can negotiate benefits, file appeals, and even file a claim for bad faith [it means the other party is using underhanded tactics].

7. Find Other Sources of Funding. There may be specialized state-funded programs for educational training, preparation for independent living, and residential placement. There is no good source of information on this. You must research heavily or use experts. If the person is injured before high school graduation and is in a public school, the public school system is responsible for providing an Individual Education Plan that addresses the student's needs. If the person is over 21 [*sic*], he or she may be eligible for Medicaid.[7]

The important thing is not to give up after a closed head injury. Your brain is constantly working to build new pathways, even around the damaged pathways and function may continue to come back. Don't let the paperwork get you down either.

42

Spina Bifida

Opportunities to find deeper powers within ourselves
come when life seems most challenging—
Joseph Campbell

Spina Bifida is a condition of the spinal cord that develops at birth instead of from injury or accident. I am going to discuss it very briefly.

Spina Bifida is Latin for "split spine."[1] It is a condition where the bones in the lowest part of the spinal column do not develop properly. This allows the spinal cord to be unprotected, and part of the cord may actually be outside the body at birth. It is a condition that is unfortunately may be becoming more common instead of less. It is theorized that a combination of vitamin deficiency, genetics, and environmental factors cause Spina Bifida. Spina Bifida also comes in different forms with different levels of severity of disability.[2]

The following factors may increase the chances of having a baby born with Spina Bifida (not in any particular order):

1. Insufficient Folic Acid, a type of B-Vitamin before and during early pregnancy
2. Family history of Spina Bifida even a distantly related relative (strongly increases chances)
3. Mother with insulin-dependent diabetes
4. Mother's use of some anti-seizure medications
5. Mother with diagnosed obesity
6. Caucasian or Hispanic ancestry raises risk (some evidence that Irish ancestry increases risk)
7. Exposure to high temperature during early pregnancy (hot tub or sauna use or prolonged fever)
8. Agent Orange exposure in the Father[3]

Agent Orange is a chemical originally developed for military use. It causes the leaves to fall off plants. It was used during the Vietnam War to clear areas of jungle in Vietnam. Agent Orange breaks down into very toxic chemicals.

Spina Bifida is surgically corrected immediately after the baby is born. Unfortunately disability from Spina Bifida cannot be reversed.

With advances in modern medicine, it may eventually be possible for doctors to operate on the baby before the baby is born, and correct the damage before birth.

What the Future Holds

43

Prognosis After a Complete Spinal Cord Injury

In a universe of ambiguity, this kind of certainty comes only once, no matter how many lifetimes you live.—
Robert James Waller

I am covering prognosis after complete spinal cord injury, incomplete spinal cord injury, and Central Cord Syndrome in three separate chapters. This is because the possible outcomes differ so greatly.

In a complete injury there is no function or feeling below the level of injury. A complete injury always affects both sides of the body equally. There is very little in life that is certain, but unfortunately the prognosis after a complete spinal cord injury is predictable. [1] Often, people with incomplete spinal cord injuries are initially diagnosed with complete injuries, but with time recover sensation and are rediagnosed as incomplete.

A person with a complete injury will not recover function or sensation below the level of injury.

This does not mean that a person with a complete injury has nothing to look forward to in life. Many people with complete spinal cord injuries still lead very full and happy lives.

44

Prognosis After an Incomplete Spinal Cord Injury

The prognosis for recovery is great.—
Terry Hoeppner

There are too many variables and too many unknowns when trying to predict the prognosis for recovery after an incomplete spinal cord injury. The Arkansas Spinal Cord Commission offers some general guidelines on what to expect for recovery:

> 1. The severity of the original injury determines whether or not recovery will occur. Unfortunately, there is no test available at this time to measure this severity and predictions must be based on what has happened to others in the past with similar neurological [nerve function] findings.
> 2. Incomplete injuries have a better chance of further recovery than complete injuries, but even with incomplete injuries there is no guarantee that any further recovery will occur.
> 3. Most of the recovery that will occur starts early (within the first few weeks). Therefore, each day that goes by without any return of function means that the chances for recovery is less!
> 4. No amount of hard work will make the nerves return. If hard work was all it took, very few people would end up with permanent paralysis.
> 5. Whether or not you have surgery and whether or not you go to therapy are not what determine how much recovery you will have. These things are done for other reasons.
> 6. Rehabilitation will not affect the degree of recovery. The purpose of rehabilitation is to improve function in self-care activities (such as dressing, transfers, and wheelchair (mobility) using whatever is available to work with. Since most recovery that will occur tends to start within the first few weeks after injury and by coincidence this is usually the same time therapy is being done, there is a tendency to think the recovery is due to the therapy. It should be clearly understood that the therapy did not cause the recovery.

> 7. Just because one nerve cell recovers does not mean that others will. Patients often get very excited when they see some small improvement in sensation or increase in strength, but only time will tell i[f] [*sic*] anything else will come back.[1]

Number three above is no longer true. The late Christopher Reeve experienced recovery eight years after his injury. Doctors believe that Reeve's long-term dedication to his rehabilitation program was responsible for his recovery.[2]

Christopher Reeve used a very structured program of rehabilitation. He used a bicycle with functional electrical stimulation (FES), weekly body-weight supported treadmill walking, and aqua therapy (therapy in a swimming pool).[3]

Functional Electrical Stimulation (FES) is a technique that uses electrical currents to activate nerves innervating extremities [arms and legs] affected by paralysis from spinal cord injury (SCI), head injury, stroke or other neurological disorders, restoring function in people with disabilities. This therapy works mainly on the Peripheral Nervous System.[4]

I, myself, have seen recovery up to two years after surgery for a spinal cord injury.

One experimental surgery is being performed to help incomplete quadriplegics with shoulder function, but without hand function to use one hand. A system of an electrical generator with a controller implanted in the shoulder can allow quadriplegics to use one hand. There are electrodes implanted to stimulate the appropriate nerves which control the hand.[5]

45

Prognosis After a Central Cord Syndrome Spinal Cord Injury

Life's challenges are not supposed to paralyze you,
they're supposed to help you discover who you are—
Bernice Johnson Reagon

The prognosis after a Central Cord Syndrome injury differs from that of the other Spinal Cord Syndromes included under an incomplete injury. It also differs from that of a complete injury, so I am covering it in a separate chapter.

Let me start with a brief observation made in a journal article on Central Cord Syndrome. One set of doctors who researched Central Cord Syndrome stated that "atypical variations are more common than the existing literature suggests...."[1]

Another set of doctors, who performed a long-term follow-up on patients with incomplete spinal cord traumatic injuries, had some very specific and perhaps surprising observations on patients in their study with Central Cord Syndrome. It appears that patients with Central Cord Syndrome are prone to additional complications of their condition long after the initial injury. They called this chronic Central Cord Syndrome.

The symptoms of chronic Central Cord Syndrome are increased spasticity and reduced function in the lower body. The long-term study showed some of Central Cord Syndrome patients were able to walk after their recovery, but by the time of the follow-up study required wheelchairs. Although several theories exist as to the deterioration with Central Cord Syndrome, none of the theories has been proven to be accurate.

The long-term prognosis for Central Cord Syndrome has been stated in these words: "Therefore, progressive neurologic deterioration with occasional ascending cord symptoms seems to be the rule in these unfortunate cases."[2]

An Australian study of a small group of Central Cord Syndrome patients found more positive long-term outcomes for the patients involved. This study found that Central Cord Syndrome patients under the age of seventy showed an increase in functionality over time after their initial injury.[3]

However, it is unclear reading the articles how seriously injured the patients were and if they required surgery. The Australian study indicated that none of its Central Cord Syndrome patients underwent surgery. This may account for the more positive outcomes experienced by the study participants.

If you have a Central Cord Syndrome injury you should be aware of the possibility of long-term complications years after your initial injury.

46

Rehabilitation After A Spinal Cord Injury

They (patients participating in support groups) are more likely to be complying with their medications, less likely to be depressed and actually in some studies people have quicker rehabilitation.—
John Miller

Rehabilitation after a spinal cord injury is critical in the recovery of the injured person. This is something I can only discuss from reading books by other spinal cord injurees, and by talking to others who have been through the rehabilitation process. I have never had any rehabilitation related to my spinal cord injury other than a couple of visits to a chiropractor in the attempt to give me more range of motion in my neck by releasing the tightened soft tissues.

I could write for weeks on the subject of rehabilitation for spinal cord injuries. But I won't. I want to discuss some basics of rehabilitation that a person who has been injured (and their family) should know. If you should want to read individual stories of rehabilitation experiences, then see the Additional Reading and Movies chapter. Two of the movies I have listed are very good stories of rehabilitation experiences.

The first is that the purpose of the rehabilitation process is to restore as much sensation, ability to move, and bodily function as possible. It involves many weeks of working with physical therapists, occupational therapists, and other professionals.

You are going to have three basic choices for a rehabilitation facility. You can either use one that is close to where you live or close to where the accident happened. Or you can use another facility of your choice located far away from your home or accident location.

There is a group of fourteen facilities in the United States that are called Model System of Care facilities. These fourteen facilities are the most progressive in their care of spinal cord injuries. The facilities that are designated Model System of Care facilities change over time. I am not specifying which institutions are the fourteen Model System of Care facilities because the institutions change quite frequently.

I have provided a list below of spinal cord injury hospitals and rehabilitation centers by state according to http://www.sci-info.pages.com. This list does not include all rehabilitation centers in all states. Check your local telephone directory as well if you need a rehabilitation center close to home.

Alabama
Spain Rehabilitation Center
University of Alabama at Birmingham (UAB)
UAB Model SCI System
Office of Research Services
619 19th Street South, SRC 529
Birmingham, AL 35249-7330
1-205-934-3293
sciweb@uab.edu
http://www.spinalcord.uab.edu

California
CareMeridian (10 facilities throughout California)
1-800-852-1256
gwakefield@caremeridian.com
http://www.caremeridian.com
There is a contact form on the website

Casa Colina Centers for Rehabilitation
255 East Bonita Avenue
P.O. Box 6001
Pomona, CA 91769-6001
1-909-596-7733
1-800-926-5462
Fax 1-909-593-0153
TDD-TYY-Q 1-909-596-3646
rehab@casacolina.org
http://www.casacolina.org

Rancho Los Amigos National Rehabilitation Center
7601 E. Imperial Highway
Downey, CA 90242
1-562-401-7111
TDD/TTY 1-562-401-8450
http://www.rancho.org

Santa Clara Valley Medical Center
Rehabilitation Research Center for TBI & SCI
Santa Clara Valley Medical Center
751 South Bascom Avenue
San Jose, CA 95128
1-408-793-6433
Fax 1-408-793-6434
http://www.tbi.sci-org

Stanford Hospital & Clinics
300 Pasteur Drive
Stanford, CA 94305
1-650-723-4000
Stanford Referral Center 1-800-756-9000
http://www.stanfordhospital.com
contact form on website

Colorado
Craig Hospital
3425 S. Clarkson Street
Englewood, CO 80113
1-303-789-8000
Spinal Cord Injury Admissions Karen Mathias 1-303-789-8437
admissions@craighospital.org
http://www.craighospital.org/Research/SCIModelsystems.asp

Spalding Rehabilitation Hospital
900 Potomac Street
Aurora, CO 80011
1-303-367-1166
http://www.spaldingrehab.com

University of Colorado Hospital
Aurora/Anschutz Medical Campus
University of Colorado Hospital
Anschutz Inpatient Pavillion
12605 E. 16th Avenue
Aurora, CO 80045
1-720-848-4011
http://www.uch.edu

University of Colorado Hospital
9th & Colorado
4200 E. Ninth Avenue
Denver, CO 80220
1-303-372-0000
http://www.uch.edu

Delaware
Regional Spinal Cord Injury Center of Delaware Valley
Thomas Jefferson University Hospital
Spinal Cord Injury Center
Main Building, Suite 375
132 South 10th Street
Philadelphia, PA 19107
1-215-955-6579
Fax 1-215-955-5152
http://www.spinalcordcenter.org

Magee Rehabilitation Hospital
1513 Race Street
6 Franklin Plaza
Philadelphia, PA 19102
1-215-587-3000
1-800-96-MAGEE
http://www.spinalcordcenter.org

District of Columbia
National Capital Spinal Cord Injury Model System

National Rehabilitation Hospital/Medstar Research Institute
102 Irving Street, NW
Washington, DC 20010
1-202-877-1000
http://www.ncscims.org

Florida
South Florida Regional Spinal Cord Injury Model System
Mailing Address
Leonard M. Miller School of Medicine University of Miami
South Florida Spinal Cord Injury Model Systems
P.O. Box 016960
Mailing Locator D-48
Miami, FL 33101

Building Location
Leonard M. Miller School of Medicine University of Miami
Department of Rehabilitative Medicine
1611 N.W. 12th Street
Rehab Center-Basement Floor
Miami, FL 33136
1-305-585-1339
Fax 1-305-585-1340
Appointments 1-305-243-6605
Consult Line 1-305-585-7112
http://www.sci.med.miami.edu

Georgia
Georgia Regional Spinal Cord Injury Care System
Shepherd Center, Inc.
2020 Peachtree Road, NW
Atlanta, GA 30309
Referral (Admissions) 1-404-350-7345
Main Line 1-404-352-2020
http://www.shepherd.org/research/model.asp

Illinois
Midwest Regional Spinal Cord Injury Care System

Northwestern University Feinberg School of Medicine
Department of Physical Medicine and Rehabilitation
Rehabilitation Institute of Chicago
345 East Superior Street
Chicago, IL 60611
1-312-238-2870
Fax 1-312-238-1219
r-bailey@northwestern.edu
http://www.medschool.northwestern.edu

Indiana
Hook Rehabilitation Center
Mailing Address
Community Health Network
1500 North Ritter Avenue
Indianapolis, IN 46219
1-317-355-1411
1-800-777-7775
http://www.ecommunity.com

Rehabilitation Hospital of Indiana—RHI
4141 Shore Drive
Indianapolis, IN 46254
1-317-329-2000
http://www.rhin.com

Maryland
Kernan Hospital
2200 Kernan Drive
Baltimore, MD 21207
1-410-448-2500
TTY 1-410-448-1967
Appointments 1-800-492-5538
University Rehabilitation Referral Service 1-410-328-8680
http://www.umm.edu/kernan
http://www.kernanhospital.com

Massachusetts
New England Regional Spinal Cord Injury Center
Boston University Medical Center Hospital
One Boston Medical Center Place
Boston, MA 02118
1-617-638-8000
http://www.bmc.org

Spaulding Rehabilitation Hospital
125 Nashua Street
Boston, MA 02118
1-617-573-7000
TTD/TTY 1-800-439-2370
http://www.spauldingrehab.org

Michigan
Center for Spinal Cord Injury Recovery
Rehabilitation Institute of Michigan
261 Mack
Detroit, MI 48201
1-866-SCI-CENTER
Brian F. Sheridan, OTR
CSCIR, Program Supervisor
bsherida@dmc.org
http://www.centerforscirecovery.org/

Mary Free Bed
235 Wealthy SE
Grand Rapids, MI 49503
1-616-242-0300 or
1-800-528-8989
Spanish or Vietnamese interpreters available
info@maryfreebed.com
http://www.maryfreebed.com

University of Michigan
University of Michigan Model Spinal Cord Injury Care System
1500 E. Medical Center Drive

Ann Arbor, MI 48109
1-734-936-4000
http://www.med.umich.edu/pmr/modelsci/index.htm

Minnesota
Gillette Children's Specialty Healthcare
2000 East University Avenue
St. Paul, MN 55101
1-651-291-2848
1-800-719-4040
TDD/TTY 1-651-229-3928
http://www.gillettechildrens.org

Mayo Clinic-Rochester
200 First Street, S.W.
Rochester, MN 55905
1-507-284-2511
Fax 1-507-284-0161
TTD/TTY 1-507-284-9786
http://www.mayoclinic.org

Miller-Dwan Medical Center
502 East Second Street
Duluth, MN 55805
1-218-727-8762
TTD/TTY 1-218-720-1950
webfeedback@smdc.org
http://www.miller-dwan.com

Missouri
Rusk Rehabilitation Center
315 Business Loop 70 W.
Columbia, MO 65203
Department 1-573-882-3101
Clinic 1-573-884-0033
http://www.muhealth.org

Nebraska
Immanuel Rehabilitation Center
Immanuel Medical Center
6901 North 72nd Street
Omaha, NE 68122
1-402-572-2121
http://www.alegent.com

Madonna Rehabilitation Center
5401 South Street
Lincoln, NE 68506
1-402-489-7102
1-800-676-5448
http://www.madonna.org

Nevada
CareMeridian
1-800-852-1256
gwakefield@caremeridian.com
http://www.caremeridian.com

New Hampshire
Northeast Rehabilitation Hospital
70 Butler Street
Salem, NH 03079
1-603-893-2900
webmaster@northeastrehab.com
http://www.northeastrehab.com

New Jersey
Kessler Medical Rehabilitation Research and Education Corporation
300 Market Street
Saddle Brook, NJ 07663
1-201-368-6000
1-888-KESSLER
Fax 1-201-368-6262
http://www.kmrrec.org/nnjscis/

Kessler Rehabilitation Corporation & NNJSCIS
1199 Pleasant Valley Way
West Orange, NJ 07052
1-973-731-3600
1-888-KESSLER
1-973-243-6819
http://www.kmrrec.org/nnjscis/

New York
Burke Rehabilitation Hospital
The Burke Rehabilitation Hospital
785 Mamaronek Avenue
White Plains, NY 10605
1-914-597-2500
web@burke.org
http://www.burke.org

Helen Hayes Hospital Center for Rehabilitation Technology
Route 9W
West Haverstraw, NY 10993
1-888-70-REHAB (73422)
Fax 1-845-947-3097
TTD/TTY 1-845-947-3187
info@helenhayes.org
http://www.helenhayeshospital.org

Mount Sinai Spinal Cord Injury Model System
Mailing Address
One Gustave L. Levy Place
New York, NY 10029
Department of Rehabilitation Medicine Faculty Practice
1-212-241-6335
1-212-241-6321
1-212-241-3981
http://www.mssm.edu/rehab/spinal

Sunnyview Rehabilitation Hospital
1270 Belmont Avenue

Schenectady, NY 12308
1-518-382-4500
1-877-REHAB-SV (1-877-734-2278)
http://www.sunnyview.org

Ohio
Northeast Ohio Regional Spinal Cord Injury System
MetroHealth System
2500 MetroHealth Drive
Cleveland, OH 44109
http://www.metrohealth.org/body.cfm?id=346&oTopID=345

Ohio State University Medical Center
410 W. 10th Avenue
Columbus, OH 43210
1-800-293-5123
http://www.medicalcenter.osu.edu

Pennsylvania
Regional Spinal Cord Injury Center of the Delaware Valley
Thomas Jefferson University Hospital
Spinal Cord Injury Center
Main Building, Suite 375
132 South 10th Street
Philadelphia, PA 19107
215-955-6579
Fax 215-955-5152
http://www.jeffersonhospital.org/rehab/

Magee Rehabilitation Hospital
1513 Race Street
6 Franklin Plaza
Philadelphia, PA 19102-1177
215-587-3000
1-800-96-MAGEE
SCI Follow-Up System
215-587-3394
MossRehab Hospital

60 East Township Line Road
Elkins Park, PA 19027
1-215-663-6000
1-800-EINSTEIN
http://www.einstein.edu

MossRehab Hospital
1200 West Tabor Road
Philadelphia, PA 19141
1-215-456-9000
1-800-EINSTEIN
http://www.einstein.edu

Shriners Hospital for Children, Philadelphia
3551 North Broad Street
Philadelphia, PA 19140
1-215-430-4000
Fax 1-215-430-4079
http://www.shriners.com

University of Pittsburgh Model Center on Spinal Cord Injury
200 Lothrop Street
Pittsburgh, PA 15213
1-412-647-UPMC (8762)
1-800-533-UPMC (8762)
http://www.upmc.-sci.org

University of Pennsylvania Health System
Hospital of the University of Pennsylvania
3400 Spruce Street
Philadelphia, PA 19104
1-215-662-4000
http://www.pennhealth.com

Rhode Island
Shake-A-Leg
P.O. Box 1264
Newport, RI 02840

1-401-849-8898
1-888-SHAKEALEG
Fax 1-401-848-9072
http://www.shakealeg.org

Texas
Texas Model Spinal Cord Injury System
The Institute for Rehabilitation and Research
Inpatient Rehabilitation Services
1333 Moursund
Houston, TX 77030
1-800-44REHAB
tirr.referals@memorialhermann.org
http://www.texasmscis.org

Virginia
VCU Rehabilitation and Research Center
P.O. Box 980661
Richmond, VA 23298-0661
1-804-828-0861
Fax 1-804-828-5074
beagle@hsc.vcu.edu
http://www.rrc.pmr.vcu.edu

Washington
NextStepsNW
4162 148th Avenue NE
Redmond, WA 98052
1-425-869-9506
Fax 1-425-869-9482
http://www.nextstepnw.org

Northwest Regional Spinal Cord Injury System
Mailing Address
Northwest Regional Spinal Cord Injury System
University of Washington
Rehabilitation Medicine, Box 356490
Seattle, WA 98195

Fax 1-206-685-3244
http://sci.washington.edu

Wisconsin
Better Days, Inc. (a non-profit corporation)
Hillsboro, WI 54634
Stanley Nofsinger 1-608-489-2628
1-608-489-2141
1-608-489-3569
http://www.betterdayinc.com [*sic*]

47

Aging with a Spinal Cord Injury

The great thing about getting older is that you don't lose all the other ages you've been.—
Anonymous

Aging with a spinal cord injury at first sounds like an awful thing. It's better than not aging with a spinal cord injury. You've got to start every day with the idea that you are on *this side* of the grass, and not the other side.

Aging to most people means getting older, adding another birthday notch to your belt as it were. Aging to doctors means "the decline of biological systems resulting from functional deterioration or death of individual cells."[1] In this chapter I am going to discuss what happens to the body of a spinal cord injury survivor, as the person gets older and the body systems decline.

Another quotation I found on aging in a book on spinal cord injury and aging breaks down the process into three distinct processes: "Aging involves at least three major lifelong developmental processes, all overlapping, but all distinctly different (a) physiologic changes of the body; (b) changing social roles, and (c) issues of self-realization."[2]

The book goes on to clarify that "physiologic changes are the most commonly discussed manifestation of aging.... sociological events include leaving home, marrying, parenting, losing one's parents, and/or losing a spouse. Self-realization.... includes the issues of developing values, ethics, morality, and ultimately finding meaning in life."[3]

Everyone experiences "normal" physiologic changes as more time passes since they were born. These include loss of muscle mass with resultant decrease in strength, decreased range of motion and osteoarthritis leading to pain and decreased function, and increased urologic and bowel problems.[4]

Here's where things start to get tricky. What is not known is what the physiologic changes listed above do when a person has a spinal cord injury. Does getting older worsen spinal cord injury symptoms and dysfunction? Does getting older make the deterioration of the body from a spinal cord injury speed up?[5] Are there other chemical changes that take place as well? What about psychological changes with a spinal cord injury? [6]

Have you ever written something on paper with a pencil, erased what you have written, and then written something different? A spinal cord injury does exactly that to the systems of the body. It "erases" your original body chemistry, organ systems balance, and anything else it can get its hands on and "rewrites" everything.[6] Something like having the files on your computer getting corrupted.

One article I found has this to say about spinal cord injury: "It [spinal cord injury] typically results in initial paralysis, but because there is an effect on essentially every body system, it has other initial and long-term effects as well."

Before World War II, spinal cord injury survivors didn't live long. Nobody thought about the aging process after a spinal cord injury. But as modern medicine has improved, aging with a spinal cord injury is an issue that almost every person with a spinal cord injury now faces. So less is known about the aging process with a spinal cord injury, both physiological and psychological, than some other areas of medicine.[8]

There are two questions when it comes to aging and spinal cord injury: do spinal cord injury survivors think about the aging process, and the decades to come differently or sooner than their non-disabled peers, and whether the aging process that spinal cord injury survivors experience is different from that of people who are not disabled? The conclusion is that "it's difficult to say."[9]

In my opinion the answers to the above two questions are both a no-brainer for anyone with a spinal cord injury. We, as spinal cord injury survivors, think about the aging process and think about it sooner than a non-disabled person because we have been forced to face our own mortality.

I also believe we experience a different aging process from other people because we have already sustained more damage. Many of us are already in severe pain, as if we had reach our "golden years." Our bodies take punishment from pushing manual wheelchairs and wearing out our joints. Our skin breaks down similarly to that of the very elderly.

We are more aware of our health problems than the non-disabled population. Again, the way we would be if we were much older. We have different medical problems than people who do not have spinal cord injuries. The orientation of the healthcare system in the United States is also set up to treat intermittent acute health problems, not ongoing chronic medical problems that spinal cord injury survivors must deal with.[10]

I have another suggestion on aging with a spinal cord injury. Scientists with The Miami Project to Cure Paralysis reported that damage from a spinal cord injury continues for some ten years after the original injury.[11] Some of the damage that doctors are attributing to the aging process may be damage from the original injury still.

Another issue related to aging with a spinal cord injury that I want to mention, but I don't want to spend a lot of time on is that women with a spinal cord injury and men with a spinal cord injury will have some differences in the aging process. Women live longer than men do, with or without a spinal cord injury.[12]

Another thought on aging, with or without a spinal cord injury. Stay active. The more active you stay, mentally and physically, the better off you will be.[13]

If you have a spinal cord injury, there is one encouraging thought. If you live long enough, your contemporaries will be in about the same shape you are.

48

Life Expectancy After a Spinal Cord Injury

Life expectancy would grow by leaps and bounds if green vegetables smelled as good as bacon.—
Doug Larson

"*What effect is a spinal cord injury going to have on my life expectancy?*" This is a question that can only be answered with a lot of assumptions and generalizations.

A basic assumption that will be true in almost all cases is a spinal cord injury will shorten the life expectancy of the injured person to some degree. By how much will be dependent on many different factors.

For purposes of this discussion I am assuming that the injured person has survived the first twenty-four hours after the accident. I am also assuming that the injured person has survived the first year and the second year after the injury.

I said in a previous chapter that women live longer than men. American women live longer than American men. The information that immediately follows is for individuals without a spinal cord injury.

White American women have an average life expectancy of 80.5 years. Black American women have an average life expectancy of 76.1 years. White American men have an average life expectancy of 75.4 years, and black American men have an average life expectancy of 69.2 years.[1]

If you are in a country other than the United States, please research the life expectancy information for your country on your own. If I were to provide life expectancy information for all the countries for which it is available, I would bury you and myself in statistics (please pardon the pun given the subject of this chapter).

There are several other factors that are consistent in estimating life expectancy with a spinal cord injury:

> 1. The life expectancy of a spinal cord injured person who is ventilator dependent will be shorter than the life expectancy of a spinal cord injured person who is not ventilator dependent.
> 2. The life expectancy of a spinal cord injured person with a complete injury will be shorter than the life expectancy of a spinal cord injured person with an incomplete injury.
> 3. The life expectancy of a spinal cord injured person with a high quadriplegia/tetraplegia (C1-C4) will be shorter than the life expectancy of a spinal cord injured person with a low quadriplegia/tetraplegia (C5-C8)
> 4. The life expectancy of a spinal cord injured person with a quadriplegic/tetraplegic injury will be shorter than the life expectancy of a spinal cord injured person with a paraplegic injury.[2]

The two other consistent trends in estimating life expectancy with a spinal cord injury are:

> 1. A person who sustained his or her injury "through personal violence" (I believe the researchers of the article mean being stabbed or being shot) will have a shorter life expectancy than a person who sustained his or her injury through an accident. [3]
> 2. The older a person is when he or she sustains the spinal cord injury, the less effect the injury will have on his or her life expectancy.[4]
> Life expectancy with a spinal cord injury has increased over time over the last 30 [*sic*] years, but is still below the life expectancy of a person without a spinal cord injury. The primary cause of death for spinal cord injuries has changed over the years, however. In the mid twentieth century the primary cause of death for individuals with a spinal cord injury was kidney failure. Currently the primary causes of death for individuals with a spinal cord injury are pneumonia, blood clot in the lungs, and blood poisoning (systemic infection).[5]

Each of the articles I have referenced below, with the exception of the first citation, has tables to help estimate life expectancy depending on age at injury, presence of motor function, ventilator dependency, and level of injury. The tables are slightly different from each other, but the basic trends are the same. For more specific information, consult the articles.

The advice I can give is for you to take care of yourself. Don't smoke. If you do smoke, then quit (I know, easier said than done). Smoking will soften your bones, and you don't need this after a spinal cord injury. Exercise regularly, even if you only do breathing exercises. See your doctor regularly. Have a pneumonia shot every five years. Reduce your stress levels (as best you can). Eat right. Maintain an optimal weight for your estimated or actual standing height. Having a positive outlook on life will also add to your life expectancy (easier said than done, I know).

All those numbers were fine and dandy, but you're probably asking, "How much longer am *I* going to live?" If I had the exact answer to that question, I could make a fortune.

49

Quality of Life After a Spinal Cord Injury

The quality of life is more important than life itself.—
Alexis Carrel

For a list of all the ways technology has failed to improve the quality of life, please press three.—
Alice Kahn

Let's start with a definition. What is "quality of life?"

The World Health Organization has defined "quality of life" as meaning "the individuals' perception of their position in life in the context of the culture and value systems in which they live, and in relation to their goals, expectations, standards, and concerns."[1]

That sounds like a definition a bureaucracy would come up with. I think I can do better than that. Quality of life boils down to the simple question of how does your life compare with your expectations of what your life should be? This can be in terms of health, love, family, friends, money, work, material possessions, or any other method you want to measure your life by.

One important factor in measuring your life against your expectations of your life is how reasonable your expectations are. If your expectations are very high, you may find yourself disappointed by your quality of life when you cannot achieve your expectations.

You had pre-injury expectations for quality of life, and you will have post-injury expectations for quality of life. They may be the same or they may be different. Depending upon what your pre-injury expectations were, you may find yourself disappointed that you cannot achieve them post-injury.

I found a very interesting article on spinal cord injury and quality of life. I would like to share the information from that article with you in this chapter.

This is a study that was performed by Craig Hospital, one of the major rehabilitation hospitals in the United States.

The article begins by discussing the wealth of research in existence that shows people with spinal cord injuries have a high quality of life. This seems to go against all common sense. Everybody knows that spinal cord injury survivors have many problems in almost all areas of their lives. Yet they seem to be happier than the general population.

The article goes on to discuss three reasons why the measured results among spinal cord injury survivors are different from what we would expect:

> 1. Researchers *think* they know *what* contributes to people's quality of life and life satisfaction—things like good health; challenging jobs; financial security and material comforts; control over their lives; romantic relationships; happy marriages, and even just satisfying relationships with others.
> 2. Researchers tell us these are things that SCI survivors often *do not have* or *are not satisfied with*, compared with nondisabled people.
> 3. At the same time, SCI survivors, as a group, tell researchers that they're happy and their quality of life is good. In fact, in one study, SCI survivors rated their quality of life *higher* than a similar group of *non*-disabled people! [italics present in original quotation][2]

The article goes on to discuss a British study of spinal cord injured men. This was a long-term study that measured their quality of life, specifically using factors that contributed to quality of life in nondisabled people. The list was as follows:

> 1. Health and personal safety
> 2. Material comforts
> 3. Relationships with family
> 4. Relationship with spouse or partner
> 5. Having and raising children
> 6. Having close friends
> 7. Helping and encouraging others
> 8. Work
> 9. Learning
> 10. Understanding oneself
> 11. Expressing oneself in a creative manner
> 12. Socializing with others
> 13. Reading, listening to music, watching sports events, and other entertainment
> 14. Participating in active recreation
> 15. Participating in activities relating to local and national government[3]

The results of the study turned out to be very interesting. And quite possibly, very unexpected. Fewer of the men surveyed thought material comforts, having and raising children, work, and participating in government were very important. More of the men felt relationships with their relatives, learning, creative expression, and reading and other quiet leisure activities were important.

The study did find that what the men thought was important was also directly related to what they had already accomplished in their lives. These men thought health was important, but they didn't see health or work as being critical to their quality of life.

They thought socializing, recreation, having a spouse or lover, having friends, and finally material comforts were important. Similar studies have shown consistent results among spinal cord injured men from other countries. [4]

Putting all the studies together gives some pretty consistent results. These three factors are evident:

1. People with spinal cord injuries may change their life priorities after their injuries. They may also change their life priorities as time passes after their injuries.
2. People with spinal cord injuries may use different criteria to judge their quality of life than nondisabled people.
3. You need to give careful consideration to what is important to you in life after your spinal cord injury. [5]

Instead of using all the "fancy" words and conclusions, let's just be blunt. We, as spinal cord injury survivors, do one of two things. We either spend the rest of our lives feeling sorry for ourselves. Or we don't take being alive for granted like so many nondisabled people do. For those of us not feeling sorry for ourselves, we know that we could easily be six feet under the ground. We are grateful to be alive. Even if we can't do the things we could do before.

50

The Importance of Hope After a Spinal Cord Injury

What seems to us as bitter trials are often blessings in disguise.—
Oscar Wilde

You may think this is an odd subject to have in a book about spinal cord injury. I have my reasons for including it.

Hope is a word used quite commonly, yet many people are not sure exactly what it means. The formal definition of hope is "a belief in a positive outcome related to events and circumstances in one's life."[1] The dictionary definition seems somehow shallow and devoid of life. I prefer a different definition from the same source: "Hope is often the result of faith in that while hope is an emotion, faith carries a divinely inspired and informed form of positive belief." [1] And yet, even that definition does not give us a good grasp of what hope really entails.

Jerome Groopman, in his book, *The Anatomy of Hope*, says that hope has two parts: a cognitive part and an affective part.[2] More fancy words, but a good grasp of what hope is. You take in information. You process it over time. The information you have taken in and processed causes you to change your opinion. Rather than expecting a negative outcome or result, you expect a positive outcome or result.

Spinal cord injury survivors who write their own stories of survival give hope to other spinal cord injury survivors.

You may be reading this chapter (or having someone read it to you) and thinking, "How in the world is there hope for me? I have a complete injury from the neck down." Or I have an incomplete injury from the neck down. Or a complete injury from the waist down. You are depressed. You are angry. You are frustrated. You are feeling many negative emotions.

What do you have to lose by hoping?

What is your goal in hoping? To be fully functional exactly the way you were before the accident? To be happy again? Both? Or something else?

It is well known in medicine that patients who have a positive attitude about their recovery recover faster and more thoroughly than those with a negative attitude. It is also well known that seriously ill patients who believe they are going to die usually do.

Advances are being made in medical science with increasing rapidity. What was impossible thirty years ago is now commonplace.

The main advice I can give you is don't give up on yourself. Keep looking for alternatives. It can be difficult to wait for your life to take a new direction. When it is the right time for it to do so after your injury, it will.

Have faith. Which leads me to the next chapter.

51

Religion and Faith After a Spinal Cord Injury

Faith isn't faith until it's all you're holding on to—
Anonymous

I am one of those individuals who has found comfort in religion after my injury. But it has been a long time coming.

Religion was not something I grew up with. My mother was raised a devout Catholic. My father was Protestant. My grandfather on my father's side was a minister. My father's brother also became a minister. But religion was not something the family on either side talked about much.

My grandparents on my mother's side of the family attended church regularly. Every Sunday they were in church. My grandfather loved the music in church. He would sing every hymn. You could hear his voice booming above the rest of the congregation during the singing of the hymns. This is not the same grandfather I mentioned early in the book who was a minister.

After my grandmother died my grandfather continued to attend church. He decided to try to broaden his understanding of religion. I believe it was his way of trying to come to terms with my grandmother's death. He began to attend church on Sunday at not only the Catholic church, but also to any other services he could find. He even attended the Jewish Synagogue. For those in the New Haven area of Connecticut, you may remember my grandfather. His name was Anthony J. Suraci.

I can remember my mother being very upset with the Catholic church during the Vietnam War. The priest at our local church was out protesting against the war along with the college students at Southern Illinois University. My mother felt this behavior was inappropriate for a priest. She never again set foot in a church from that time until the day she died.

My father was never much of a religious sort. In his later years before he retired he started attending church again on a regular basis. But he never spoke about religion.

So I grew up not attending church regularly. I remember going to church as a very young girl. But having to sit in hard church pews listening to sermons in Latin was not my idea of fun at age four or so. The black patent leather shoes, only worn once a week, rubbed blisters on my heels. So as soon as I had the opportunity not to go to church, I stopped going.

It's not that I didn't believe in a divine being. I just didn't know what direction to take my beliefs. I was doubly unsure after my spinal cord injury. I didn't understand how a just God could allow this injury to happen to a person.

It wasn't until many years after my accident that I began to seek solace in religion. That I discovered the comfort of prayer. And even then only very recently.

If you are comfortable in your faith and beliefs, then praying will not be difficult for you. Spinal cord injury is a situation that can raise doubts in a person's faith, however.

In pondering what I wanted to say in this chapter, I started thinking about all the various things a person could pray for after a spinal cord injury. A person could pray for the ability to afford the medical expenses from the injury. Praying to be able to find a good, reliable paid caregiver would be something else to request in one's prayers.

Let's not forget the basic prayer of having as much of a full recovery as is possible from the injury. Asking for family harmony to be restored after such a stressful situation is a thought. Perhaps being able to find a job after recovery is a subject for prayer. How about asking for guidance in making the right choices on equipment, such as a wheelchair? Perhaps you could ask for being able to find an accessible place to live? Praying for acceptance of the injury and the new life it is going to grant you is another idea. Praying for forgiveness in a situation where you lost your temper or did not have enough patience is a choice as well.

How to pray is also a good question for someone who is not comfortable with religion. Some people believe all that is necessary is just to say a prayer. Some people kneel to pray. This is probably not going to be an option after a spinal cord injury. I don't think it matters how you pray. If you feel the need to pray, then just pray. I think religion, faith, and hope all tie in together.

So that left me with the problem of having originally written this chapter from a very detached point of view. What do I do with this chapter? Do I leave it only as a personal message of my own faith? Do I edit out the parts of the chapter I had originally written which dealt with religion after a spinal cord injury as more of an academic exercise?

I have decided to present religion and faith from both perspectives, the personal and the academic. The beginning of this chapter dealt with my own views on religion. And how I have used religion and faith to start my recovery from my spinal cord and closed head injury. The remainder of this chapter is the chapter as I originally wrote it, dealing with religion and faith after a spinal cord injury from a more scholarly perspective. I hope you will find both outlooks useful.

The question of the role of religion and faith, whatever denomination or belief system you have, after a spinal cord injury may be one of the most interesting questions related to a spinal cord injury.

I say this for two reasons. The first is how a person's view of religion and faith can change after a spinal cord injury. The second is looking at spinal cord injury survivors as a group, and looking at the role that religion and faith play in their daily lives.

I will start with the question of how a person's view of religion and faith can change after a spinal cord injury. I can see the following combinations of religion and faith before and after possible:

1. Non-religious person before, religious person after

2. Non-religious person before, same degree of non-religiousness after

3. Non-religious person before, increased degree of "non-religiousness" after

4. Religious person before, same degree of religiousness after

5. Religious person before, increased degree of religiousness after

6. Religious person before, a non-religious person after

I found a discussion of religion and spirituality after a spinal cord injury in the book *Wheeling and Dealing: Living with Spinal Cord Injury*. The author of the book mentions one individual who indicated that his religious convictions were an important element in his recovery and his constant striving to better himself. He (the individual) said, "I could not possibly have gone as far as I have without religion. Every day I pray and meditate and I believe God has a reason I'm still here."

Another individual said that his religious convictions and his belief in God served as a "coping mechanism for everything." The author of the book said she interviewed many survivors who had been active in their churches before their accidents, and who continued to be active at the same level after their injuries.[1]

She notes that religion can be used to make sense of a spinal cord injury. There are supernatural theories about the causation of spinal cord injury that say that the person was being punished by their God for violating rules, being injured by spirits for violating rules, or through witchcraft, a hex, an "evil eye."[2]

Some of the author's interviewees said they had been angry with their God before their accidents, but after their accidents, their anger had gradually dissipated.[3] One participant said he was agnostic before the accident, and he was still agnostic after his accident.[4]

The book's author continues her discussion of religion and spinal cord injury by saying:

> While individuals with disabilities often turn to religious institutions for support and comfort, they are sometimes treated with hostility by churches, synagogues, and other religious establishments. Religious and cultural attitudes vary widely across time and place, and individuals with disabilities have been viewed as saints, sinners, and almost everything in between.[5]

The late Christopher Reeve has a chapter on religion in his book, *Nothing is Impossible: Reflections on a New Life*. Reeve discussed in the chapter that many people were expecting him to be a deeply religious person. Reeve talks about his introduction to Scientology, a popular Hollywood "religion," and his later disillusionment with it.

Reeve makes these two statements about his religious beliefs: "The truth is that I only found a religion very recently that I can reconcile with a lifelong quest for the meaning of spirituality" and "The end of my encounter with Scientology marked the beginning of an ongoing search for the meaning of spirituality in my life. It would take many years, many well-intentioned but misguided detours, and ultimately a near-fatal accident for me to find the answer."[6] Reeve never says which particular religion he found in his search. I can only guess that he felt the decision was too personal to discuss.

As for spinal cord injury survivors as a group, in reading the various books I have on interviews with spinal cord injury survivors; I found that many of them indicated they had an increased belief in the God of their denomination and faith. I searched for information specifically on atheists and how their spinal cord injuries had affected them. I was unable to find information beyond what I have discussed.

I have presented you with much to think about in this chapter. I hope it will be helpful to you.

Emotional Baggage

52

Survivor Guilt I: "What Did I Do To Deserve This?"

Guilt upon the conscience, like rust upon iron, both defiles and consumes it, gnawing and creeping into it, as that does which at last eats out the very heart and substance of the metal—
Bishop Robert South

"What did I do to deserve this?" is a common question both thought and expressed by spinal cord injury survivors shortly after their accidents. I want to explore this feeling in more detail in this chapter. I believe survivor guilt is such an important topic related to spinal cord injury that I am breaking it into four chapters for easier understanding.

I want to start off by discussing survivor guilt in general. Then I will discuss survivor guilt as it relates to spinal cord injury in more detail. Survivor guilt or survivor syndrome is the mental condition that results from the appraisal that a person has done wrong by surviving traumatic events. It is most commonly used to describe feelings experienced after an event that affects a group of people such as combat, natural disasters, or surviving a lay-off in the workplace.[1] [2] Survivor guilt/survivor syndrome used to be a unique diagnosis in and of itself, but has since been recategorized as a part of posttraumatic stress disorder.[3] Let me translate briefly. You feel guilty because you lived over something that somebody else didn't. It's as simple as that.

Posttraumatic stress disorder (PTSD) is a term for certain severe psychological consequences of exposure to, or confrontation with, stressful events that the person experiences as highly traumatic. These events usually involve actual or threatened death, serious physical injury, or a threat to physical and/or psychological integrity, to a degree that usual psychological defenses are incapable of coping with the impact. Post-traumatic stress disorder is only diagnosed if the condition is present for more than three months after the triggering event.[4]

In plain English, if the event is stressful enough that the emotional effects don't pass on their own within a reasonable time, you've got posttraumatic stress disorder.

I've shoved a lot of fancy psychological terms at you so far in this chapter. I still need to explain how it all relates to a spinal cord injury. Most of the ways in which people get spinal cord injuries are traumatic as the result of external circumstances. I'm leaving out spinal cord injuries from disease and surgical complications. These are traumatic; but not in the same way as car wrecks, diving accidents, sports accidents, and being shot.

The traumatic external circumstances causing the spinal cord injury are sufficient to cause posttraumatic stress disorder. Survivor guilt is a part of posttraumatic stress disorder, as I said above.

Psychologists believe that guilt serves four functions. It defends against helplessness. It serves as self-punishment. It inhibits impulses. Finally, it prevents an event from being meaningless.[5]

The main reason I wanted to write this chapter is to raise awareness of the issue of "what-did-I-do-to-deserve-this?" survivor guilt among spinal cord injury survivors. It is something I experienced. I suspect this is something that is widely experienced by SCI survivors, but I can't prove it.

I only found one article that discussed this feeling as it was experienced by one quadriplegic. This article stated that the individual experiences this feeling repeatedly. The article's author was hopeful that the individual would have fewer days with this feeling because he had just undergone successful experimental surgery so he would no longer need a ventilator to breathe. He was also able to talk normally again and to smell normally again.[6]

I want to end this chapter with a quick guide on how to get over this type of survivor guilt:

1. Talk, talk and then talk some more. [not possibly though if you are on a ventilator].
2. Restore a sense of safety and stability. Return to routines as soon as you can [difficult if you are a spinal cord injury survivor in the hospital for a long period of time].
3. Challenge irrational thoughts.
4. Take an asset/strength inventory. What qualities or strategies have helped you through times of stress or crisis before?

> 5. Connect with your support network. Remind yourself of the things and people that are important in your life.

I especially liked a quotation from the previous article on survivor guilt: "guilt is the penance one pays for the gift of survival." The article continues:

> rather than focus on the burden of guilt, remind yourself that you and your loved ones have been given a gift—the gift of your survival. Embrace your will to survive and fight the forces that challenge your way of being.[7]

I could not have said it better myself.

53

Survivor Guilt II: "I Did Something Stupid To Get Hurt"

Guilt is anger directed at ourselves—
Peter McWilliams

More long psychological terms in this chapter? Fear not. There are no citations in this chapter. No long psychological terms. I'm just going to pose a question for you to think about.

I want to address the situation where a person has done something "stupid" that resulted in a spinal cord injury. I am curious about the psychological aspects of recovery in given situations.

Let's start with the situation where the person who has the spinal cord injury did something "stupid" or lacking in common sense that resulted in the injury. Often small groups of people are involved in the situation also. These can be friends, family members, or a mix of friends of the injured person and people he or she doesn't know or doesn't know well. Often alcohol is involved.

I've read about and heard of all sorts of scenarios. Diving into shallow water while drunk. Riding a four-wheeler while drunk. Driving while drunk. Being on a tree limb to thin to hold your own weight while trying to trim a tree. Participating in horseplay while drunk. Fighting while drunk. The list can go on and on.

Does a person experience guilt when their injury was sustained in one of the scenarios where their own actions were the cause of the injury?

Let's move on to a different situation. Let's say the person who was injured got hurt because of the stupidity of another person. It could be an auto accident where someone is hurt because they were in an accident where the driver of the other car was drunk. Or simply made a stupid decision while driving.

Does a person experience guilt when his or her injury was sustained in one of the scenarios where the stupid actions of another person were the cause of the injury? I think it is human nature that we try to figure out what we could have done differently in the situation.

But in which situation is the guilt worse? Is it easier to go on if you are responsible for the accident? Is it easier to go on if someone else is responsible for the accident?

I haven't seen these issues addressed. I couldn't find anything on the Internet about it. So I have written this chapter to get you to think about the idea. Maybe someone will decide to research the ideas in this chapter.

If you do, please let me know what you learn.

54

Survivor Guilt III: "My Actions Unintentionally Killed or Seriously Injured Another Person"

The worst guilt is to accept an unearned guilt—
Ayn Rand

The topic of this chapter is rarely discussed in the mainstream. It is as if there is some sort of taboo about the idea. I am hoping that this chapter will help those in the situation.

What if your actions caused someone to be killed or suffer a spinal cord injury? In the context of this chapter I am assuming that you did not intend to kill or cause the person to have a spinal cord injury.

I personally know of two situations where this happened. I did not know any of the people involved in the two accidents. The first was a situation that happened many years ago. A young man had just gotten a new sports car. Young men typically want to show off their sports cars to their friends. This one did so to his best friend. I don't remember if alcohol was involved. Not surprising they decided to take it out onto a rural highway, and try it at high speed. The driver lost control, and ran into a telephone pole. The driver was knocked unconscious, and only suffered minor injuries. His best friend was killed.

To make matters worse, a hotshot county prosecuting attorney decided to make an example of the driver and charge him with murder. Fortunately, the driver hired an excellent attorney, and the driver was found not guilty. The young man was given an opportunity to start his life again after the accident. He didn't have to spend years in jail. But he was emotionally unable to do so. He could not get over the guilt of having done something stupid that caused his best friend to die. He began to drink heavily. I don't know if he ever recovered.

The second situation is a work-in-progress at the time of this writing. It involves, again, two young men. This situation involved alcohol. These two individuals were getting ready to graduate from high school. They were clowning around, engaging in horseplay, as young men who have been drinking have been known to do. One of the young men involved was a track star. The other young man involved was a wrestler. They were best friends.

The lighter of the two, the runner, head-butted his friend in the chest. The heavier of the two, the wrestler, responded on instinct as a wrestler by picking up his friend under the armpits, raising him into the air upside down. With no place for the vertebrae in the runner's neck to go, being firmly held against the wrestler's chest; they could not withstand the stress and broke. His neck was broken at C4 and C5. Bone fragments were on the runner's spinal cord.

Emergency surgery was performed. Initially (as is often the case), the runner was labeled as having a complete injury. The young man went through the routine of bedsores, infections, and a collapsed lung. Close to eight weeks after the injury, the young man was relabeled as an incomplete injury.

Fortunately the injured young man started to improve physically and emotionally. He received a phone call from someone on the Paralympics Rugby Team who heard about the accident. They spent a long time on the phone. It seemed to be just what the injured young man needed. Last I heard, he was looking forward to the future again.

The wrestler, though, had emotional problems dealing with the situation. He felt terribly guilty over what happened. The situation was not his fault, by any means. It was just one of those things that happened. He was put on suicide watch. His parents did not risk leaving him alone. Whether he is able to overcome the circumstances, and go on with his life remains to be seen.

I only know of two situations where this happened. I am sure there must be hundreds, if not thousands of them, that happen every year worldwide. No one wants to talk about situations where this happened. I could find no references on the Internet. It is as if some taboo exists about the situation.

Everyone is always concerned about the injured or dead person. Rightfully so after a spinal cord injury or a death. But often no one seems to be concerned about the emotional stability of the survivor.

And yet the emotional stability of the survivor may be more important than dealing with the aftermath of the other person. Emotional stability can be very fragile. And if the person cannot get over the guilt, his or her future and possibly actual survival is at risk.

This is another chapter of food for thought. Maybe someone will start researching this problem and more information will start appearing in psychological literature. We see plenty on survivor guilt for large-scale events. There needs to be more on survivor guilt for events that only involve a few people.

If you research this issue, please let me know what you find out.

55

Survivor Guilt IV: "Why Wasn't I Hurt Worse or as Badly as So-and-So?"

Guilt: punishing Yourself Before God Doesn't—
Alan Cohen

I'm going to go out on a limb in this chapter. Proverbial since I can't do it physically. I am going to raise the idea that incomplete spinal cord injury patients experience a specific type of survivor guilt. I don't have anything but stories to base my hunch on. But it will have to be enough proof to raise the question.

In a larger-scale disaster such as a plane crash, this scenario would be covered by general survivor guilt. People wonder why they survived and this, that, or the other passenger sitting in this, that, or the other seat did not. Maybe they were spared, and the person they were sitting next to was killed.

As more and more people are experiencing spinal cord injuries, the variation in injuries increases. Incomplete spinal cord injuries are more common than complete injuries. I read that somewhere. The citation isn't important for purposes of this chapter. Take the information on faith.

With more incomplete spinal cord injuries there are more spinal cord syndrome injuries. More "walking quads." More "walking paras." More people who "shouldn't be able to do what they are doing" with the particular type of spinal cord injury they each have.

Spinal cord injury survivors see other SCI survivors at support group meetings. We may see them in the hospital or doctors' offices. We may meet them in rehab. We see other people with complete injuries. We see other people with incomplete injuries worse than our own incomplete injuries.

And we feel guilty. When we have absolutely nothing to feel guilty about. But yet we still feel guilty. We ask ourselves why we weren't hurt as badly as "So-and-So."

It doesn't matter that we are twenty years post accident, and they are a year post accident.

It doesn't matter that we fell down a flight of stairs, and they were in a plane crash.

It doesn't matter that we were in an auto accident, and they had a motorcycle wreck where they had less metal around them to protect them.

It doesn't matter that we were in an auto accident in something like a large SUV, and they were in an auto accident in a tiny vehicle like a Fiat.

And it doesn't matter that we had our seatbelts and shoulder harnesses fastened and they didn't. We still feel guilty.

I discovered I had this problem when I first joined a spinal cord injury support group. It had been some eleven years since my accident before I joined a support group. I realized I still had some issues. Especially since my condition was deteriorating.

What I wasn't counting on was experiencing survivor guilt when comparing myself to the other people around me who had a SCI, and were in chairs. You may see or hear the word "wheelchair" referred to as "chair" in the spinal cord community. Some were complete. Some were incomplete, and had less movement than I do. They were in wheelchairs. I am not.

"*Why wasn't I hurt as badly as So-and-So*?"

I can't answer this question. For myself. Or for anybody else who feels the same way I do. I can only raise it.

I'm not alone in feeling this way. A posting on the National Spinal Cord Injury Association Forum under Central Cord Syndrome by a lady went like this:

> well hello!
> I am what they call a "walking quad". (C2-7) while I do not have the function you have, my upper is indeed weaker or worse than my lower.
> I can only stand and move a bit at a time.... but I can.
> I am indeed, extremely lucky, and especially when first hurt, felt guilty over my function. It simply "shouldn't be" according to the docs.[1]

Logically it is an easy question to answer. The mechanics of the accident were such that the damage to my spinal cord were not as severe as those other people experienced. Every person who is asking himself or herself the question above can rationally say this.

I can certainly say the mechanics of my accident were such that the damage to my spinal cord was not as severe as those other people experienced. Most people who are complete or incomplete have broken their necks or broken their backs. They have damaged the vertebra or vertebrae to the point where they have broken and the bones are on the spinal cord, on the spinal nerves, or the fragments have severed the spinal cord completely or incompletely.

I didn't break my neck. I only destroyed (pulverized might be a better word) the cervical discs that were between the vertebrae. One doctor says I have osteoarthritis, where my bones are harder than normal. This is why my neck didn't break. Who would have ever thought a condition like that would come in handy?

My accident was at relatively low speed. I was only doing thirty-five mph (miles per hour), and the other driver couldn't have been doing more than twenty mph. He had just pulled out from a stop sign.

Why do we feel guilty the way we do? Do we feel the need to punish ourselves for something? Are we special in some way that the supreme being we believe in decided to spare us to some degree? Is it just that we cannot comprehend the idea so many different factors go into determining how badly a person is hurt with a spinal cord injury that we cannot understand all the different factors and make sense of how they interact?

Maybe medical professionals will start to recognize that we go through this and try to help us get through it. Maybe they will start researching and recognizing this type of survivor guilt.

Let me know if you do.

56

Depression After a Spinal Cord Injury

Depression is the inability to construct a future—
Rollo May

What is depression? Depression is a condition that causes feelings of sadness and hopelessness. Depression may be short-term or long-term. Sometimes a situation can cause depression. Like having a death in the family. Sometimes a lack of sleep can cause depression. Hormonal imbalances can cause depression. Many different things can cause depression.

What are the signs of depression? They are:

1. Eating too little or too much
2. Feeling hopeless or worthless
3. Not caring about how you look, like not bathing, changing clothes, brushing teeth, or using deodorant
4. Not caring about things you used to enjoy, like sports or movies
5. Sleeping too much or too little
6. Thinking about or trying to commit suicide
7. Being unable to cope with normal daily activities[1]

The University of Washington Northwest Regional Spinal Cord Injury System (NWRSCIS) adds:

1. Changes in sleep
2. Diminished energy or activity
3. Difficulty concentrating or making decisions[2]

One study of two hundred one spinal cord injured patients found 28.9% of them to be depressed.[3] Another study found thirty-five percent of the sixty patients studied to be suffering from depression.[4] Another source states that between twenty-three and thirty percent of spinal cord injury patients suffer from depression.[5] Another source says estimated rates of depression among people with SCI range from eleven percent to thirty-seven percent.[2] Still another study says that from twenty-two percent to over thirty percent of spinal cord injured patients are depressed.[6]

Here's a "great" quotation: "most people with SCI are not depressed. They adjust and gradually feel better about their lives."[5]

I think these "experts" are so caught up in their numbers they aren't looking at the picture with common sense. It would be human nature to be depressed after a spinal cord injury. It would be almost impossible not to be just a little depressed. A person not even a little depressed after a spinal cord injury would be a truly admirable person. Or not completely sane.

And why shouldn't we be depressed? Even just a little bit. We have just experienced a life-changing event that impacts every single aspect of our lives. We can no longer physically move at will the way we used to. We no longer have the same degree of coordination. We no longer have control over our bodily functions the way we used to.

We have lost our earning power. We are accumulating large medical bills. Friends and family react to us differently now than they did before the accident. We must use adaptive equipment, which is often very expensive. We are thrown into a bureaucracy of paperwork, bills, insurance, and fighting insurance denials. Plans that were made now have to be rescheduled or cancelled completely. We no longer feel attractive or sexy. We feel that others no longer view us as being attractive or sexy. We can no longer participate in activities we used to enjoy.

We are stuck in a hospital for an extended period of time sometimes with doctors who cannot empathize with our situation. Some doctors have no experience or training with spinal cord injuries. Some doctors who have had training in spinal cord injuries treat us as an academic exercise or a "diagnosis."

These "experts" are also part of a society that has decided if someone is depressed for more than two weeks, then we need to pump them full of expensive pills to cheer them up. They are also missing the fact that pain causes depression.[7] Spinal cord injuries can be intensely painful. Other injuries that happen at the same time as spinal cord injuries, like broken bones, can also be intensely painful.

We don't need to be treated for depression initially. We need grief counseling. Grief counseling is a concept made famous by Dr. Elisabeth Kübler-Ross. The five stages of grief are denial, anger, bargaining, depression, and acceptance. The stages last for different periods of time. They are not linear. This means you don't go through each stage in order.

You don't automatically go from stage one to stage two to stage three. You may go from stage one to stage two and then back to stage one again. But you can't get to a stage unless you have gone through the stage(s) before it.

Everybody is different. We each heal emotionally at our own pace. There is no "set" time to get over grief.

Denial helps us survive the loss. We process only as much as we can handle. Gradually the denial fades, and then we become angry. Letting out the anger allows us to let out the emotional pain. Then the anger gives way to bargaining. This is where we experience the "what if," the "if only," and bargaining with God if the current situation will only change.

After bargaining comes depression. Depression is very normal in the situation after a spinal cord injury. Once you have finished with depression, then you can have acceptance. You don't have to be happy with something to accept it. Acceptance means that you start having more good days than bad days. You realize that the future is not going to be the same as the past.[8]

I want to stress that life after a spinal cord injury does have meaning. It is very possible to have a full and emotionally satisfying life after a spinal cord injury.

As strange a concept as it may be, many spinal cord injured people find their lives after their injury are more emotionally rewarding than they were before the injury. They find life directions they never would have without their injuries. Many of them find spirituality becomes more important to them than it did before their injury. They get pleasure from this. They meet people they never would have without their injuries that have a positive effect on their lives. And they learn more about themselves, what kind of "inner stuff" they are made of.

If you (or your family member) had a tendency to be depressive or were on prescription antidepressants before the accident, make sure your doctor is aware of this.

If I hadn't had a spinal cord injury, I wouldn't have written this book. Writing this book has helped me accept my injury.

So you never know.

57

Addiction After a Spinal Cord Injury

Starved.... laughter is the best medicine.
I know from my recovery in all areas of addiction that humor
is a tremendously, tremendously important antidote to recovery.—
Eric Schaeffer

I wish I didn't have to follow a chapter ending on an upbeat note with a chapter on a downbeat note. But I cannot help you get through your situation if I don't discuss some of the more unpleasant things that can happen after a spinal cord injury.

Addiction after a spinal cord injury is unfortunately all too common. Addiction is very common after any traumatic event. People are using some form of behavior to relieve their symptoms of anxiety, irritability, and depression. The addictive behavior compensates for deficiencies in endorphin activity following a traumatic experience.[1]

This addiction can happen to the spinal cord injury survivor, any member of his or her family, and his or her friends. If someone near to the spinal cord injury survivor feels responsible for the injury, this person may be especially prone to addictive behavior.

Endorphins are biochemical compounds produced in the pituitary gland and the brain. They resemble drugs because they provide pain relief and a sense of well-being.[2]

I performed a search on the Internet to figure out the different things people can be addicted to. The list I came up with is: 1) alcohol 2) prescription drugs 3) illegal drugs 4) sex 5) exercise 6) video games 7) sports 8) pornography 9) shopping 10) chocolate 11) eating 12) gambling 13) caffeine and 14) tobacco (nicotine).

Almost anything that is enjoyable people can become addicted to. Exercise addiction is probably not as likely after a spinal cord injury as some of the other items in the list.

A hobby or pastime becomes an addiction when someone has to do it "just to get by" or "just to feel or function normally." A spinal cord injury survivor may technically be addicted to his or her prescription medication, and also needs to it to function normally.

On the eating addiction, some medications commonly prescribed for spinal cord injury symptoms, such as Lyrica®, have weight gain as a side effect.[3] I want to clarify something here because the company that makes Lyrica® is unclear on how it causes weight gain. Does the medication itself cause weight gain? Or does the medication cause hunger in the patient? Or is a person seeking emotional comfort by eating? It makes a big difference.

Some prescriptions may cause behavior like excessive gambling. I saw an ad for something on TV last night, but I can't remember what medication it was for. So you may need to explore whether your addictive behavior is a side effect of your medication, or if it is an addiction separate from prescription medicine. That is, if you think you have addictive behavior.

An addiction takes as little as days or as long as months or years to develop. Each individual is different and it depends on what they are addicted to.[4]

If your dependency on something becomes detrimental to you being able to lead a normal life, then you are addicted. If you suspect you are having a problem, please seek help from a medical professional. If you don't recognize you have an addiction, hopefully a friend or family member will realize it for you and urge you to get help.

Support groups exist for just about everything these days. Don't hesitate to get help if you need it.

How Often Does Spinal Cord Injury Happen and How?

58

Spinal Cord Injury Statistics

Facts are stubborn, but statistics are more pliable.—
There are lies, damned lies and statistics—
Mark Twain

In a perfect world, there would be no spinal cord injuries. And all existing spinal cord injuries would be completely curable. In a perfect world statistically speaking, all states in the United States would have official spinal cord registries with identical rules for inclusion. As long as I'm wishing statistically speaking, I might as well wish that all countries kept good records on spinal cord injuries. I think I'll save my wishes for Christmas.

This book started out as an idea for a journal article. I had this "grand idea" I was going to be able to compare how many people in each state for every 100,000 people living in the state had a spinal cord injury during the course of a given calendar year. I had health issues and by the time I finished the basic research for the article, all the information I had collected was older than I cared for.

I learned that trying to compare spinal cord injury statistics between states is like trying to compare apples and oranges. I found a statement from the Center for Disease Control (CDC) while I was doing the original research that I have not been able to locate again. I am going to repeat its basic idea.

The CDC feels it is not scientifically valid to compare data from one state to another because every state is different in the way it collects its data, if it collects it at all. I found this was quite true. I had the problem of calendar years, fiscal years, fatal spinal cord injuries, non-fatal spinal cord injuries, unavailable state data, estimating figures from hospital discharge statistics, comparing hospital discharge data to official state spinal cord registry data, and comparing states with spinal cord registries with more restrictive terms for inclusion to states with less restrictive terms for inclusion. And then having my data get "old."

The CDC feels that estimating spinal cord injury incidence from hospital discharge data only six out of ten spinal cord injury cases identified are true cases.[1] I think you can see why I decided not to write the article. Let me share with you some quick basic numbers from my original research:

1. There are about 200,000 people in the United States who have a spinal cord injury-related disability.
2. About 10,000 people every year have a spinal cord injury (new injuries).
3. Nationwide, there are about 4 spinal cord injuries for every 100,000 people.
4. If you are under the age of sixty-five and have a spinal cord injury, you most likely got it from an auto accident. If you are over the age of sixty-five, you most likely got it from a fall.
5. Sports and recreational activities cause about one-fifth of spinal cord injuries in the U.S.
6. Males are more likely than females have spinal cord injuries.
7. Blacks are more likely than whites to have spinal cord injuries.
8. More than half of the people who have spinal cord injuries are 15 to 29 [*sic*] years old.[2]

One quick observation I was able to make about the causes of injury by state is that in the states with more traditional colder winter weather, falls were a greater contributing factor to spinal cord injuries than in states with warmer winters. I also suspect that in states with higher elderly populations, falls are more of a contributing factor to the rate of spinal cord injury.

Here are the actual figures. Some states did not collect the data. Other states I contacted never provided information to me, despite repeated attempts to obtain the information. States for which I was unable to obtain actual data are estimated.

This is a very non-scientific survey and the results should be used as general guidelines only.

State	***Incidence per 100,000 Population***
1. Hawaii	77.60
2. Ohio	45.86
3. Michigan	40.48
4. Georgia	26.14
5. Washington	25.15
6. Tennessee	23.85
7. Ohio	14.56
8. Iowa	11.87
9. Kansas	10.98
10. Delaware	10.50
11. Mississippi	9.30
12. Maryland	9.28
13. Indiana	8.32
14. Alaska	8.30
15. Missouri	7.70
16. Nevada	6.69
17. Idaho	5.72
18. New Hampshire	5.68
19. Rhode Island	5.48
20. Louisiana	5.40
21. Pennsylvania	5.30
22. Maine	5.29
23. Texas	5.00
24. Oklahoma	4.93
25. Wisconsin	4.90
26. Minnesota	4.78
27. District of Columbia	4.52
28. North Carolina	4.51
29. Massachusetts	4.40
30. New York	4.30
31. Alabama	4.05
32. Arizona	4.00
National U.S. Average	4.00
33. Montana	3.74
34. Arkansas	3.60
35. Kentucky	3.60
36. Illinois	3.58

37. Colorado	3.52
38. California	3.41
39. New Mexico	3.40
40. Florida	3.37
41. Connecticut	3.30
42. Utah	3.27
43. New Jersey	3.14
44. South Dakota	3.10
45. Nebraska	2.80
46. Virginia	2.64
47. North Dakota	2.55
48. West Virginia	2.50
49. Wyoming	2.04
50. South Carolina	1.41
51. Vermont	0.673

Sources for actual data obtained are in the Endnotes. The methodology for each state's data that had to be estimated is provided in the Appendix—Methodology.

As for some quick worldwide comparisons, a conservative annual incidence worldwide is 1.4 cases per 100,000 population. Canada has an estimated 2.7 cases per 100,000 population incidence. The United Kingdom has an estimated 1.2 cases per 100,000 population incidence. Germany has an estimated 1.85 cases per 100,000 population. Italy's estimated incidence per 100,000 population is 1.2. The estimate for Sweden is 1.5 to 2.0 cases per 100,000 population. Australia's estimate is 1.36 cases per 100,000 population. The rate in France is 3.2 per 100,000. South Africa's rate is 1.12 cases per 100,000 population.[4] [5] As above, the national U.S. average is approximately 4.00 cases per 100,000 population.

For my money, I don't think we should be as concerned about counting spinal cord injuries as we should be in educating people and preventing them. Funny how that leads me right into the next chapter.

59

Spinal Cord Injury Prevention

Dream as if you'll live forever, live as if you'll die today.—
James Dean

Obviously injury prevention is not an appropriate subject for a spinal cord injured person. It is too late. But spinal cord injury prevention is an issue for the uninjured family members, friends, and everybody else.

The Foundation for Spinal Cord Injury Prevention, Care & Cure (FSCIPCC) is a non-profit educational group. It exists for the prevention, care and cure of spinal cord injuries through public awareness, education, and funding research. It is an organization for anyone interested in learning more about spinal cord injuries. The organization is headquartered in Michigan. Its website contains informational links on a variety of subjects related to spinal cord injury.[1]

The FSCIPCC has proposed a "Wipeout Spinal Cord Injury" program. The goal of this program is to reduce spinal cord injuries by ten percent each year. The organization is using the following tactics to accomplish its goal:

1. Educational programs for elementary and secondary school students
2. Nationwide mandatory spinal cord injury reporting programs
3. Public service announcements on TV and radio
4. Billboard public service announcements
5. Informational brochures and flyer, such as "Diving is Deadly"
6. Prevention messages on pizza box tops
7. Messages on grocery store bags
8. Placements at fast food restaurants with SCI prevention messages[2]

Trampolines are considered so dangerous by the FSCIPCC it has a special section on its website about them. Trampolines have resulted in a dramatic increase in serious injuries in the eight-year-old to adult age groups. The injuries sustained using trampolines are broken necks, spinal cord injuries, and disabling head injuries. The injuries are causing permanent paralysis and even death.[3]

I discuss injury prevention in hockey, baseball, and football in the chapter on sports as a cause of spinal cord injury. I found two articles on swimming pool accidents. The first article indicates that the majority of the spinal cord injuries obtained by the study group occurred because of a lack of good judgment and common sense. Intoxication and pool structural deficiencies were not contributing factors. Contributing factors that were noted were the lack of appropriate first-aid and extrication [being removed from the pool in a medically-approved manner restricting neck movement and back movement through immobilization], and the absence of uniform treatment and care received by the majority of patients.[4]

The second article was a study involving diving accidents. The study was more specific if the individual injured had been injured in a swimming pool. Approximately two-thirds of the initial group injured in a diving accident were injured in a "natural aquatic environment" (river, lake, ocean). One-third were injured in swimming pools. Of those who were injured in a swimming pool, approximately two-thirds were injured in a below-ground pool. Approximately one-third were injured in an above-ground pool.

Most of the people injured in a pool were performing a normal diving maneuver, but in shallow water. About half the injuries took place during a party, and about half of the people injured during a party indicated they had been drinking. Often it was the person's first visit to that particular pool, or the person's first dive into the pool.

Other factors that were involved in the accident:

1. No warning signs posted in 87% [*sic*] of the cases.
2. No water depth indicators present in 75% [*sic*] of the cases.
3. No lifeguard on duty in 94% [*sic*] of the cases.
4. Dives generally occurred from the side of the pool rather than a diving board or other diving device.
5. No artificial lighting available in 53% [*sic*] of cases. When lights turned on, the amount of light provided was inadequate in about half of the cases. [5]

A national initiative exists in the U.S. called Healthy People 2010. The purpose of this initiative is to reduce the number of annual injuries, including spinal cord injuries. The group's goal is to reduce the incidence of non-fatal spinal cord injuries nationally in the United States from 4.8 hospitalizations per 100,000 population in 1997 to 2.6 hospitalizations per 100,00 population. This would be a forty-six percent improvement.[6] I am assuming they would like to reduce the incidence of fatal spinal cord injuries per 100,000. There is an injury prevention agency or program in virtually every state in the United States.

The Center for Disease Control's National Center for Injury Prevention and Control offers these tips for preventing a spinal cord injury:

Cars
1. Always wear a seat belt.
2. Secure or buckle children into age- and weight-appropriate child safety seats.
3. Never drive under the influence of alcohol or drugs.
4. Do not ride in a car with a driver who is impaired by alcohol or drugs.
5. Prevent others from driving while impaired by alcohol or drugs.

Homes
1. Secure banisters and handrails at all stairwells.
2. Use a step stool with a grab bar to reach objects on high shelves.
3. Place non-slip mats on the bathtub and shower floor.
4. Install grab bars in the shower and bathtub.
5. Exercise regularly to keep muscle tone and balance.
6. Wear sturdy non-slip shoes.
7. Where possible, reduce the use of medications with the side effects that increase the risk of falling.
8. Perform a home safety check and remove things that may be tripped over.
9. Use safety gates at the bottom and top of stairs when young children are around.
10. Install window guards in windows above the first floor.

Sports and recreational activities
Always wear a helmet when:
1. Riding a bike, motorcycle, scooter, or skateboard
2. In-line skating and roller-skating
3. Skiing or snowboarding
4. Horseback riding
Wear a helmet during the following sports activities:
5. Football
6. Ice hockey
7. Batting and running the bases in baseball and softball
8. Make sure the water is deep enough before you go in headfirst.
9. Wear the appropriate safety gear when engaging in sports activities
10. Avoid head-first moves, such as tackling with the top of your head or sliding head-first into a base.
11. Insist on spotters when performing activities that can put you at risk, such as new gymnastics moves.[7]

Additional safety tips for pools are:

1. Be familiar with the pool where you swim.
2. Know the water depth in the pool before you dive.
3. Avoid drinking alcohol when swimming or diving.
4. Do not swim or dive in pools that are poorly lit.
5. Do not swim alone.
6. Know proper diving techniques.
7. Do not swim in a public pool without a lifeguard present.[8]

For in-home gun safety the National Rifle Association recommends that 1) Always keep the gun pointed in a safe direction, 2) Always keep your finger off the trigger until ready to shoot, and 3) Always keep the gun unloaded until ready to use.[9]

Finally, for hunter safety the Ohio Department of Natural Resources offers these tips:

1. Treat every gun as if it was loaded
2. Always point the muzzle in a safe direction
3. Be sure of your target *and beyond* [*sic*]
4. Never point a gun at anything you don't want to shoot
5. Unload guns when not in use.
6. Store guns and ammunition separately.
7. Be sure the barrel and action are clear of obstructions.
8. Never climb a fence or tree, cross a log or a stream, or jump a ditch with a loaded gun.
9. Never shoot a bullet at a flat, hard surface or water.
10. Never use alcoholic beverages or drugs when handling a firearm.
11. Guns should be kept unloaded and secured in a scabbard or holder designed for this use while riding an ATV.
12. Never put a loaded gun on the bottom of a moving boat, especially when dogs are aboard.
13. For most species of game hunting, hunters should wear hunter orange (blaze orange)
14. Never use home-made tree stands and tree stands made from wood.
15. Never use wood steps that are attached to a tree with nails or spikes to get to a tree stand.
16. Never use a single safety belt as a fall restraint system.
17. Always use a haul line (rope) to raise your weapon to the tree stand.[10]

All-Terrain Vehicles (ATV's) are another cause of spinal cord injury. The ATV Safety Institute offers these tips for safe ATV operation:

1. Always wear a helmet and other protective gear.
2. Never ride on public roads—another vehicle could hit you.
3. Never ride under the influence of alcohol or drugs.
4. Never carry a passenger on a single-rider vehicle.
5. Ride an ATV that's right for your age.
6. Supervise riders younger than 16; ATV's are not toys.
7. Ride only on designated trails and at a safe speed.
8. Take an ATV RiderCourse; Call Toll-Free at 1-800-887-2887 or go to http://www.atvsafety.org[11]

In case you think number three under All-Terrain Vehicles doesn't cause spinal cord injuries that often, I know someone who is now a paraplegic because he went riding on an ATV while he was intoxicated. He has had a t-shirt printed up that says, "I am a bad example," and has volunteered to speak on injury prevention for the Arkansas Spinal Cord Commission. Similarly, snomobiling can cause spinal cord injuries.[12]

Injury prevention efforts fall into one of three categories: primary, secondary, and tertiary. Primary prevention "seeks to reduce susceptibility, eliminating or minimizing behaviors and environmental factors that increase the risk of injury. Environmental, legislative, and educational activities are examples of primary prevention."[13]

Secondary prevention is "the effort aimed at reducing or halting the progression of the disabling condition after the initial injury has occurred (for example, specialized emergency medical services for those who sustain an SCI)."[14]

Tertiary prevention refers to "preventing or limiting conditions associated with the SCI such as ducubitus ulcers (pressure sores), and contractions. Secondary and tertiary levels of prevention work in concert to prevent the disabling condition from becoming a handicap."[15]

There are three broad approaches to primary prevention: environmental modification, legislation, and education. An example of environmental modification is seat belts and shoulder harnesses in cars. Legislation would include lowering blood alcohol level definitions to qualify for driving under the influence. Education is aimed directly at individuals to teach them about the different types of injury, how injuries occur, how people can minimize the risks of injury, and why they should do so.[16]

The American Association of Neurological Surgeons and the Congress of Neurological Surgeons sponsor a national program with chapters in forty-seven states called Think First. It is a program directed and middle school students and high school students to reduce the incidence of injury.[17]

Unfortunately, no matter how much money is spent on injury prevention, accidents will always happen. But any accident that can be prevented is a victory.

60

Sports as a Cause of Spinal Cord Injury

Games played with the ball, and others of that nature, are too violent for the body and stamp no character on the mind.—
Thomas Jefferson

This is one of those "numbers chapters." If you don't like numbers, feel free to skip ahead.

Depending upon which source you believe, sports injuries account for between eight and eighteen percent of spinal cord injuries in the United States.[1 2 3 4] According to the Spinalcord [*sic*] Injury Information Network, the incidence of spinal cord injury from sports is declining over time.[5]

The estimate that gives sporting injuries as the cause of eight percent of sporting-related injuries says that diving accidents account for two-thirds of sports injuries.[6] Among males, diving accidents rank fourth as a cause of spinal cord injury. Among females, medical/surgical complications rank fourth, and diving accidents rank fifth. Sports and recreation-related SCI injuries primarily affect people under age twenty-nine.[7] The highest risk athletic activities are: football, rugby, wrestling, gymnastics, diving, surfing, ice hockey, and downhill skiing.[8]

Several factors in recent years have reduced the number of spinal cord injuries in high school and college football. The first is the ban of spear tackling or head tackling by the National Collegiate Athletic Association (NCAA) and the National Federation of State High School Athletic Associations in 1976.[9]

Another factor is the recognition that some athletes have a developmental narrowing of the cervical spinal cord and are more likely to have a severe spinal cord injury because of the lack of room for the spinal cord to expand upon injury.[10 11]

In ice hockey coaches are increasingly teaching players to keep their heads up. According to the Michigan Amateur Hockey Association, neck injuries occur when a player's head makes contact with the boards, goal posts, or with another player when a player's neck is slightly flexed (chin near chest). This sets up a series of events that can result in a burst fracture of a vertebrae. This can happen even at walking speed.

Coaches are also being advised to teach players to cushion their collision with the boards or goal posts with any part of their body other than their head. If a collision between the boards or goal posts and the head is unavoidable, players are being advised to keep their heads up so the forehead or facemask takes most of the force of the collision.

Checking from behind in ice hockey is also a very dangerous practice. Hockey rules have been changed so checking from behind is a major penalty and game misconduct. Goal lines are also being moved out to give extra distance behind the goal net to reduce the chances of contact with the boards. Neck strengthening and flexibility exercises are also thought to reduce the chances of spinal cord injury.[12]

Baseball is another sport where spinal cord injury can occur, although not as frequently as in contact sports. There is little research on the incidence of spinal cord injury in baseball. I did find a study of high school and college baseball over a twenty year period. Players were injured through fielding and base running collisions and headfirst slides. Baseball coaches are urged to teach proper techniques to avoid player collisions and to eliminate headfirst slides.[13]

As sports continue to grow in popularity, it is increasingly important to teach proper techniques to prevent spinal cord injuries.

What to Expect Physically After a Spinal Cord Injury

61

Breathing Problems After a Spinal Cord Injury

Whenever I feel blue, I start breathing again—
L. Frank Baum

Some people may not see the humor in the quotation I used in this chapter. This is because of the effect spinal cord injury can have on a person's ability to breathe. I felt it was important to use a humorous quotation despite the seriousness of the subject. If you are not familiar with the effects that a spinal cord injury can have on the ability to breathe, then you need to read this chapter.

Human beings need oxygen to survive. We inhale air to obtain oxygen. We exhale to remove carbon dioxide from our bodies. We have a respiratory system specifically for this purpose. The respiratory system is also called the pulmonary system.

We inhale air through our mouths and/or noses. Each of us should only have one nose, despite the construction of the previous sentence. Oxygen travels down our windpipes into our lungs. Each person has two lungs. Our lungs filter out the oxygen. The oxygen then goes into our bloodstream, and to the rest of the body. We exhale and the carbon dioxide leaves the body; back through the windpipe and nose or mouth or both. [1]

Exhaling requires no effort from the muscles in the body. Inhaling does. We use four groups of muscles when we inhale: the diaphragm, the intercostal muscles, the neck muscles, and the abdominal muscles. The diaphragm separates the abdominal and chest cavities. It is the main muscle used to inhale. The intercostal muscles are located between the ribs. The neck muscles are, of course, in the neck. The abdominal muscles work in coordination with the other sets of muscles.[2]

A normal person does not have to think about breathing. It happens automatically. The brain signals the body to inhale and exhale as needed.

Then there is a spinal cord injury. If your injury is below T12, you generally won't lose any control over the muscles needed to breathe. Above T12 can be a different story.

If your injury is above T12, how much control you lose depends on the level of injury. And whether the injury is complete or not. As with most other bodily functions related to a spinal cord injury, the higher the injury the more you lose. [3]

Let's assume you have a complete injury above C3. You will lose all control of the muscles you need to breathe. You will need a ventilator (breathing machine) to breathe full-time. Like Christopher Reeve did. But he eventually reached the point where he could survive using the ventilator part-time.

How about a complete injury between C3 and C5? You will lose all control of the muscles you need to breathe. You will need a ventilator to breathe either full-time or part-time. Sometimes a complete C4 will be able to breathe eventually without a ventilator. The occasional C3 may have this happen as well.[4]

What of a complete C6 to C8? You will lose some of your diaphragm muscle control, intercostal muscle control, and abdominal muscle control. T1-T12? You will lose some of your intercostal and abdominal muscle control. At this level your diaphragm control should not be affected.

Incomplete cervical injuries will result in some loss of diaphragm muscle, intercostal muscle, and abdominal muscle control. Incomplete upper back injuries will result in some intercostal and abdominal muscle control loss. Incomplete lower back injuries will result in some abdominal muscle control loss.[5]

When I had the injury to my spinal cord at the C3 level, I kept trying to tell the doctors that it was taking more concentration that it should to breathe. It was no longer something "I didn't have to think about."

Respiratory problems after a spinal cord injury can be very serious. For new injuries, pneumonia (a bacterial infection of the lungs) is the most common cause of death; no matter what level the injury. Within the first year of injury, a blood clot in the lungs is the leading cause of death.[6]

Symptoms of pneumonia are shortness of breath, pale skin, fever, feeling of a heavy chest, and an increase in congestion. "Walking pneumonia" may have no symptoms at all.

Our risk of dying from respiratory problems, as spinal cord injury survivors, remains much greater than that of the general population through our entire lives.[7]

Sleep Apnea is another possible complication after a spinal cord injury. This condition causes a person to stop breathing while they are asleep, sometimes for several seconds or minutes. It can happen a few times an hour or several times an hour. It is a dangerous condition. It is diagnosed through a sleep study in a special laboratory. There is no cure for sleep apnea; but it can be controlled through medication and through the use of a special breathing machine while you sleep.[8]

It is highly recommended that you receive a pneumonia shot while you are in the hospital or in rehabilitation.

> Recommendations for long-term respiratory health include:
> 1. Maintain proper posture and mobility. Don't allow congestion to build up.
> 2. Cough regularly.
> 3. Wear and abdominal binder to help assist your intercostal and abdominal muscles.
> 4. Follow a healthy diet and manage your weight.
> 5. Drink plenty of water.
> 6. Do not smoke.
> 7. Live sensibly by avoiding people with a cold or the flu and avoid areas with dust, smog or other air pollutants.[9]
> 8. See a doctor at least once a year.
> 9. Exercise even if it is just breathing exercises.
>
> Breathing Exercises:
> Do these at least twice a day.
> 1. Take a deep breath and hold it for a few seconds before slowly breathing out.
> 2. Take a deep breath bringing in as much air as you can and as fast as you can before pushing the air out as fast as you can.
> 3. Take a deep breath and hold it, take another breath and hold it, and take one more before slowly breathing out.
> 4. Take a deep breath in then breathe out counting as long and as fast as you can.
> 5. If you have a spirometer, use it to both exercise and keep a measurement of your progress.[10]

A spirometer is a device to measure how much air you breathe in and breathe out.[11]

This is serious stuff. This chapter is not just another bit of "medical wisdom" to do with what you will. I can tell you first hand just how important your lung function is after a spinal cord injury.

My doctor has ordered me to exercise regularly to strengthen my diaphragm muscle, because it is no longer strong enough to allow me to cough properly. I have to be able to cough properly to clear congestion from my lungs.

Coughing during and after a cold, flu, virus, asthma, or any other respiratory disorder is vitally important. Our bodies do it for a reason.

Don't think of coughing as just an irritating symptom after a respiratory illness. It could save your life.

62

Blood Flow Problems After a Spinal Cord Injury

He is so old that his blood type was discontinued.—
George William Curtis

Oh boy. Another chapter with an anatomy lesson. Bet you are just thrilled. I learned a lot researching this chapter, and I hope you will learn a lot reading it.

Inside each of our bodies is the circulatory system. The circulatory system consists of the heart and blood vessels. It is also called the cardiovascular system. There are many different types of blood vessels. Each has a specific purpose.

Let's start with the heart. The heart is a muscle. It is also an organ. Its purpose is to move blood through your body. The heart speeds up and slows down while pumping, depending on your body's need for oxygen at any given moment. You have felt your heart beating harder in your chest when you are doing something that requires exertion.

I'm going to really simplify the function of the heart. It's not that the heart isn't very important in your body. It's that for the purposes of this chapter you only need a basic understanding of how it works.

One side of the heart takes in blood from the body that needs oxygen. The other side of the heart takes the blood that has come back from the lungs full of oxygen, and sends it out to the rest of the body. It's that simple. The heart uses a combination of chambers to do this. There are also valves that keep the blood where it belongs.

Veins carry the blood that all the oxygen has been taken out of back to the heart. They are the blood vessels that look blue under your skin. They look blue because the blood in them doesn't have oxygen in it.

The blood vessels that take blood away from the heart are called arteries. Arteries are very thick. Their walls have muscles in them to keep the blood moving away from the heart. You certainly don't want blood flowing backwards anywhere in your body. Arteries are very elastic.[1]

Arteries branch into arterioles. These are the smallest arteries. Arterioles branch into capillaries. Capillaries aren't really arteries because their function is to exchange gases, sugars, and other nutrients into tissues. They are very tiny. Arteries and arterioles move blood. The word arteriole always sounds to me like an insult that you would call somebody. You arteriole!

According to Wikipedia, "Arterioles have the greatest collective influence on both local blood flow and on overall blood pressure. They are the primary "adjustable nozzles" in the blood system, across which the greatest pressure drop occurs."[2]

Wasn't that a mouthful? It means that your arterioles are charged with the duty of making sure oxygenated blood gets to all parts of your body. And that your blood pressure is appropriate for what your body happens to be doing at the time.

A spinal cord injury enters the picture. Your brain and spinal cord control your autonomic nervous system (ANS). Suddenly the communication between your brain, your spinal cord, and the rest of your body has been interfered with or lost completely.

If you have a spinal cord injury in the low back, you are not as likely to have some of the circulatory problems a spinal cord injury can cause. You are less likely to have low blood pressure, a slow heartbeat, or autonomic dysreflexia.[3] See the chapter on Autonomic Dysreflexia for more information on this condition.

However, if you have a higher spinal cord injury, such as in the upper back or neck, you are more likely to have the problems listed above.

Let's do a little more anatomy. Your sympathetic nervous system (SNS) controls the rate at which your heart beats and your blood vessels contract. This is related to your autonomic nervous system (ANS). If your spinal cord is damaged high enough and especially if it is a complete injury, your body's ability to control your sympathetic nervous system (SNS) is lost.[4]

Studies have shown that circulation in the lower parts of the body is decreased after a spinal cord injury by about fifty to sixty-seven percent of normal since your body can no longer control the autonomic nervous system (ANS).[5] One study suggests "since there are strong reasons to suspect that this circulation [to the legs] is reduced in these patients [patients with spinal cord injuries in wheelchairs]. Not only is atrophy [wasting away] of the muscles associated with a diminished number of small blood vessels, but patients with SCI have increased risk factors for arteriosclerotic changes."[6] If you can feel your feet, every wonder why they get cold? Now you know. They're not getting as much blood as they should.

So this puts you at risk for pressure sores (see the chapter on skin problems after a spinal cord injury) and blood clots. Oh those doctors. They just can't leave well enough alone and talk like the rest of us. Doctors call blood clots deep vein thromboses (DVTs).[7]

Anybody can have a blood clot. People sometimes get them after surgery. You can get one sitting for a long time in the same position on an airplane. Blood clots can lead to a blocked artery in the lungs. You can even get a blood clot sitting at a desk all day in an office if you don't move around enough.

If you get a large blood clot and it goes to your lungs, you're dead. If you get a large blood clot and it goes to your heart, you have a heart attack. You may or may not survive. That's it. Goodbye Charlie. Fortunately there are medications and devices to prevent blood clots. For example, in travel equipment/clothing mail-order catalogs, you can buy special socks to prevent blood clots.

Blood clots cause inflammation. Inflammation causes symptoms. If you have the following symptoms in your legs, see your doctor immediately or go to the emergency room:

1. Swelling at the site of the clot
2. Gradual onset of pain at the site of the clot (if you can feel pain)
3. Redness
4. Warm to the touch
5. Worsening leg pain when bending the foot
6. Leg cramps, especially at night
7. Bluish or whitish discoloration of the skin

Some people have no symptoms when they have a blood clot. This does not make a blood clot any less dangerous.[8]

You may have heard people talk about how long their pressure sores take to heal. The prolonged healing is the result of a spinal cord injury.

I found one article that states specifically that "slow healing of any injury to the paralyzed limb" is a complication of spinal cord injury.[9]

I have a variation of the slow healing process I would like to share with you. In May 2007, I was locking my front door. My house has a large step as the first step going up to the front door. The second step is narrower than the first. The third step is very narrow.

I was standing on the top step, locking my door. I turned around to step down. When I put my right foot on the second step, I only caught the edge of the step. My right foot rolled off the edge of the step, and I landed with great force on my right leg on the first step.

"You say, ouch, betcha that hurt." Indeed it did and still does. One of those things that adds insult to injury. Or maybe better injury to injury.

My ankle and foot swelled like crazy. They turned all sorts of colors. I went to the doctor after a few days to make sure I hadn't broken anything. I hadn't. He said give it about six weeks, and if it hadn't healed, come back. Six weeks went by. It was better, but it was still swollen and my foot did not want to take weight.

I went back to the doctor. He decided to refer me to an orthopedic specialist. I saw the orthopedic specialist about two weeks later. He took more x-rays, and nothing was broken. He told me that because of the spinal cord injury, the severe sprain I had suffered to my ankle and foot was going to take longer to heal than it would in a normal person. He said to expect another two months at least. That will mean this injury is going to take at least five months total to heal.

The same injury in a person without a spinal cord injury would probably take about three months to heal. This gives you some idea of how much additional time an injury can take to heal after a spinal cord injury.

63

Digestive System Function After A Spinal Cord Injury

Happiness is a good bank account, a good cook,
and a good digestion.—
Jean-Jacques Rousseau

*Sh** Happens.... or not—*
Carolyn Boyles

I can discuss this chapter in very technical terms, or I can discuss it in simple terms. I have chosen to discuss it in simple terms. I will refer you to a publication if you want a more technical discussion.

If you want a very technical and thorough discussion of bowel function and dysfunction after spinal cord injury, Paralyzed Veterans of America publishes a booklet called "Neurogenic Bowel Management in Adults with Spinal Cord Injury." The contact information for the Paralyzed Veterans of America is in the Resources chapter of this book.

The University of Alabama at Birmingham publishes a nice fact sheet on bowel management. It starts off by explaining the functions of the human body related to digestion. The digestive system, like almost all other systems in the body, is connected to the brain via the spinal cord. A spinal cord injury disrupts the digestive system's ability to communicate with the brain.

From birth until we are toddlers, bowel functions occur automatically. If the brain senses that the bowel is full, it signals the body to tense certain muscles and relax others for defecation to occur. At roughly the age of two, our parents teach us voluntary control over the bowel so that defecation occurs when we choose.[2] [If you don't know what defecation means, you can probably make a good guess based on the subject of this chapter.] Unless a person is experiencing severe diarrhea, bowel control is voluntary under normal circumstances.

Unlike other problems after a spinal cord injury, bowel dysfunction only has two possible options. If your spinal cord injury is above the T12 level, you have what is called an upper motor neuron injury. If your spinal cord injury is below the T12 level, you have what is called a lower motor neuron injury.[3] Fancy names, huh?

The difference is important. If the injury is above T12, the message from your bowels is not getting *through the spinal cord*. If the injury is below T12, the message from your bowels is not getting from the nerve branches *to the spinal cord*.[4]

With an injury above T12, your bowels will empty themselves automatically when they are full. With an injury below T12, your bowels will have a much more difficult time trying to empty than normal. And may not be able to do so even when you want them to. Your doctor may describe either disorder as a motility disorder. You may also hear the condition described as a neurogenic bowel.[5]

There are a lot of "fun" problems that can happen after a spinal cord injury related to the digestive system: constipation (where you don't "go" as often as you normally do); diarrhea (loose, watery stools); gas (a foul smelling airy noisy discharge from the rectum); hemorrhoids (enlarged veins in the rectum and anus); rectal bleeding (abnormal bleeding in the rectum which can be caused by many things).[6]

If you have bowel movements when you don't want to, then you must teach your body to have bowel movements on a set schedule so there are no "accidents." Your doctor may teach you how to stimulate the anal area with your finger to encourage your body to defecate. You may also need to use laxatives, stool softeners, suppositories, or enemas. Suppositories either stimulate the nerve endings in the rectum or draw water into the stool to stimulate evacuation. Enemas and mini-enemas soften the stool, lubricate the bowel, and draw water into the stool to stimulate evacuation. Laxatives and enemas are available both over-the-counter and by prescription.

Impaction is another problem that can occur. It is the result of chronic constipation. It is a mass of hard, dry stool that can develop in the rectum. Sudden, watery diarrhea in someone who has chronic constipation is usually an indication of fecal impaction.[7]

You may hear about a product called the Magic Bullet. This product is widely discussed among spinal cord injury survivors as a very reliable suppository, which relieves constipation. I have supplied the contact information for this product in the Resources Chapter.

Another excellent product that I have used is called Colosan. Colosan works by oxygenating the digestive system. It is composed of magnesium compounds. It initially causes diarrhea but this is a sign it is working. It tastes kind of chalky. It comes in a powder or capsules. I have only used the powder. You add the power to a glass of water and drink it. Then you drink lemon juice (or vinegar) to activate it in your stomach. You can drink a mixture of lemon juice and honey if this is easier for you. I have provided several sources for Colosan in the Resources chapter.

If you are unsure whether or not you should use either product, check with your doctor. A good bowel program can be very important for regaining your self-confidence after a spinal cord injury.

64

Autonomic Dysreflexia (Hyperreflexia): A Life-Threatening Condition After a Spinal Cord Injury

There are more things to alarm us than to harm us,
and we suffer more often in apprehension than reality.—
Seneca

Wasn't that title a mouthful?

This is a condition that you need to know about. Nobody told me about it. I had to discover its existence through researching for this book. Only then did I know what was happening to my body.

In an earlier chapter I discussed that spinal cord injuries fall into three categories: cervical (neck), thoracic (chest), and lumbar (lower back). In this chapter I'm going to give you a different set of categories that are important.

Let's start with that mouthful of words. Autonomic Dysreflexia or Hyperreflexia. The doctors' "fancy" definition is:

> a syndrome characterized by abrupt onset of excessively high blood pressure caused by uncontrolled sympathetic nervous system discharge in persons with spinal cord injury.[1]

> Autonomic dysreflexia means an over-activity of the Autonomic Nervous System. It can occur when an irritating stimulus is introduced to the body below the level of spinal cord injury.… The stimulus sends nerve impulses to the spinal cord, where they travel upward until they are blocked by the lesion [the injury to the spinal cord] at the level of injury. Since the impulses cannot reach the brain, a reflex is activated that increases activity of the sympathetic

> portion of the autonomic nervous system. This results in spasms and a narrowing of the blood vessels, which causes a rise in blood pressure. Nerve receptors in the heart and blood vessels detect this rise in blood pressure and send a message to the brain. The brain sends a message to the heart, causing the heartbeat to slow down and the blood vessels above the injury to dilate [open wider]. However, the brain cannot send messages below the level of injury, due to the spinal cord lesion, and therefore the blood pressure cannot be regulated.[2]
>
> Autonomic Dysreflexia (AD), also known as Hyperreflexia, is a potentially dangerous complication of spinal cord injury (SCI). In AD, an individual's blood pressure may rise to dangerous levels and if not treated can lead to stroke and possibly death. Individuals with SCI at the T-6 level or above are at great risk. AD usually occurs because of a noxious (irritating stimulus below the level of injury....
>
> AD occurs primarily because of an imbalance in the body systems which control the blood pressure. The human body is an incredibly complicated and beautifully balanced machine. There are balances to each system of the body, including the blood pressure. One of the major ways the body controls blood pressure is by tightening or relaxing little muscles around the blood vessels. When the muscles contract, the blood vessels get smaller and blood pressure increases. Imagine a garden hose with water streaming through it; when you put your thumb over the opening of the hose, reducing the opening for the water to flow through, the water shoots out at a higher pressure. Similarly, when the blood vessels are smaller, the blood rushes around your body at higher pressure.
>
> When a noxious stimulus occurs, a reflex is initiated that causes the blood vessels to constrict and raises the blood pressure. In an intact spinal cord, this same stimulus also sets in motion another set of reflexes that moderates the constriction of blood vessels. However, in someone who has SCI at the T-6 level or above, the signal which tells the blood vessels to relax cannot get through the spinal cord because of the injury. Some of the nerves at the T-6 level also control the blood flow to and from the gut, which is a large reservoir of blood. Uncontrolled activity of these nerves may cause the blood from the gut to flow into the rest of the blood system. The result is that blood pressure can increase to dangerous levels and the increase in blood pressure must be controlled by outside means.[3]

Whew! That was almost as bad as the name of the condition!

In plain English, your body now has its own "alarm system." Like a smoke alarm. It can go off in the middle of the night and wake you up, just like a smoke alarm. It can go off and you can't figure out why it's going off, just like a smoke alarm. But unlike a smoke alarm, its batteries never go dead. It is always there. Twenty four hours a day. If it can't go off, then you are already dead.

But it doesn't happen to everybody with a spinal cord injury. If your spinal cord injury is at the level of T5 or above, you *need* to know about this condition. If your spinal cord injury is at the level of T6-T10, you *may need* to know about this condition. If your spinal cord injury is below the level of T10, you *do not need* to know about this condition, unless you have friends with a spinal cord injury above T10.

You now know the condition exists. You need to be aware of the symptoms (you may not have all the symptoms at the same time):

1. Pounding headache (caused by the elevation in blood pressure)
2. Hypertension/high blood pressure (blood pressure greater than 200/100)
3. Goose pimples/goose bumps/goose flesh *below* the level of injury
4. Sweating *above* the level of injury
5. Nasal congestion/stuffiness
6. Slow pulse (slower than 60 beats per minute)
7. Blotchiness of the skin *above* the level of injury
8. Restlessness
9. Nausea
10. Cold, clammy skin *below* the level of injury
11. Flushed, reddened face[4 5 6]

Next, let's go over the list of triggers for Autonomic Dysreflexia/Hyperreflexia (any one of the following can cause Autonomic Dysreflexia/Hyperreflexia):

1. Skin irritation
2. Pressure sore(s)
3. Wounds
4. Burns
5. Broken bones
6. Pregnancy (females only)
7. Ingrown toenails
8. Appendicitis (in individuals who have not had their appendix removed previously)

9. An overfull bladder
10. Blockage in the urinary drainage device (catheter, collection bag)
11. Bladder infection (cystitis)/urinary tract infection
12. Inadequate bladder emptying
13. Bladder spasms
14. Bladder stones
15. Kidney stones
16. Not following the intermittent catheterization program
17. Constipation/impaction
18. Distention during bowel program (digital stimulation)
19. Hemorrhoids or anal fissures
20. Infection or irritation of the digestive system (gastric ulcer, colitis)
21. Labor or delivery (pregnant females only)
22. Over stimulation during sexual activity (stimulus to the pelvic region which would be painful if sensation were present)
23. Menstrual cramps (females only)
24. Tight or restrictive clothing
25. Pressure to skin from sitting on wrinkled clothing
26. Development of bone in abnormal areas, usually in soft tissues (if this happens, it will happen within the first four months of spinal cord injury)[7]
27. Sunburn[8 9]
28. Yeast infection
29. Asthma or acute asthma attack (in individuals with asthma)
30. Nerve pain

I have added yeast infection, asthma attack, and nerve pain from my own personal experience. Another way to know if something is wrong is to experience an increase in spasticity, especially if the location of the spasms is adjacent to the area of the body where the problem exists. I will discuss spasticity in a separate chapter.

Yeast infection can occur in/on the genitals of either sex. It can also occur in the mouth, throat, or esophagus. I had an increase in spasms once when I contracted a yeast infection as a side effect of steroid inhalers. I did not know I had a yeast infection until I happened to have an upper GI scoping for other reasons.

Over time, you will learn your own body. If you are a caregiver, you will learn the body of the injury person, and know what typically sets off the symptoms of autonomic dysreflexia/hyperreflexia.

I have trouble sometimes remembering the name of this condition, so I think of it as its initials, A.D., meaning "Alarm Detonation."

Make sure you get emergency treatment if you have this condition. Don't ignore it because ignoring it could kill you.

65

Skin Problems After a Spinal Cord Injury

Beauty may be skin deep, but ugly goes clear to the bone.—
Redd Foxx

Skin is something we all take for granted. Until something goes wrong with it. Spinal cord injuries can cause potentially life-threatening skin problems. So let's learn more about skin, what it is, and how best to take care of it after a spinal cord injury.

Skin is actually an organ in your body (bet you didn't know that!). It is actually the body's largest organ (apologies to the male readers out there). It covers the entire outside of the body and by itself weighs about six pounds.

Skin is a protective shield against heat, light, injury and infection. It serves to regulate body temperature; store water, fat, and vitamin D; and sense pleasant and unpleasant sensation (something like an early warning system to the body).

What we normally think of as one layer of skin is actually three separate layers. Each layer performs a distinct function. The thin outer layer of skin is called the epidermis. The middle layer of skin is called the dermis. The deepest layer of skin is called the fat layer or subcutis. [1]

The epidermis, dermis, and subcutis each have layers within them. The top layer of the epidermis is constantly shedding dead skin cells. The middle layer of the epidermis has living skin cells. These help provide the skin with its needs so it can protect the rest of the body. The deepest layer of the epidermis creates new skin cells that eventually make their way to the top layer of the epidermis to replace the skin cells that have died. [2]

The middle layer of skin, the dermis, contains blood vessels, lymph vessels, hair follicles, sweat glands, and pain and touch receptors. The deepest layer of skin contain protein and fat cells. This layer helps conserve body heat and protects the internal organs from injury by absorbing sudden movements.[3]

It is pretty common knowledge that people with spinal cord injuries often have skin problems. The reason for these skin problems is somewhat complicated. It results from changes to the circulation of blood to the skin. I cover blood flow problems after spinal cord injury in another chapter.

The most common skin problem after a spinal cord injury is pressure sores. Pressure sores are areas of injured skin and tissue. Doctors always have to have fancy words for things. They call pressure sores skin ulcerations or decubitus ulcers. Pressure sores are also called pressure ulcers.

Ok, your circulation to your skin after your injury is no longer normal. It is not getting as much blood flow as it was before your injury. Areas of your body that are padded with lots of skin, like your thighs, are going to have more blood flowing to them than areas that are mainly bony, like your elbows, heels, hips, ankles, shoulders, back, low back, and the back of the head.[4 5]

Pressure sores can happen to anyone. Even a normal person. They are caused when blood supply is reduced to an area of the body that has had too much weight on it. The elderly are prone to them when bedridden for an extended period of time. Even younger people can get pressure sores if they are in bed for long periods of time. Like recovering from surgery or a serious illness. People in wheelchairs are subject to pressure sores. [6]

When the skin in an area of your body has had the blood flow cut off to it, it dies. The skin turns red or dark purple. The darker your skin, the darker the area of the pressure sore. The area may feel warmer to the touch than the surrounding skin. [7] You would think it would feel colder.

Pressure sores can be mild or can be severe. More severe pressure sores can go into the muscle. Very severe pressure sores can go into the bone. The stages of a pressure sore start with reddened skin. If the pressure sore gets worse, the reddened skin forms a blister. The blister then forms an open wound. The open wound can become a crater. Each of these stages has a number. The less severe stage is number one. The most severe stage is number four. Stage Four pressure sores often require surgery.[8]

You need to be aware of the signs of infection so you can seek proper medical care. The signs of infection are:

1. Thick yellow or green pus
2. A bad smell from the sore
3. Redness or warmth around the sore

4. Swelling around the sore
5. Tenderness around the sore

The signs that the infection has spread to the rest of the body are:

1. Fever or chills
2. Mental confusion or difficulty concentrating (more than normal if you have mental confusion or difficulty concentrating already)
3. Rapid heartbeat
4. Weakness[9]

If you have autonomic dysreflexia then you may experience extremely high blood pressure and other symptoms of autonomic dysreflexia.

If a pressure sore is not kept clean and free of dead tissue, it will not heal. You or your caregiver can rinse the area with a solution of salt and water (this will probably sting!). Then the pressure sore needs to be covered with a bandage or dressing. Depending on the type of bandage or dressing, you may have to change it as often as daily or as little as once a week. Placing wet gauze bandages on the sore and letting them dry is another way to remove dead tissue. [10]

Be prepared that cleaning and maintaining pressure sores is a painful process. You may need to take some form a painkiller half an hour to an hour before the cleaning process.[11]

Pillows and foam pads can be your best friends when it comes to reducing the weight of your body on a pressure sore. If you don't have extra pillows or foam pads, get some. There are also special mattresses, mattress covers, and seat cushions which serve to lessen weight on an affected area.[12]

Whether you're in bed or in a wheelchair, change your position no less than every two hours. If you are in a manual wheelchair, someone should have taught you how to perform manual pressure releases. If you are in an electric wheelchair that tilts back, you can perform a pressure release electronically.[13] If you don't know how to do pressure releases, make sure you learn. Find out from another spinal cord injury survivor or a medical professional.

Because pressure sores are such a common problem, people who have found successful cures from sores that are hard to heal are quite willing to share the information with others through letters to the editor in magazines for the disabled and on Internet forums. It is similar to finding a cure for hiccups that really works.

I did a search of the magazines and the Internet to see what I could find out about cures for pressure sores. I found a letter to the editor in *New Mobility* magazine indicating that after months of unsuccessful treatment, Betadine ointment worked.[14] If you are allergic to iodine, you should not use any form of Betadine product. Another product that people have raved about is Miracle Mist Plus. It is an all nature product intended to heal pressure sores and other skin problems.[15]

The Sci-Info-Pages website has an excellent section on skin management after spinal cord injury. It advises not smoking to maintain good skin quality. It also advises eating a well-balanced diet that includes plenty of protein foods, fresh fruits and vegetables and liquids. It also advises if you have a skin problem to increase your intake of protein (lean meats, dairy foods and beans), carbohydrates (breads and cereals), vitamins A, B6, C, E, and zinc. If you are anemic, be sure to take extra iron.[16]

The Sci-Info-Pages website also advises the following to maintain good skin quality:

1. Avoid using soaps labeled "antibacterial" or "antimicrobial." These tend to reduce the skin's acidity. The skin's acidity acts as a protection against infection.
2. Keep the skin clean and dry. Wash with soap and water daily. Rinse and dry thoroughly.
3. Wash skin folds and creases (groin area and underarms) more frequently, twice a day.
4. Tapes, soaps, fabrics or other irritants can cause rashes. Food or drug allergies can cause total body rashes.
5. Don't use harsh soaps or alcohol-based products because they dry the skin.
6. Lubricate dry skin with moisturizing creams or ointments. Use care in applying creams over bony areas because they may promote skin breakdown.
7. Soiled skin can break down easily. If you have a bowel or bladder accident, be sure to clean up immediately.
8. Avoid using talc powders. They may support yeast growth. They can also absorb moisture and keep it close to the skin which will cause skin breakdown.
9. If you get calluses on your feet and hands be sure to soak frequently in warm water and towel briskly to remove dead skin. Moisturizing creams can help soften calluses. If you have limited sense of touch, do not use callous files sold in discount stores and drug stores. You may continue filing past the dead skin and into the living skin. I have done this and it is painful.
10. Take special care of your fingernails and toenails. Soak them and rub gently with a towel to remove dead skin and decrease the chance of hangnails. Cut your nails after soaking. Cut nails straight across to avoid ingrown nails and short nails are safer.[17]

Make sure you or your caregiver inspect your skin frequently. If there are areas you cannot see, use a mirror. Anemia, vascular disease, and diabetes can contribute to skin problems. For additional recommendations on skin care, see http://www.sci-info-pages.com.

I have been fortunate that I have never experienced a pressure sore. I assume it is because I am a "walking quad" and thus I can change my position on a regular basis. What I do have problems with is chronically itchy skin. I did not have chronically itchy skin before my spinal cord injury.

I was curious if I was the only person who has experienced chronically itchy skin. I found a posting on the National Spinal Cord Injury Association Forum that my buddy "Poster7" also has problems with chronic itchy skin.[18] Interestingly enough, in the same place I do, the right shoulder joint.

Another oddity I'm going to mention in this chapter is something I've seen discussed after a spinal cord injury. I've experienced it, and I see it talked about from time to time in spinal cord injury magazines. Some people have noticed that their fingernails and hair grow faster after a spinal cord injury. This is not directly related to skin problems after a spinal cord injury, but it's the best place I could find to discuss it.

Take care of your skin. You won't regret it.

66

Fatigue After a Spinal Cord Injury

Fatigue is the best pillow—
Benjamin Franklin

Oddly enough, I could find very little information on fatigue after a spinal cord injury. In this chapter I am talking about physical fatigue, not psychological fatigue.

But that does not mean it isn't a very important consideration after a spinal cord injury. While you (or your family member) are in the hospital, you are going to be exhausted. It takes a lot of energy to recover from a serious traumatic injury. Although your fatigue is going to get better, you may find it with you for the rest of your life.

If you are a spinal cord injury survivor who does not use a wheelchair, crutches, walker, or cane, then your fatigue will fall under invisible disability. See the chapter on invisible disability for more information.

Let's talk about why we, as spinal cord injury survivors, are so tired all the time. Not all of us are, but I would venture a guess that more spinal cord injury survivors experience increased fatigue after their injuries than those who don't.

First, if you are a woman, you are more prone to fatigue than men. Doctors don't have an answer to this one. It could be hormonal. It could be nutritional. It could be the busy lifestyles that women lead today with trying to work and raise children.[1] It could be undiagnosed asthma. Adult women are more likely to have asthma than adult men.[2]

If you have asthma and your doctor has prescribed inhalers for you to use, be sure to use them as your doctor has prescribed. That feeling of not being able to think could be your asthma. If you are having difficulty breathing or feel like you have an elephant sitting on your chest, see your doctor.

Prescription medication can cause fatigue. Pain can cause fatigue. Pain after a spinal cord injury? Never heard of it. Yeah, right.

There is one basic fact when it comes to energy levels and spinal cord injuries. It takes more energy to perform a task after a spinal cord injury than it did before the injury. Tasks can take longer. Tasks can be harder. Because it takes longer to perform basic tasks, we may get less rest as a result.[3]

There are some things you can do to reduce the amount of fatigue you experience. Pay attention to whether you have more energy in the mornings, afternoons, or evenings. Perform your most demanding tasks, if possible, during the time of day when you have the most energy.

Nap if you feel fatigued, and your schedule will allow it. Don't do so while driving. Rearrange your schedule to perform your errands that require driving so you can do them all in one trip.

Talk to your doctor about getting more help or by getting a lighter or electric wheelchair. If there are any activities that you can eliminate from your schedule, do so.

Go to bed earlier at night. If you are not exercising regularly, start doing so.[4]

Fatigue is going to be part of your life, but this does not mean you cannot lead a full and happy life after a spinal cord injury.

67

Nutrition After a Spinal Cord Injury

Nutrition makes me puke.—
Jimmy Piersall

Nutrition. It's a word we hear or see several times a day. News broadcasts. TV commercials. Magazine and newspaper advertisements. E-mail messages. Eat more bread. Eat less bread. Eat less fat. Eat more fat. Avoid trans-fat. Increase trans-fat.

"Just what is this *nutrition* stuff and why is it important to me as a spinal cord injury survivor?"

Nutrition is the science that studies the relationship between diet and health.[1] It is important because, as a spinal cord injury survivor, you need to be doing everything you can to maintain your health and extend your lifespan.

According to Vickeri Barton, associate director of nutrition at Harborview Medical Center in Seattle, Washington, people with spinal cord injuries have unique nutrition issues. Barton explains the reasons are changes in body composition and metabolism, changes in activity level, and because of the barriers to preparing meals, shopping, etc.[2]

Nutrition and weight management are important after spinal cord injury for the following reasons:

1. There is an increased risk for diabetes, elevated cholesterol and obesity
2. Weight gain affects mobility and independence
3. Weight gain can increase expenses
4. There is a risk of getting pressure ulcers
5. There is an increased risk for osteoporosis (brittle bones)

6. Additional fiber may be needed for individuals with a neurogenic bowel.[3]

Weight charts exist for the general public, but not specifically for spinal cord injury survivors. Normal weight charts can be adjusted for SCI survivors. These charts must be adjusted to compensate for the loss in muscle mass. A general rule of adjustment is to subtract five to ten percent for paraplegia and ten to fifteen percent for quadriplegia/tetraplegia.[4]

Body mass charts have become popular among the general population in recent years. However, these charts are not recommended for use among the spinal cord injured population because they underestimate body fat in SCI survivors.[5]

"So how do I know how much I am supposed to eat every day?" Don't fret. There is a formula to estimate what your ideal calorie intake should be. First, find a weight chart for the general public and perform the adjustment recommended depending upon if you are a paraplegic or quadriplegic/tetraplegic. If you don't have use of your arms/hands or are not good at math, have a friend or family member do it for you.

Now you know what your ideal weight should be. The next step is to calculate what your actual body weight is in kilograms. I know, I tried the metric system in school too and didn't like it. One kilogram is the same as 2.2 pounds. Divide your body weight in pounds by 2.2 to get your weight in kilograms.

If you have paraplegia, then multiply your body weight in kilograms by 27.9 to get your ideal caloric intake. If you have quadriplegia/tetraplegia, then multiply your body weight in kilograms by 22.7 to get your ideal calorie intake. The above formula, however, does not consider whether you are male or female; active or a couch potato, or whether you are sixteen or sixty. It will take a bit of trial and error to see what works best for you.[6]

Barton also offers some general nutrition guidelines:

1. If you have a wound that is healing, increase your protein intake
2. Stay as active as possible
3. Eat regular meals
4. Be aware of portion sizes
5. Eat a variety of foods
6. Eat low fat, high fiber foods

7. Watch beverage calories
8. Know how to read a food label.[7]

The University of Alabama has developed a twelve-week diet program specifically for people with a spinal cord injury. This video and workbook can be ordered off the Internet for a small charge. The program does require writing down everything you eat every day. This may be a problem for quadriplegic/tetraplegic incomplete injurees, and individuals with a complete injury. See if someone will help you record the information on a daily basis if you are unable to yourself. Maybe a family member, paid caregiver, or friend will volunteer. See the Resources chapter for more information.

There is a lot of controversial information when it comes to eating right. Many sources recommend the use of artificial sweeteners for individuals who are trying to lose weight. Some sources say artificial sweeteners actually make you gain weight. However, there are no long-term studies on the health effects of some artificial sweeteners. Some sources claim artificial sweeteners are very bad for you, and should not be consumed under any circumstances. This is a matter of personal choice whether you consume artificial sweeteners or not. If you are diabetic, your choices are more limited.

Controversy also exists as to the consumption of "so called" trans-fats. Some states have even banned the use of trans-fat in their states. Decisions about what kind of oil you are going to use in your diet are personal choices. You may be a hardcore lard user. You may prefer canola oil. If you use fats that tend to add calories, then adjust your calorie consumption elsewhere. If you use fats that don't tend to add calories, then you may not have to adjust your calorie intake elsewhere. See what works best for you.

Typical weight management programs are designed for "normal" people, not spinal cord injured people. Your metabolism has been slowed down, not only by the injury, but by many of the prescriptions medications you must take. You are not as active as you were before, so you are not burning calories the way you used to. If you have an injury or pressure sore, you will need to change your diet temporarily while you are healing and consume more protein. You may also find that some foods you could eat without problems before your injury you can no longer eat. They may cause constipation, diarrhea, gas, indigestion, or other problems.

One final note I want to add is that sustaining a spinal cord injury is a life-changing event, as we all know. It can be depressing as well. Some people react to depression by eating. Aging adds pounds to our weight. The combination of aging and coping with depression by eating poses the risk of substantial weight gain after a spinal cord injury.

Please take care of yourself whether you are an injury survivor, friend, family member, or medical professional.

68

Pain After a Spinal Cord Injury

Pain is such an uncomfortable feeling that even a tiny amount of it is enough to ruin every enjoyment—
Will Rogers

I am having a really bad day today. I cannot get the pain to stop today. I have taken the maximum amount of all my medicines for pain and spasms, and I'm still hurting. So I decided to write about pain today. I am not going to go into the triviality of defining pain. We all know what pain is.

It is common for men to say that the pain from kidney stones is worse than labor. Women say that labor is worse. I've never had labor pains, but I have had kidney stone pain. Spinal cord pain is worse.

Doctor Ron Tasker, a neurosurgeon, has described spinal cord pain, more specifically central cord pain (more on this later), as "the worst pain known to man."[1] Refer back to the chapter on Central Cord Syndrome for more information how the spinal cord is injured to cause this type of pain if you need to.

Nobody ever seems to agree on anything when it comes to spinal cord injury. The SpinalCord [*sic*] Injury Information Network at the University of Alabama says that one-third of spinal cord injured people have severe pain which doesn't go away.[2] An article in *PN* magazine says that an estimated eighty to ninety percent of people with spinal cord injury have persistent annoying pain.[3] A third article says that more than fifty percent of spinal cord injured people have pain.[4]

Doctors always like to get so technical about things. Especially when discussing pain after a spinal cord injury. There are five different types of pain that can be felt by those with a spinal cord injury:

1. Central pain

2. Root pain

3. Mechanical pain

4. Syrinx pain

5. Referred pain

More information exists on the Internet about central pain than any of the other types of pain. This is because central pain is the most problematic type of pain experienced by spinal cord injury survivors. Central pain interferes with the quality of a person's life. It may be a constant pain or a periodic pain.

One oddity about central pain is that is can be present where you have no sensation. Try explaining that to a normal person and get them to understand! Central Pain Syndrome can be felt as a burning pain, a pins and needles pain, or numbness at or below the level of injury. This type of pain starts weeks or months after a spinal cord injury.[5] Central pain has also been described as throbbing or tingling.[6] Central pain has been described as "the pain beyond pain." This is what I am having today.

The website PainOnline.com describes central pain as "a pain syndrome which occurs when injury to the Central Nervous System is insufficient to cause numbness, but sufficient to cause central sensitization of the pain system."

PainOnline has a nice explanation of how Central Pain Syndrome happens (if there is such a thing as a "nice" explanation of pain). Injured pain nerves carry more signal than normal pain nerves. Eventually they gain the ability to "persuade" neighboring uninjured nerves to transmit pain signals to the brain. The thalamus is the area of the brain that registers pain. Eventually after enough transmission of pain, the thalamus becomes overloaded and shuts down. The entire pain system starts acting like a nerve ending. With the thalamus shut down, the cortex of the brain starts receiving constant, unregulated pain signals.[7]

Some of the articles also mention a sensation of cold along with the sensation of pain. They also mention that touch or the rubbing sensation of clothing on the skin may worsen central pain.

The second type of pain experienced by spinal cord injured individuals is root pain. Root pain is felt at or below the level of injury. It can start days or weeks after the initial injury. It can get worse over time. It can be felt as a stabbing pain or a sharp pain or a band of burning pain where normal feeling stops. Light touch can worsen this pain.[8] Root pain is also called segmental pain. Another way to describe this pain is it is a kind of pain where things that normally wouldn't be painful cause extreme pain.[9]

Mechanical pain happens where you still have normal sensation. It can be a sudden sharpness. It can be a dull ache. A lot of physical activity can make mechanical pain worse. Muscle overuse, muscle damage, unstable bone fractures, infection, or deforming changes in bones (osteoporosis) and joints (arthritis) causes this type of pain.[10]

Paraplegics who use manual wheelchairs commonly experience mechanical pain. Wheelchair propulsion and transfers from one place to another are the most common ways paraplegics become injured.[11]

Another cause of spinal cord pain is syrinx pain. Fortunately, this type of pain is rare. A syrinx is a hollow, fluid filled cavity that sometimes forms in the spinal cord as it heals. Think of it as a pimple on your spinal cord. It can enlarge over time, causing pain and loss of feeling.[12]

Referred pain is the fifth type of pain after a spinal cord injury. This type of pain is different from the other types of pain because it is felt in a location other than where the pain is actually coming from.[13] Let me give you an example. I sometimes have pain in my neck. I actually feel the pain between my shoulder blades in my back. It feels like I have a knife stuck in my back. But I know the pain is actually in my neck. If you can't feel pain in an area, you may experience increased spasticity instead of pain. Referred pain is not well understood.[14]

I'm going to add to what I've already said on the different types of pain. I found another source that expands the types and causes of pain. Muscle spasms are another kind of mechanical pain. These, as we injurees well know, are involuntary movements of the body in areas that have lost some or all motor function.

Mechanical instability of the spine in another type of mechanical pain. It is caused by damaged ligaments or bone fractures. Usually it happens after injury, but it can happen later. If it happens, it takes place around the area of injury.[15]

There is another type of pain that spinal cord injury survivors experience. It is called visceral pain. It usually starts shortly after the injury. It is a constant burning, cramping pain. It takes place in the area of the stomach. Depending on where the injury is, it is either above or below the injury. I have this problem. It is very uncomfortable.

Now I want to talk about things that make pain after a spinal cord injury worse. This has been studied and the conclusions are pretty consistent from study to study. Factors that worsen pain are:

1. Urinary Tract Infections (UTIs)
2. Viral Illnesses (cold, flu etc.)
3. Changes in your sleep cycle

4. Changes in your daily activity
5. Menstrual cycle (women only)
6. Upset stomache [*sic*] (heartburn or constipation)
7. Other sources of pain (musculoskeletal)
8. Prolonged sitting
9. Fatigue
10. Muscle spasms
11. Cold weather
12. Sudden movements [17] [18]

In one study five sets of factors magnified pain: negative mood (depression), prolonged nerve transmission by spinal cord nerves (bowel management, bladder management, etc.), weather, voluntary physical activity, and periodic nerve transmission by spinal cord nerves.[19]

I've talked about what makes the pain worse. Now I want to talk about what can make the pain better. Doctors used to advise their patients with nerve pain not to exercise. Now doctors are advising these patients to exercise within reason using low-impact exercises. Examples of low-impact exercises are: riding a recumbent stationery bike, riding an elliptical trainer, walking, and water aerobics.[20]

Another option for people who hate the "e" word (exercise) is hypnosis. With hypnosis, the goal is to eliminate the "emotional overlay" of pain. According to Dr. Bruce Eimer:

> Living with Chronic Persistent Pain can be a terrible energy drain and distraction. In addition to the "physical hurt" of the pain, there usually is a component of "emotional suffering." This emotional component, or "emotional overlay" to the physical pain can make the pain hurt more, and it can also interfere with pain treatment. Emotional suffering makes physical pain worse.[21]

I have had hypnosis done for pain management. It has made it somewhat easier to deal with the pain. I cannot say how much it has reduced the pain. If you are going to use hypnosis for pain management, make sure you find a state-licensed hypnotist. Don't use a friend or brother-in-law who is dabbling in hypnosis.

Many people avoid hypnosis because of the fear they will lose control. I've been hypnotized several times and have never done anything I didn't want to do. I didn't dance around the room acting like a chicken either (not that I can after my spinal cord injury). It wasn't that I couldn't do it physically that kept me from doing it. I didn't have the urge to.

Another little-known method of dealing with pain is a TENS unit. TENS stands for Transcutaneous ("through the skin") Electrical Nerve Stimulator. It is an electronic device that produces electrical signal used to stimulate nerves. It uses electrodes on unbroken skin. It has been used most often for labor pain but it also used for nerve pain.[22] I have a TENS unit, and it has been effective for me in controlling the nerve pain in my legs at times.

The final method for controlling pain I want to discuss is painkillers. Painkillers come in two categories: addictive and non-addictive. Because doctors are still learning about how spinal cord injuries cause pain, current prescription pain pills are often not effective in reducing or eliminating pain.

Another problem in pain control for spinal cord injury survivors is the unwillingness of doctors to prescribe strong pain medication for some categories of patients. It is understandable in patients with a history of drug abuse or addiction. But women often have difficulty getting doctors to prescribe pain medication sufficiently strong to actually provide some relief. I have certainly had this problem. If you are young, you may also have experience this problem. Doctors always give the excuse of "I don't want to get you addicted."

Some people have told me they have the opposite problem. Doctors are too willing to push strong painkillers at them that they do not want.

It is your decision whether or not to take medication for pain. If you need to drive and are still capable of doing so, then avoid the use of prescription pain medicine until it is safe for you to take it.

69

Kidney and Bladder Problems After a Spinal Cord Injury

To Pee or Not To Pee—
Various

One of the most problematic complications after a spinal cord injury is the effect on the urinary system (kidneys, ureters, bladder, sphincter muscles, and urethra). Let's start with what the urinary system is, and its role in the body in a normal human. The internal parts of the urinary system are almost identical in men and women.

The urinary system is quite complicated in its function. It has several parts. The first is the kidney. A normal human has two of them. They are located below the ribs toward the middle of the back. The kidneys have three functions: to remove liquid waste from the blood in the form of urine, to keep a stable balance of salts and other substances in the blood, and to produce a hormone that aids the formation of red blood cells. Kidneys are a very complex filtering system.

The next part of the urinary system is the ureter. This is a narrow tube that runs from the kidney to the bladder. There is one for each kidney. The muscles in the ureter walls force the urine from the kidneys to the bladder, and prevent urine from backing up into the kidneys.

The bladder is a triangular-shaped, hollow organ located in the lower abdomen. The bladder is an expandable organ. The bladder expands to hold urine, similar to the way the uterus in a woman expands to hold a baby when she is pregnant. The walls of the bladder relax to hold urine and contract to empty the bladder.

At the base of the bladder are two sphincter muscles. These help keep urine from leaking around the opening of the bladder. Another part of the urinary system is the nerves in the bladder. These alert a person when the bladder is full.

Finally there is the urethra. This is the tube that allows urine to flow from the bladder out of the body.

Urination is the process of expelling urine from the bladder out of the body. In a normal person, the process is as follows: the bladder has become full with urine, the nerves in the bladder tell the brain that the bladder is full and needs to be emptied. The brain tells the bladder muscles to tighten, and then urine is squeezed from the bladder. The brain telling the bladder muscles to tighten doesn't do any good unless the sphincter muscles are alerted at the same time to relax, which happens automatically. All the signals must happen in the right order for a person to urinate or "pee."[1]

Now comes the "fun" part. What can go wrong with the urinary system after a spinal cord injury?

You may remember I spoke in a previous chapter about how there are nerves at the end of the spinal cord. These are the nerves that control the urinary system. They also control the digestive system. Any spinal cord injury will affect the urinary system because no matter what the level of the spinal cord injury, it is above the level that controls the urinary system.

I'm going to assume that you know the difference between boys and girls because I really, really don't want to explain it. It's going to matter later in this chapter in some types of bladder management.

The urinary system can't get messages properly anymore after a spinal cord injury. So it gets really confused. It gets confused in two different ways. Which way depends on whether your spinal cord injury is in the neck or in the back.

Would you rather have a "floppy" bladder or a "spastic" bladder? I know what you're thinking. Neither one sounds like a good choice. They each have advantages and disadvantages.

Let's say you have a "floppy" bladder. This is also called having a flaccid bladder. If your injury is below T12/L1 you're going to have a "floppy" or flaccid bladder. In this situation, you can't feel when your bladder is full.

There are two problems with a "floppy" or flaccid bladder. The first is the risk of your bladder overstretching from getting filled beyond its normal capacity. The second is the risk of urine backing up into your kidneys once your bladder has overfilled.

What if you have a "spastic" bladder? This is also called having a reflex bladder. If your injury is above T12, you will have this condition or a variation of it. This situation is like your pre-potty training days. When your bladder is full, it empties when it wants to. It may also leak urine instead of getting full. "Fun," huh?

Another variation of the "spastic" or reflex bladder is when the bladder is full, but the sphincter muscles don't get the message from the brain at the same time the bladder is trying to empty. Doctors have a fancy word for this. It is called dyssynergia.

People with a spinal cord injury with either type of bladder problem are more likely to have urinary tract infections, bladder stones, kidney stones, urinary debris, and just slightly more likely than the general public to develop bladder cancer. If urinary debris clump together they become kidney stones or bladder stones.[2] Unclumped, they remain as debris.

Don't despair. There are ways to cope with spinal cord injury bladder problems. Many quadriplegics and paraplegics lead full, busy lives including working full- or part-time. Many advances in bladder management after a spinal cord injury have been made in recent years.

You've got one of two problems after a spinal cord injury: you either need to get the urine out of your bladder and can't. Or you need to keep the urine from coming out of your bladder when you don't want it to.

Developments in the field of plastics have made bladder management much easier today than it was immediately after World War II. Bladder management often uses a catheter. A catheter is a tube that is inserted into a body cavity, duct, or vessel.[3] In bladder management the catheter is a plastic tube inserted into the bladder through the urethra. Catheters come in various sizes.

A catheter can be inserted into the bladder and remain there. It drains the bladder constantly so the bladder is never full. This is called a Foley or Suprapubic Catheter. It is a Foley Catheter if it is inserted into the urethra (the opening leading into the bladder from the outside) and a Suprapubic Catheter if it is permanently inserted through the abdomen.[4]

External catheters are available for males and females. The anatomy of males makes the design of external catheters much easier. Female external catheters exist but are not as "foolproof" as the male versions for reasons of the design of the anatomy itself. Catheters for either sex require a prescription from a doctor because the exact size of the catheter must be determined to fit the individual. They are sized by circumference of the plastic tube under the French system. You may hear the term French Catheter in bladder management.

Males wear either condom catheters ("Texas condoms") or an External Continence Device (ECD). Both systems use a collection bag, typically worn on the leg. Without getting embarrassingly technical, condom catheters cover more "male territory" than ECDs.

Female external catheters are called Female Urinary Pouches. They are typically used in situations where the person is confined to bed. It is more difficult to keep a Female Urinary Pouch attached to the body, so they are not recommended for active females. [5]

External catheters are also marketed for healthy men and women by BioRelief under the names Stadium Pal and Stadium Gal. They are intended for use at sporting events, Mardi Gras, long road trips, flying in small planes, and other such situations where restrooms are not readily available.[6]

Adult diapers are another option for bladder management. These do not require a prescription, and are readily available in discount stores, buying club stores, supermarkets, and drug stores in the United States.

Intermittent Catheterization is another option for bladder management. With intermittent catheterization. a person inserts a catheter into his or her bladder to drain the urine at set intervals during the day to prevent the bladder from either becoming full or leaking urine. The catheter does not stay in the bladder between catheterization sessions.

There are also methods to stimulate bladder emptying. The Crede method involves manually pressing down on the bladder. Tapping involves tapping the area over the bladder with fingertips or the side of the hand, lightly and repeatedly, to stimulate appropriate muscle contractions and urination. The Valsalva method involves increasing pressure inside the abdomen by bearing down as if you were going to have a bowel movement. Anal or Rectal Stretch involves using an abdominal corset and the Valsalva.[4]

There are also surgical procedures for more complicated problems, but I am not going to discuss them in this chapter.

One advance in the area of bladder management has been the development of prescription drugs to aid in bladder management. These drugs were originally developed for urinary management in men with prostate problems, but are commonly used in spinal cord bladder management as well. The drugs used are: Cardura®, Flomax®, Hytrin®, Minipress®, and Uroxatral®.[7]

Learning tools exist for those new to intermittent catheterization. The first is Shadow Buddies. These are male and female dolls used to train children and adults in self-catheterization.[8] The second learning tool is for females to learn the proper positioning of the intermittent catheter. This is because female anatomy is not as convenient as male anatomy for some urinary issues. This tool is called Asta-Cath. It is available by prescription only.[9]

Intermittent catheterization can be performed by an individual on him- or herself if he/she has sufficient coordination. A complete spinal cord injury survivor would not be able to self-catheterize. Catheterization can also be performed by a spouse, family member, friend, or caregiver.

Anyone needing to perform a catheterization must be properly taught in sterile procedure to avoid introducing germs into the urinary system unnecessarily. The use of sterile gloves is necessary. It is also vital to sterilize the area around the urethra to avoid unnecessary bacteria. Intermittent catheterization can be performed with drainage into a leg bag, a toilet, an empty two-liter soda bottle, a portable urinal, or any other appropriate container.

Here are two more scenarios. The first is where you can empty your bladder normally with the use of medication, but you have difficulty getting up from a sitting position and sitting down from a standing position. The second is that you cannot empty your bladder completely in a sitting position. You need to be standing to be able to empty your bladder.

If you are male and have either of the above problems, then a portable urinal is an option for you. For both the above scenarios if you are female, you many need either a portable urinal or a Female Urinary Director (FUD). Female Urinary Directors were originally developed for women who like to spend time out of doors with hobbies such as camping or hiking and for women during long flights in small aircraft. Female members of the military have also adopted the use of FUDs. Female Urinary Directors are available in both disposable and non-disposable form. See the Resources chapter for more information.

You may be embarrassed at first to discuss your urinary issues with medical professionals, family members, friends, paid caregivers, or support group members. You will get over the embarrassment as time goes on. It is very important to consult medical professionals when you have kidney and bladder problems. Infections can be very serious. Do not hesitate to get emergency care if you use a permanent catheter, and it becomes blocked.

Your urinary health is very important to your continue good health. Don't jeopardize your health because of embarrassment.

70

Spasticity After a Spinal Cord Injury

These feet which kick furiously, legs which bend in to protect a tender stomach. This flesh which is but a mass of spasms, starts, and shakes—
Dr. Frederick Leboyer

Does anyone remember the cartoon where Wile E. Coyote swallowed a whole bottle of Earthquake Pills?)—
"BRIGHTSIDE", NSCIA Discussion Forum

Spasticity is something that you and your family member(s) may already be familiar with by the time you have reached this chapter. It would be nice if it were something only experienced by a small percentage of spinal cord injury survivors. But medical science has not reached that point yet.

In this chapter I'm going to talk about what spasticity is and the most common forms of treatment. Wikipedia has this to say about spasticity:

> Spasticity is a disorder of the body's motor system in which certain muscles are continuously contracted. This contraction causes stiffness or tightness of the muscles and may interfere with gait [walking], movement, and speech. The person with the spastic muscles may or may not feel it, know about or want to do something about it. The human motor system is not always linked with the sensory systems, nor the voluntary-muscle systems.
>
> Spasticity is usually caused by damage to the portion of the brain or spinal cord that controls voluntary movement. Symptoms may include hypertonia (increased muscle tone), clonus (a series of rapid muscle contractions), exaggerated deep tendon reflexes [in plain English, you kick really hard when the doctor taps your knee with a rubber mallet], muscle spasms, scissoring (involuntary crossing of the legs), and fixed joints. The degree of spasticity varies

> from mild muscle stiffness to severe, painful, and uncontrollable muscle spasms.
>
> The condition can interfere with rehabilitation in patients.… and often interferes with daily activities. Over the years, it may increase in its effect, so more severe treatments may be needed later. Cold weather and fatigue can trigger spasms more severely than other times. Multi-tasking (such as walking, talking, eating and other activities) can also trigger more severe spasticity.[1]

Spasticity is only supposed to occur in people with a spinal cord injury above a T10 level.[2] I have found that this is untrue in real life. I know paraplegics with injuries below T12 that suffer from spasticity.

Spasticity can also cause unusual posturing [tendency to assume a body position] or holding a shoulder, arm, wrist, and [or] finger at an abnormal angle.[3] I have heard of severe cases of spasticity resulting in individuals being unable to move from a fetal position.

I wanted to provide an explanation in simple English about the causes of spasticity. I found that doctors don't have a good understanding of what specifically goes wrong to cause spasticity. I also found that the simplest explanation was far too complicated for me to understand completely.

I can briefly summarize that damage occurs to the spinal cord. Days to weeks later spasticity evolves. Depending on the level of injury to the cord determines how long it takes for spasticity to develop. At this point I would have liked to have been able to say "if your injury is between levels x and y, it takes a days for spasticity to develop," and "if your injury is between levels y and z, it takes b weeks for spasticity to develop." I could not find this information.[4]

Spasms can be caused by a variety of different medical conditions. They can be caused by injury to the neurological system or by disease. Spasticity from spinal cord injury is different from spasticity from other causes. In spinal cord injury, the spasms more typically cause body parts to contract and be drawn toward the body. In other types of spasticity, the spasms more typically cause body parts to be pushed away from the body.[5]

This is not to say that spinal cord injury survivors don't have extensor spasms. Anybody who has ever been thrown out of a wheelchair by his or her legs straightening and becoming rigid knows this is true.[6]

All that being said, spinal cord spasms do serve some beneficial functions. Perhaps the beneficial functions are the reason they exist. Spasticity can help with:

1. Walking

2. Standing
3. Transferring (stand pivot transfers)
4. Maintaining muscle bulk
5. May help prevent blood clots
6. May prevent pressure sore formation over joints[7]

In addition, spinal cord spasms may also function as an "early warning system." Spasms may help alert a person to medical problems that a person might otherwise not be aware of. Bladder and kidney infections can increase spasms. Pressure sores can increase spasms. Pain can increase spasms.[8 9] I have also had spasms warn me that I was ill when I didn't know it.

Exercise can also be useful in preventing spasms. Regular range of motion exercises performed on a daily basis are often useful.[10]

Various options exist for the temporary treatment of spinal cord spasms. There are five commonly used medications for treating spasticity: Diazepam (Valium®), Dantrolene (Dantrium®), Baclofen (Lioresal®), Tizanidine (Zanaflex®), and Gabapentin (Neurontin®).[11]

Baclofen is probably the most widely used drug and the one most familiar to spinal cord injurees. It is a versatile treatment because it comes in pill form or it can be administered through the use of an implanted pump. Baclofen, as with any prescription medication, has side effects. The use of the implanted pump is supposed to reduce the side effects because it delivers a small dose of the medicine directly to the spinal cord.[12]

The potential advantages of the pump are claimed to be:

> 1. Effectively reduces spasticity and involuntary spasms, promoting a more active lifestyle, better sleep, and reduced need for oral medication.
> 2. Continuously delivers baclofen [*sic*] in small doses directly to the intraspinal fluid, increasing the therapeutic benefits and causing fewer and less severe side effects than that seen with oral medication.
> 3. Can be individually adjusted to allow infusion rates that vary over a 24-hour [*sic*] period. It can be turned on or off or programmed to infuse different levels of medication through the day, depending on your needs. For example, people who find their spasticity helpful in maintaining leg extension for standing or walking can have a lower infusion rate during the day.
> 4. Can be turned off if spasticity reduction has show no benefits.[13]

The side effects of Baclofen are dizziness, drowsiness, headache, nausea, and weakness. Problems with the infusion pump can cause either overdose or sudden withdrawal of baclofen [*sic*].[14]

I found one article on the Internet by a mother whose son had the Baclofen pump implanted who advises people considering the pump implant to proceed with caution. Her son only had improvement with his spasticity for two months (he is not an SCI survivor, but instead has a neurological disease). She found out the pump is actually more effective with the problem of ridigity.[15]

Rigidity is an increase in muscle tone, leading to a resistance to passive movement throughout the range of motion.[16] It means the muscles contract to the point where they cannot be moved voluntarily.

Her son with the implanted pump ended up having to have surgery to repair the pump a few months after it was implanted. When his pump was refilled, the dosage was set wrong and he overdosed on Baclofen. He went into cardiac arrest and stopped breathing. His parents chose the option of letting the Baclofen gradually work its way out of his system. It seems the antidote had a significant risk of heart attack.[17]

Another treatment option is to temporarily paralyze the muscles that spasm or the nerves causing the spasm. This is done through chemical nerve blocks.[18] The most common chemical used is a variation of the bacteria that causes botulism, an often fatal type of infection found in food. The chemically altered substance is completely safe. This product is marketed under the name BOTOX®.[19] The downsides to BOTOX® are the cost and its limited duration of effectiveness of four to six months.[20]

The treatment of last resort for spasticity is to surgically cut the nerves, which are causing the spasticity. It permanently eliminates all reflexes, including those that are helpful.[21]

Another drug that is reputed to have beneficial effects on spasticity is marijuana.[22] Here we have the problem that marijuana is still illegal under federal law. Twelve states, however, have legalized marijuana for medical use. These states are: Alaska, California, Colorado, Hawaii, Maine, Maryland, Montana, Nevada, New Mexico, Oregon, Rhode Island, Vermont, and Washington.[23]

I am neither recommending nor arguing against the use of marijuana for treatment of spasticity. This is a decision that each individual must make for him- or herself; depending upon effectiveness of prescription medication for spasticity treatment, and the state in which the individual lives.

Researchers at the University of Florida have made a discovery about spasticity by studying rats with spinal cord injuries. A little humor here before I go on. I assume that researchers induced the spinal cord injuries in the rats. The article did not mention how the rats sustained their spinal cord injuries. I get this mental image of these rats driving tiny little cars and having auto accidents, thus suffering spinal cord injuries. Or images of rats diving into shallow pools and being injured. You get the idea.

Anyway, the researchers discovered that spasticity set in during the first week after the rats' injuries. It improved somewhat during the second and third weeks. It became permanent in the fourth week. They are investigating methods of treatment to be used during the second and third weeks after injury in humans when spasticity improves for a brief period of time.[24]

Hopefully, with the advances in modern medicine, spasticity will soon be a thing of the past for spinal cord injury survivors.

71

Chronic Dizziness After a Spinal Cord Injury

Dizzy, I'm so dizzy my head is spinning
Like a whirlpool it never ends—
"Dizzy" by Tommy Roe

This is a symptom after a spinal cord injury that is rarely discussed. It is something I don't want to spend a lot of time on but I felt it should be mentioned briefly. I have suffered from chronic dizziness since my accident. The doctors are unsure if it is a result of my closed head injury or the spinal cord injury or both.

I'm going to give you a short explanation of dizziness. It has three categories. The first is called vertigo. You may have heard of vertigo. Vertigo is the feeling that either you or your surroundings are spinning. This is what I have. The other two types of dizziness are syncope and nonsyncope nonvertigo. Syncope is the second type. It is basically fainting. It includes a brief loss of consciousness or by dimmed vision, feeling uncoordinated, confused, and lightheaded. Syncope happens when you stand up too fast. Syncope is related to the loss of blood flow to the brain. If you have nonsyncope nonvertigo dizziness, you have the problem that you cannot keep your balance.[1]

You can have dizziness for minutes, hours, days, or weeks. How long depends on what is causing the dizziness. Your brain, your eyes, and your inner ear are all involved in the process of keeping your balance. Damage to your autonomic nervous system can cause dizziness. This is the part of your nervous system that controls involuntary functions like breathing.[2]

Your doctor may refer you to an ear, nose, and throat specialist (ENT) to determine what is causing your dizziness. Your ENT may order a hearing test to make sure your hearing is normal for your age.

There are several standard tests to determine the cause of dizziness. If your doctor orders these tests, be sure to check with your medical insurance, Medicare, or Medicaid in advance because not all these tests are covered. These tests are called vestibular tests. They test the function of your inner ear to see if it is the cause of your dizziness.[3]

Depending on your age, some or all of your dizziness may be caused by a disorder with a long and complicated name, Benign Paroxysmal Positional Vertigo (BPPV). I'm not sure which is worse, having it or trying to say it. The older you are, the more likely you are to have BPPV. I'll give you a quick translation on this disorder. You have fluid in your inner ear, which controls your balance. Inside this fluid are little tiny rocks. If the rocks get knocked into a part of the ear where they don't belong, you get dizzy.

There is a very effective treatment that can be done in a trained therapist's office, which involves putting you in certain specific positions to move the rocks that are out of place into a location in your ear where they will not signal misinformation to the brain. This therapy is not commonly known in the United States.[4] I have had it performed, and it was very effective for me. I have a friend without a spinal cord injury who also found the treatment very effective.

Once your ENT has ruled out a disorder or disease of the inner ear, problems with blood flow to the brain (through other tests), and BPPV, by process of elimination, your dizziness is likely being caused by damage to your involuntary nervous system. I still had dizziness after the BPPV treatment, so my ENT concluded it was due to damage of the nervous system.

One treatment for nervous system dizziness is a very low dose of Desyrel® (Amitriptyline) daily. The dose is actually lower than what would be prescribed for depression, which puzzles the doctors. At this dosage, the medicine should theoretically have no effect. But it works to control dizziness.

This drug should not be given to anyone under eighteen. A teenage patient being given this medicine should be monitored very closely for suicidal tendencies.[5]

Hopefully, dizziness is not a symptom you will have to deal with after a spinal cord injury, or from any other cause.

72

Transitional Syndrome aka Adjacent Segment Disease

The human body is the only machine for which there are no spare parts.—
Hermann M. Biggs

This is a very difficult chapter for me emotionally. I have experienced what I am going to discuss in this chapter. If I had known what I know now about possible complications from spinal fusions, I would have made many decisions differently than the way I made them at the time.

Let me start by saying spinal fusion surgery has become so common that it is now performed on an outpatient basis in most cases. Most people have one or two discs fused and recover quite nicely. This is not always the case.

"There can be no question but that rigid instrumented spine fusion can be, for the right patient, a truly beneficial treatment" [*sic*] says an article I found on the Internet.[1] The article continues in fancy doctor language to say that putting a rigid structure into what was once a flexible structure puts extreme stress on the areas adjacent to the spinal fusion.

So what ends up happening in some people is the soft discs adjacent to the fusion deteriorate, and eventually need to be fused as well. They can deteriorate upward from the fusion or downward from the fusion. I imagine they can deteriorate both ways as well at the same time.

There are basically three types of spinal cord injury patients with fusions. There is what is called a Type A transition zone patient. This patient has no pre-existing preoperative disease at the level, which ultimately degenerated. There is the Type B transition zone patient. These are people with pre-existing degenerative disease at the level, which ultimately failed adjacent to the fusion. Finally you have the Type C transition zone patient. These people develop the transition zone problem as the result of damage during the fusion surgery to adjacent bony vertebrae or soft discs.[2] So basically either the adjacent soft discs can fail or the bony vertebrae can break.

Let me change subjects briefly here, and explain something before I go on. If you are going to have a surgical procedure of any kind, the physician and hospital will require you to sign an informed consent form. This is a legal document. You must have an appropriate state of mind and the mental ability to be able to understand the risks involved in the procedure you are about to have. You cannot sign any kind of legal document if you are under the influence of alcohol or drugs, legal or illegal. If you have been given the initial medication before surgery to sedate you, but you are still conscious, a family member will have to sign for you.

Basically it means that you understand that some things can go wrong during an operation and you are still agreeing to have the operation. If one of the things that can go wrong does go wrong, then the doctor and the hospital are not legally liable.

According to one author, "Failure of a surgeon to explain to the patient the possibility of a transitional syndrome developing means that the surgeon has not provided the patient with adequate informed consent."[3]I was not told about transitional syndrome before my first operation, which consisted of a double disc fusion.

One article I found states that "more than twenty five percent of patients will develop adjacent segment disease of the cervical spine within ten years of anterior cervical fusion procedures."[4]

73

Range of Motion After Neck Disc Fusion

Spinnin' a rope is fun,
if your neck ain't in it.—
Will Rogers

This is a common concern of patients before they undergo surgery after their accident. Let's start with some basics about the function of a normal neck. Most of the information in this chapter is for people who will be having disc fusion surgery on an out-patient basis. Some of the information will also apply to people who have emergency surgery.

Picture a circle. A circle is 360 degrees. If you are a cartoon character and something outrageous happens to you, your neck spins all the way around 360 degrees. The normal range of motion for a neck is seven degrees on average.[1]

Now let's talk about the up and down motion of your neck. Like when you nod your head. You have a range of motion, on average, moving your head up and down of seven degrees.[2]

Let's assume you have had a spinal cord injury in the neck at one level. Your range of motion is no longer normal. This is as a result of muscle spasms and pain. You have spinal disc fusion surgery on one level. You will recover most of your normal range of motion because you are no longer having muscle spasms and pain. The range of motion you lose from having one level fused is equivalent to the range of motion you lost from the muscle spasms and pain, more or less.[3]

Now let's assume you have had a spinal cord injury in the neck at two levels. You will lose a little more motion than if you had had a fusion at one level. I can talk about this from personal experience. My first fusion was at two levels. I lost quite a bit of range of motion.

What if you have had a spinal cord injury in the neck at three levels? You will really start feeling stiff in your neck. I can attest to that. And you will lose more range of motion. At four levels you are pretty much solid, and have far less than normal range of motion. Boy, does my neck feel stiff and immobile now. I was one of the unlucky twenty five percent plus of people who developed Transitional Syndrome.

Let me give you some real life examples of things I don't do well anymore because I can't look up, down or sideways well anymore. I don't go to air shows because I can't look up. I can't gargle well. I don't look at the stars anymore. Flying kites is out. I don't go to fireworks shows anymore. Driving is challenging because of the lack of range of motion to both sides. Especially when trying to merge. I had to be very particular in buying a car because I needed one with lots of window area to compensate for the lack of motion in my neck. In case you are curious I drive a 2000 Subaru Forester. I can also get in it without having to climb.

What about the success rate of this particular surgery? This may be a concern for you and your family (or you and the patient in your family). You will be happy to know that disc fusion surgery in the neck has one of the highest success rates in medicine. One study found that more than eighty-five percent of the patients studied had their pain levels improve to the point where they had no pain. If you include all the functional tests as well as the level of pain indicators to determine success rate after surgery, two years after surgery more than sixty-eight percent of the patients studied were deemed successful.[4]

You may be curious about your limitations immediately after surgery. You may be placed in either a soft neck collar or a hard rigid neck collar for a period of days, weeks or months. This will depend upon your level of injury, the type of fusion you have, your doctor's preferences, whether or not you smoke, and/or have soft bones, and perhaps other factors. If your situation is such that you can still drive, you will not be permitted to drive for a period of time after surgery. You may also have lifting restrictions.

After my first surgery, I was placed in a soft neck collar. I had to wear the collar twenty four hours a day for the first month except when bathing or showering. I was not allowed to drive for the first month. After the first month, I was instructed to wear the collar while I was driving for the next three months. After my second and third surgeries, I did not have to wear a neck collar. I was not allowed to drive for one week after each surgery.

I would like to explain to you how your neck will feel different after the surgery, but it is very difficult to put the difference into words. It does feel stiffer. It feels very different, though. Almost like it is being stretched. My neurosurgeon for the second and third surgeries built me some slack into my neck since I have a narrow spinal canal. I am now about an inch taller than I was before my accident.

Another area of concern about the surgery is the effect it will have on your vocal cords. This is only an issue if your surgeon goes in from the front of your neck. Depending on your injury and the surgery that needs to be done, your surgeon may go in through the back of your neck.

I was told that it is advisable for the surgeon to go in on the left side of the neck because it reduces the risk of damage to the vocal cords. They have to be moved out of the way to perform the disc fusion surgery. My first neurosurgeon went in on the right side of my neck. My second neurosurgeon went in on the left side of my neck, and then reused the incision for the third surgery.

After being moved out of the way three times, my vocal cords have sustained some damage. I can no longer talk as loudly as I could before the surgery. I used to be one of these people who hummed music all the time. I can no longer hum. This is a small price to pay for being alive.

You may be curious how long you will be in the hospital after your surgery. This depends on your degree of injury. Disc fusion surgery in the neck at more common levels of injury (C5/6 and C6/7) is actually done now as outpatient surgery. Surgery at level C4 is also done as outpatient surgery. Surgery at level C3, which controls breathing, is done with an overnight stay in the hospital to make sure the spinal cord was not damaged during surgery. The fear is the patient will stop breathing if the cord has been damaged at this level. Or you may have a stay of a few days. Multiple-level fusions may also require an overnight stay in the hospital. If you include time in the hospital for recovery from surgery and for rehabilitation, your hospital stay may be months long.

I found an article that discusses range of motion after cervical fusion. The article states that there is very little scientific evidence that a doctor can provide a patient to predict how much range of motion the patient will lose.[5]

The study mentioned in the previous paragraph found that patients regained significant ranges of motion after fusion surgery, but not enough to match the range of motion shown by uninjured individuals.[6] The study also found that there was no relationship between the number of levels fused and the return of range of motion.[7]

Unfortunately, the above study did not answer the question of what happened to the difference in the range of motion seen by a healthy person and the range of motion seen by a fused cervical spinal cord injuree.[8]

I e-mailed the lead author of the article cited in Note eight of the Endnotes to inquire about "where the range of motion went." He indicated he and his co-authors believe the uppermost discs (occiput, C1, and C2) take the range of motion once the cervical discs have been fused.[9]

I do miss the range of motion in my neck, and way it doesn't feel like a "normal" neck anymore.

74

Changes in Sensation After a Spinal Cord Injury

It is in moments of illness that we are compelled to
recognize that we live not alone but chained to a
creature of a different kingdom, whole worlds apart,
who has no knowledge of us and by whom it is
impossible to make ourselves understood:
our body.—
Marcel Proust

I thought this was going to be an easy chapter to write. Short and basic about how a spinal cord injury affects sensations like touch. But when I started researching the chapter, I found very little material on the subject. What little I did find was written in "doctorese."

I found out that the human body is a whole lot more complicated than I thought. We as human beings do things in everyday life that we totally take for granted. We can tell if we are standing up, sitting down, or bending over. We can feel people touching us. We can tell if something is hard or soft. Warm or cold. We know where our arms and legs are relative to each other and to everything else. Until a spinal cord injury.

Changes in sensation are different, of course, between a complete and an incomplete injury. This is another one of those things where there are as many variations as there are people with spinal cord injuries. The odds of a person having exactly the same limitations as another person with a spinal cord injury are pretty low. It reminds me of the fact that no two fingerprints are the same.

Your brain and your inner ear are responsible for receiving the information being transmitted from the rest of the body about body parts positions, sensations of standing, sitting, moving, etc. If your spinal cord is damaged, the information cannot get from the body parts to the brain and inner ear properly.[1]

The list below summarizes what may change after a spinal cord injury. These abilities may be completely lost, or they may be altered from what would be normal.

1. Sense of balance
2. Ability to determine where a particular body part is in space
3. Sensation that a particular body part has moved
4. Sense of feeling pressure on the skin
5. Sense of skin temperature
6. Sense of temperature of an external stimulus (is the shower water hot or cold?)
7. Sense of texture of an external stimulus (is something hard or soft, rough or smooth?)
8. Feeling touch or pressure when none is present
9. Ability to feel vibration
10. Ability to feel pain when a painful stimulus is actually present
11. Feeling pain when no painful stimulus is present
12. Feeling pain in a location other than where the painful stimulus is present (transferred or referred pain)[2]

I want to talk more about the ability to tell where a particular body part is in space. I found a study done in Australia that talked about people with spinal cord injuries having problems telling where their body parts were within twenty-four hours of the injury. The study included this in a category called "complex sensations."

Some of the injured people thought their limbs were still in the position they were in when the spinal cord injury happened. For example, someone thinking their legs are up in the air when their legs are actually lying straight on an examination table.

The sensations seem to be unrelated to level of injury or type of cord syndrome. They seem to be related to whether the injury is complete or incomplete, with "complex sensations" being more common in people with complete injuries.[3]

Incomplete injuries can be a challenge to describe when it comes to changes in sensation. Some people experience feeling in the damaged parts of their bodies similar to the feeling when you have been resting on your hand or leg too long. You cut off the blood flow to it and it "goes to sleep." The "pins and needles" feeling. They feel like that all the time.

Other people have normal sensation except for temperature or touch sensation. Sometimes it is impossible to describe the sensation felt in the damaged parts of the body. The sensations are just *different.*

Let me give you some actual examples. My bed has a very nice mattress on it. I know the mattress is soft. But there are nights I feel like I am lying on a block of concrete. I cannot process the sensation properly of the softness of the mattress.

Sometimes different spots on my feet will go completely numb. I cannot feel touch in the numb spot at all. And the spots that are numb change location with each occurrence.

I only have partial sensation in my feet. I get calluses on my feet. I file them with one of those callous files you buy in a discount store. I cannot feel the file on my foot. It is probably not the best idea in the world for me to file the calluses because I can remove healthy skin and not know it. I would be much smarter to use moisturizing cream to soften the calluses.

I cannot reliably judge temperature below my waist. Sometimes I get into a bathtub of warm water and if the temperature of the water is close to body temperature, I cannot feel the water. I cannot sense the temperature. This is a very strange feeling. It is sort of like sitting in an empty bathtub, but you don't feel the cold temperature of the tub itself or the air on your legs.

I have problems with determining hot and cold. I have trouble with texture sensations on my legs.

Sometimes I can't feel anything below the waist. At times when the signal is not going through my spinal cord properly.

Not being able to accurate judge temperature can be a dangerous problem to have, especially when it comes to being able to sense temperature. If you cannot accurately sense temperature, don't use things like massaging foot baths you fill with hot water. Always have someone else check the temperature of anything your skin comes in contact with (shower water, for example) if there is a risk of you being burned or even frozen.

My skin is also becoming hypersensitive to stimulus. If a hair from my head has fallen onto my arm, I have to immediately get it off. I can no longer ignore it.

75

Claw Hand After a Spinal Cord Injury

Is he alone who has courage on his right hand and faith on his left hand?—
Charles Lindbergh

You may have seen a spinal cord injury survivor with his or her hands clenched in a claw position. This is known as claw hand deformity. People with medical issues other than a spinal cord injury can have claw hand. I have seen people with incomplete spinal cord injuries with this condition. I am assuming that people with complete spinal cord injuries can also have this condition.

The medical explanation for claw hand is so complicated I'm not sure I completely understand it. I'm not going to reproduce it here. For the medical professional who wants to learn more about claw hand, I suggest consulting the *Wheeless' Textbook of Orthopedics* online.[1]

In a claw hand deformity, the palms of the hands flatten and the fingers curve. All five fingers (assuming you have all five fingers) on the hand can curve or fewer than five fingers can do so. It depends on the injury or disease. There is weakness of the hand so that the soft tissues that control hand movement cannot open the fingers.

Surgery can be performed to correct claw hand deformity if the person desires.[2] I assume the benefits seen after surgery depend on the degree of injury itself.

76

Dental Care After a Spinal Cord Injury

You don't have to brush your teeth—
just the ones you want to keep.
Author Unknown

"Carolyn, have you lost your mind? I've got a spinal cord injury, and you want to talk about going to the dentist? Don't I have enough problems as it is?"

I have been accused of having lost my mind many times. But not when it comes to going to the dentist. I do so religiously (yes I do pray beforehand that I won't have a cavity). I mean I go to the dentist without fail every three months and have my teeth cleaned.

I discussed life expectancy after a spinal cord injury in a previous chapter. In this chapter I am going to provide information on another way you can improve your life expectancy.

"Ok, Carolyn, you've got my attention. Why is going to the dentist so darn important?"

Medical research in the last few years has come up with an interesting connection. People who have periodontal disease (gum disease to the rest of us) are at greater risk to have heart disease/heart attacks (dentists have to have fancy words too, don't they?).[1 2] If you already have a heart condition, going to the dentist becomes even more important for you.

Going to the dentist presents more of a challenge for individuals with a spinal cord injury for reasons beyond just the cost. The dentist's parking lot must have accessible parking spaces. There must be curb cutoffs for individuals in wheelchairs. The dentist's office must be accessible in the following areas:

1. Walkways, sidewalks, and parking facilities
2. Entrance ramps, handrails, hallways, and elevators

3. Door width and threshold height, door pressure or ease of opening
4. Adequate space around door to maneuver a wheelchair, and elevator accessibility
5. Floor surface, carpets, and rugs
6. Telephone facilities
7. Drinking fountains
8. Restroom facilities
9. Reception room design, furniture style, and lighting
10. Operatory design to allow for wheelchair transfer or in-wheelchair treatment[3]

An individual with a high-level spinal cord injury may need dental work to be performed in a hospital for closer monitoring of his or her physical condition. There may be additional medical personnel needed. There may need to be rapid evacuation of fluids in the mouth during treatment. There may need to be special monitoring of the person's blood pressure or other specific types of monitoring, especially if the person has breathing problems. [4]

For people with lower level spinal cord injuries, generally the only challenge faced in going to a dentist beyond the cost is the accessibility issue. For any patient with a bowel and bladder program, these programs should be carried out before going to a dentist appointment. [5]

Other concerns for dental visits are the transfer procedure from the person's wheelchair to the dental chair if the person is not going to be treated while in a wheelchair, the danger of pressure sore development while in the dental chair, the risk of blood clots developing while in the dental chair, and the need for premedication with antibiotics for patients with pre-existing heart problems. Individuals with blood clotting disorders may also need special considerations. [6]

Dental care for a person with a spinal cord injury should be closely coordinated with other relevant health care providers for the individual. The patient should always bring a list of prescription medications to every dentist appointment and alert the dentist to any pre-existing medical conditions. [7]

If you are unable to brush your teeth or floss between your teeth, your paid caregiver or a family member may be able to do so for you.

As for the cost of visiting a dentist, some states have programs to facilitate dental care for disabled individuals. Check with your local Department of Health or equivalent state agency for further information.

77

Eye Care After a Spinal Cord Injury

No one ever injured his eyesight by looking on the bright side of things—
Anonymous

Dealing with your eyesight is a topic I have rarely seen discussed in relation to a spinal cord injury. I don't have pages and pages to say about it. But there are a few things I want to bring to your attention.

First, if you or your family member has been diagnosed with a closed head injury in addition to the spinal cord injury, you may find your eyesight has changed. A visit to your eye care professional is advisable.

If you wore glasses or contacts before your accident (or if your family member wore glasses or contacts before his or her accident), there are a few bits of information that may be useful to you.

The next bit of information is a "no-brainer." If your injury is in the neck, then you will have limited or no use of arms, hands, or fingers. You will not be able to insert and remove your own contact lenses. You may be unable to pick up and put on your glasses as well.

Another tidbit of information for you. If you are taking muscle relaxants and/or painkillers, they may cause your eyesight to be blurry. Taking muscle relaxants and/or painkillers may also make it impossible for you to continue wearing your contacts. This is because your eyes cannot focus as they would normally, which makes wearing contacts impossible. This is what my eye doctor told me.

There is some good news for quadriplegics who wear glasses or contacts. A program called Focus On Independence was started in 2006 in which eye surgeons provide LASIK (vision correction surgery) to quadriplegics at no cost. A person must be at least eighteen years old to qualify for the program. He or she must have had a traumatic spinal cord injury. Finally, he or she must have lost use of their hands and/or arms so that putting on or taking off glasses or contacts is difficult or impossible.

The Focus On Independence program is nationwide. The goal of the program is to have the surgery available within a hundred miles of anyone who needs it. So far seven doctors across the country have volunteered their time. The program is headquartered in Los Angeles. For more information call The Maloney Vision Institute at 1-877-EYESIGHT or 1-310-208-3937 or e-mail focus@maloneyvision.com.[1 2]

78

Exercise After a Spinal Cord Injury

I do not try to dance better than anyone else.
I only try to dance better than myself.—
Mikhail Baryshnikov

"I didn't want to exercise *before* my spinal cord injury. *Now* you're telling me I need to be exercising *after* a spinal cord injury?"

I am urging you to exercise regularly. Because a spinal cord injury can reduce your lifespan, even if slightly; you need to do anything you can to put those years back into your life.

No matter what your level or degree of spinal cord injury, there is a way for you to exercise. Even if you just do breathing exercises.

Research shows that exercise after a spinal cord injury reduces the risk of urinary tract infection, pressure sores, and respiratory illnesses.[1]

But let's not stop there. Spasticity, weight gain, and chronic pain can all be positively affected by exercise and being physically active. Want a way to improve your ability to do everyday tasks? Exercise will help improve your strength and endurance.... [1]

"Oh, but Carolyn, I *hate* exercising! It's so boring!" I understand completely. On the bright side, you only need to exercise twenty to thirty minutes a day *every other day* to see health benefits. More exercise means increased benefits.[2]

Exercising on a regular basis is especially important if you have lung problems or asthma.

A field I expect to see grow in the next few years is personal training for people with disabilities. Especially for people with spinal cord injuries. If you do consult a personal trainer or rehabilitation therapist, make sure that person is experienced in dealing with spinal cord injuries. Proper certification as a therapist or trainer is very important, because a therapist or trainer who does not know what he/she is doing can seriously injure someone.

Because so many options exist for exercising with a spinal cord injury, I have listed further information in the Resources chapter rather than going into additional information in this chapter.

79

Prescription Medication After a Spinal Cord Injury

Drugs are not always necessary, but
belief in recovery always is.—
Angel Cordero Jr.

Does your pharmacist know you on a first name basis? Do you "rattle when you roll" down the street in your wheelchair? Or do you prefer to avoid prescription medications at all costs?

As you already know, your body no longer works properly after a spinal cord injury. It is often necessary for a spinal cord injury survivor to take prescription medication to make organ systems function the way they should.

In my opinion there are three different types of prescription medication:

1. "Life Necessity Emergency" prescriptions. These are medications such as stimulant pens to be used after insect stings and asthma inhalers
2. "Bodily Function" prescriptions. These are medications that are used to make organ systems function the way they should.
3. "Comfort" prescriptions. These are medications to relieve pain, swelling, spasticity, etc.

I also think prescription medications can be divided into two different categories in another way:

1. "Normal Person" prescriptions. These are medications like cholesterol medication, hormone replacement, sinus medicines, antibiotics etc. These are medications that any normal person without a spinal cord injury would take.

2. "Spinal Cord Injury" prescriptions. These are medications that spinal cord injury survivors take but uninjured people wouldn't need. An example would be strong antispasmodics that are stronger than what a normal person would take in the way of muscle relaxants. Another example would be an implanted Baclofen pump.

Some people with a spinal cord injury only take one or two prescription medications on a daily basis. Others may take twenty different prescription medications on a daily basis. This will vary depending upon what degree and level the injury is. It will also depend upon any medical conditions requiring medication the person had before the spinal cord injury, such as high blood pressure.

Be aware that prescription medications may interact with food, other prescription medications, or alcohol. If in doubt, check with your pharmacist.

There are some individuals who believe that modern medicine does more harm than good. These individuals prefer to seek "old world," natural, or alternative medicine therapies such as acupuncture.[1] Some people use Qigong (coordination of breathing patterns and postures)[2] or meditation.[3] Others use diet.[4] Some believe in laser[5] or laserpuncture therapy.[6] Vibrational healing is an option for some people.[7] Herbal medicines are an option.[8] There is dolphin healing.[9] Electromagnetic healing is a treatment advocated by some.[10] Native American healing exists as does prayer and spiritual healing.[11]

Whatever route you choose, prescription medications, alternative medicine, or both, may you feel better!

Putting Humpty Dumpty Together Again: Rebuilding Your Life

80

Caregivers

Take care of your body. It's the only place you have to live.—
Jim Rohn

Let's assume that you (or a family member) has sustained a spinal cord injury. You or the injured person spends a certain amount of time in the hospital and in rehabilitation. Finally, it is time to come home.

It goes without saying that you (or the injured family member) can no longer perform certain activities that we all take for granted in daily life. This may be bathing, dressing, feeding oneself, driving, moving from one place to another, shopping, housekeeping, or basic bodily functions. If you provide assistance to a family member or friend; even if you are not being paid for the assistance you provide to your family member, you are still a caregiver.[1]

Forty percent of all individuals with a spinal cord injury use some assistance. More than half of those using assistance receive it from a family member. Women are more likely to have a paid caregiver, and men are more likely to have a spouse or parent as a caregiver.[2]

One of the topics often discussed in spinal cord injury support groups is the difficulty of finding good paid caregivers that are well trained and reliable. Paying for a caregiver can be a source of stress for the injured person. Private insurance, long-term care insurance, Medicare, or Medicaid can pay for caregivers. If the accident was work-related then Worker's Compensation may be a source of funding.

Taking care of a person after a spinal cord injury is very stressful. Being the person needing the care is also very stressful. Both the caregiver and the person being cared for will have to adjust to the situation over time. I am unsure which situation is more stressful, having a family member as a caregiver or having a paid caregiver who is initially a stranger.

See the Resources chapter for additional information.

81

Clothing After a Spinal Cord Injury

People seldom notice old clothes, if you wear a big smile—
Lee Mildon

Depending upon your level of spinal cord injury, you may also have to make some changes in your wardrobe after your injury. This is true if you are in a wheelchair, use crutches, or have any limitation you did not have before the accident. This may be as a result of inability to regulate body temperature, pressure sores, feeling confined, or just about any other reason. For example, I can no longer wear jeans in the house in the summer even with the air conditioning on. I get too hot.

The Mississippi State University Extension Service has this to say about clothing for the disabled:

> Approximately 35 [*sic*] million American adults and children are disabled, with some physical or mental impairment that limits their activities. Their basic clothing should be functional, comfortable, and attractive. Clothing can enhance or limit independence and productivity. Tight or confining clothing can impair movement and reduce comfort. It also may cause a feeling of unattractiveness, possibly lowering self-esteem. Many people with disabilities, whether temporary or permanent, have reduced physical strength and dexterity. The more independent they can become, the more psychologically healthy they will feel.[1]

I started thinking about all the considerations that have to go into the design of clothing for the disabled and the list was incredibly long:

1. Adult or child?

2. Wheelchair user?
3. Crutch user?
4. Walker user?
5. Fitted with a cast?
6. Use braces on arm or leg?
7. Does the garment need to be waterproof?
8. Does the garment need to have built-in support slings (for paralyzed or weakened arms)?
9. What types of fasteners should be used?
10. What adaptations need to be made for bodily function adaptability/access?
11. Are there any body symmetry issues?
12. Is the garment a piece of sleepwear or day clothing?
13. Is the garment to be washed in a home washer/dryer setting or an institutional washer/dryer setting?
14. Is the person sensitive to fabric rubbing?
15. Does the person have fabric allergies?
16. Is the person autistic?
17. Is the person normal weight, underweight, or overweight?
18. What is the person's ability to control his or her body temperature to adjust to the environment?

Two main options exist for adaptable clothing: modify existing clothing or purchase new clothing. The Mississippi State Extension Service offers the following tips:

> People in wheelchairs can be uncomfortable with extra fabric or bulk across the lap and underneath them as they sit. The following garment

changes can help:

1. Fold out extra fabric across lap of pants, skirts, or dresses
2. Extend back crotch length at the waist of slacks
3. Shorten tops or jackets and cut out back seat area of skirts
4. Make pant legs wide enough to slip on easily. An alternative is to attach closures (zippers, nylon hooks, or loop fasteners) in sideseam area
5. Ponchos or capes are good for cold weather and are much easier to maneuver than coats. Do not allow edges to get caught in the wheels during movement.[2]

Clothing for people using crutches, either temporarily or permanently, demands careful consideration. The use of crutches can cause excessive rubbing against clothing, especially in the underarm and sleeve areas. Reaching and pulling also cause additional strain on fabrics. Garments tend to lift up from normal body positions when crutches are used. Clothing for crutch users should move with the wearer, and not bind during movement.

With careful planning and a few alterations or changes in design, clothing can promote ease of movement for physically or mentally challenged people. It is desirable to be able to function independently, and clothing can be an important factor in promoting independent living.[3]

Women and teenage girls may find they need to change styles of bras. This is for two reasons. Bras, such as sports bras, that were accessible before the injury may no longer be accessible. Elastic that was comfortable before the injury may be uncomfortable after the injury. This depends upon where you feel referred pain (if you do), and where skin is hypersensitive to pressure, texture, or touch. I have provided a reference in the Resources chapter for a bra that is specifically designed for women with upper body mobility issues.

Unfortunately one of the leading companies for clothing for wheelchair users, Rolli-Moden, has recently gone out of business. The company was a subsidiary of the German company, Manfred Sauer Continence Products. In the ten years that Rolli-Moden was in business in the United States, it failed to break even. This was despite discounts to the normal sale prices from the company's costs of manufacturing the products.

Research is being performed at Northwestern University to assist quadriplegics in being able to control the speed, direction, and velocity of wheelchairs through their clothing. The clothing consists of a shirt with sensors. The sensors monitor the person's shoulder, neck and head movements. The system evaluates what movements the person is best able to make.

The research is being performed with the assumption that motor skills change on a daily basis with a disability. The sensor shirt is tailor-made for each person. Shirt-wearers use a virtual reality environment to learn the skills necessary for safe operation.[4]

See the Resources chapter for disabled clothing companies.

82

Going Back to School After a Spinal Cord Injury

Intellectual growth should commence at birth
and cease only at death—
Albert Einstein

The difference between school and life?
In school, you're taught a lesson and then given a test.
In life, you're given a test that teaches you a lesson.—
Tom Bodett

Whether you've had a spinal cord injury for a year or for twenty years, returning to school is something you may be interested in doing. Many people with spinal cord injuries take advantage of the change in life's direction, and return to school with renewed interest and enthusiasm. They now have a direction that they were lacking before their injury.

If you have your high school diploma then a two-year or four-year college degree may be of interest to you. If you didn't get your high school diploma, then by all means, get your G.E.D (General Education Development test). I have included information in the Resources chapter of this book. If you are in the United States, check with your state agency on education or higher education.

I know several people who were active military when they sustained a spinal cord injury, either from a combat-related accident or through an unrelated accident. They each took the opportunity to go back to school and get a college degree.

If you have been away from school for a long time, don't worry! It is much easier to go back than it ever has been before. Years ago, the only people attending college were young. Now people of all ages are attending college. News broadcasts at graduation time almost always have a story about someone in their

60s, 70s, 80s, or 90s returning to school, and getting a degree. If they can do it, so can you!

"*But I'm disabled,*" you say. No matter. Schools all over the country have become increasingly accommodating of disabled students. Your challenge is to find the financial aid, the school, and the area of study best for you. Some degree programs are even offered completely on-line.

The higher education agency in your state may have information on financial aid available. In addition, you may find you are eligible for various scholarships and/or grants. If you have access to a computer, you can research on the Internet for loans, scholarships, and grants. You may also find that a visit to your local public library turns up information on funding ideas.

Careers & the disABLED magazine has a regular column that highlights various colleges making strides for accommodating disabled students. For example, an article in the Fall 2006 issue profiled Ball State University in Indiana, and Brevard Community College in Florida.

Ball State University was proud to release the results of a study that found a non-disabled Ball State student typically earned a degree in 4.45 years. Students with mobility, hearing, and visual impairments typically took 4.61 years. Students with cognitive or health-related disabilities typically took 4.67 years.

Brevard Community College announced it had been awarded a $47,000 grant to help college students with disabilities participate in community service and service-learning projects.[1]

I was fortunate to find two other excellent articles on disabled students in college. The February 2007 issue of *PN* magazine had an article on disabled students returning to school. I was excited when I first saw the article, which begins a full-page photo of a young man in a wheelchair making his way to class on a college campus. The photo was taken at my alma mater, the University of Illinois at Champaign-Urbana. I remember seeing a lot of wheelchair students on the campus while I was in school there. This was long before my accident.

The article adds useful information that I would not have thought of without it. For example, it mentions two-year college certificates, technical schools, and online education as options for disabled students. It also mentions non-traditional scheduling for courses such as online, evening, and distance learning. Higher education has changed a lot since this "old fart" was in school.

The article contains advice on choosing the school that is best for you. The steps it lists are:

1. Determine the criteria for potential colleges

2. List those that meet your needs (visit http://www.educationquest.org)
3. Gather information on each school
4. Narrow your list to three or four institutions
5. Apply to those that will best meet your needs

The article also mentions that you may face expenses that other students may not have and to be sure and factor these expenses into your financial ad requests. Such needs may include: services for personal use while on campus such as personal-care attendants, special-education equipment related to your disability; and its maintenance, special transportation, medical expenses relating directly to your disability and not covered by insurance.

The article continues by mentioning that you will receive services related to a disability only if you (1) contact the coordinator of disability services, (2) provide the required documentation, and (3) request those services each term.

You must document your disability for the institution of higher education to be able to determine eligibility for services and specific services needed. It is very important for you to understand that *the law does not state that all students with disabilities must receive all accommodations* [italics mine].

The article goes on by listing possible accommodations:

> 1. Note-takers, tutoring, proofreaders, and editing services [with computer word-processing programs, these services may not be as necessary as they were in the past; comment mine]
> 2. Textbooks and other educational materials in alternative forms
> 3. Access to educational materials in advance (i.e. taped lectures)
> 4. Test-taking alternatives such as extended time, taped tests, oral tests, alternative test site, elimination of computer-scored answer sheets, and use of a computer or spell-checking device for quizzes and exams
> 5. Access to adaptive equipment such as low-vision reading aids and tape recorders
> 6. Opportunity to "make up" quizzes, exams, or assignments if your absence was disability[-]related
> 7. Preferential seating in the classroom
> 8. Extension of time line for completing specific courses
> 9. Extension of time line to complete certification or degree requirements
> 10. Permission to take less than full-time credit and still be eligible for financial aid[2]

Another point I want to make is that you may be able to make some extra money working part-time on campus by providing accommodations to disabled students yourself. If you don't need visual accommodation yourself, you may be able to read to a blind student. If you have normal use of your arms, you may be able to take notes or write exams for a disabled student.

Long before my accident, I made some extra money at the University of Arkansas in Fayetteville by writing exams for a quadriplegic fellow. You may also be able to pick up some extra cash by tutoring college athletes. Check with the appropriate offices at your institution once you get there to see what opportunities are available.

If I were to return to school now, I would need to make sure my classes were either on the first floor or that the buildings had elevators in them. I would have to be able to take notes on a laptop or have someone take notes for me because I can no longer write by hand other than writing a few checks or signing my name. Thank goodness for personal computers or I would not be able to write this book.

SpeciaLiving magazine also did an article, "Finding an accessible college campus," in its Fall 2006 issue. The article focused on the requirements of the Americans with Disabilities Act (ADA) and how colleges and universities must comply.

In very general terms, because colleges and universities receive funding from the federal government, they must comply with the ADA. The article goes into some specifics on the ADA and advises to research the institution on the Internet. If you can visit the school before you enroll there, that would be ideal. If visiting is not an option for you, then find the disability services coordinator at the school and contact that person for specifics on accessibility. Look for a person with the title of ADA Coordinator or a similar title.

The article also mentions two schools, Florida University and Illinois State University, as having wheelchair ramps. It also mentions a fully accessible Disability Resource Testing and Assistive Technology facility that opened in April 2006 at Florida University.[3]

If you have use of your arms, hands, and fingers, you might also consider going to a vocational school and learning a trade.

Whatever your dream may be, don't look at your disability as an obstacle to your education. Look at it as an opportunity instead.

83

Employment After a Spinal Cord Injury

There is nothing like employment, active indispensable employment, for relieving sorrow.—
Jane Austen

There are three basic scenarios involving employment after a spinal cord injury.

The first is where you are working in a job, you become injured and recover (to the extent you are going to), and then you return to your former job. The second is where you are working in a job, you become injured and recover, and then return to work doing something different than your previous employment, The third scenario is where you were not working before you were injured, you have recovered, and you have decided you want to work, whether full-time or part time.

Your return to work may also involve a return to school. If you have not completed your high school education, you may decide to obtain your G.E.D. If you started college, whether two-year, four-year, or postgraduate study, you may decide to complete your education.

You may decide to complete your education in the same field you were studying or you may have decided to change fields of study because you have found another field that suits you more. Your spinal cord injury may have changed your life's direction.

Returning to work after a spinal cord injury involves many challenges. If you have been out of the workforce for a long period of time recovering from your injury, employers may be reluctant to hire you. Even getting an interview may be challenging, depending upon the job market in your area.

The job interview may be challenging. There are laws that govern what a potential employer may ask you about your injury during the interview. Functioning in the workplace may be challenging. There may be problems with doorways or other inaccessible areas.

You may be afraid to return to work. This involves change. You may be afraid of failure. You may be afraid of losing your government benefits.[1]

You may not know where to begin. Here is one place. Every state has a federally funded department or division of vocational rehabilitation to help people with disabilities prepare for and obtain work by providing services such as counseling, career goal development, job preparation skills, training, education, job placement, accommodations or assistive technology, and short-term medical support.[2] Check with your state agency to learn more.

You may decide to start your own business. First, get yourself well enough to meet the challenges of work. According to Urban Miyares, people start their own businesses for one of three reasons: 1) control 2) money or 3) pleasure. But for only one of the three reasons.[3]

If you want to start your own business and you need to obtain loans or grants, you need to have a good business plan. This is something you can learn to do yourself instead of hiring a fancy consultant. If you want to hire a consultant, that's fine too. There is information in public libraries and on the Internet on writing business plans. There are also plenty of books on the subject. There may even be skeleton business plans for the type of business you want to start already on the Internet. One quick word of advice: do what you know or do what you love.

Update your resume frequently. Go to local job fairs. If you live in a community of sufficient size where there are job fairs specifically for the disabled, then go to these fairs. *Careers & the disABLED* magazine is a good source of information on disabled job fairs.

Let your friends and family members know you are in the job market. Give them your resume. If you have done any volunteer work while you have been out of the job market, put that on your resume. It accounts for "missing time" in your job history. It also adds skills to your background.

The federal government offers work incentive programs for people on SSI and SSDI disability. You can earn additional money working up to a set limit based on your monthly disability payment and not lose any of your benefits. The Ticket to Work program offers many incentives for individuals wanting to go back to work. Check with your local Social Security office for details.[4]

Whatever road you want to take with employment, pursue it with the determination you had while working to get well in rehab. Don't give up. It may take time for you to land a job, or make your own business successful.

84

Service Animals

Outside of a dog, a book is a man's best friend.
Inside of a dog, it's too dark to read.—
Groucho Marx

According to the U.S. Department of Justice, the Americans with Disabilities Act defines a service animal as "any guide dog, signal dog, or other animal individually trained to provide assistance to an individual with a disability." If they meet this definition, animals are considered service animals under the ADA regardless of whether they have been licensed or certified by a state or local government.[1]

The Department of Justice continues by saying that service animals perform some of the functions and tasks that the individual with a disability cannot perform for him or herself. The three examples given that apply most directly to spinal cord injured persons are pulling wheelchairs, picking up things for persons with mobility impairments, and assisting persons with mobility impairments with balance.[2]

The Department of Justice further states that some service animals wear special collars or harnesses to alert the public they are service animals and not pets. Service animals must be allowed in businesses, in taxis, and on commercial airplanes (depending on the policy of the individual airline).[3]

Dogs are commonly used as service animals, but capuchin monkeys are also used for quadriplegics and other people with severe spinal cord injuries or mobility impairments. Helping Hands, a Boston, Massachusetts-based organization, provides service monkeys free of charge to people who need them. There is a very strict set of qualifications to determine which individuals will benefit most from the assistance of the monkey, and to insure the monkey is placed in a situation where it will receive the highest quality of care.[4]

Additional information on service animals is provided in the Resources chapter.

85

Pets as Therapy After a Spinal Cord Injury

No animal should ever jump up on the dining-room furniture unless absolutely certain that he can hold his own in the conversation.—
Fran Lebowitz

This chapter is intended for injurees who already had pets before their injury, or who are considering acquiring a pet after their injury. A pet, for purposes of this chapter, does not include service animals. Service animals are covered in the previous chapter.

I found a lengthy article on pets and stress on the Internet that compares the stress in pet owners and non-pet owners. For purposes of discussion, I am going to assume that stress is not a desired physical or emotional quantity. Stress increases the chances of having upper respiratory infections, peptic ulcers, and headaches (I don't think all at the same time, but it could happen). More stress causes more depression. A person's degree of social support has an impact on that person's risk of heart disease. The less social support, the more likely heart disease is. The less social support a person has, the more anxiety-related disorders, the person is likely to have.[1]

Studies show that people who own pets are physically healthier than people who do not own pets. Owning pets lowers blood pressure, and the beating rate of a person's heart. Owning pets reduces stress, according to research. Your immune system works better if you have a pet. Pet owners recover faster from stressful activities than non-pet owners. For the interaction with a pet to have the maximum beneficial effects, it must be a pet that the person knows.[2]

The article states that pet owners appear to be healthier overall than non-pet owners. Pet owners also recover more quickly from illness.[3] Other studies show that having a dog or a cat reduces the risk of having allergies or asthma in children who have neither.[4] It has been shown that having a pet in the house helps children adjust to the serious illness of a parent.[5] There is so much evidence on the health benefits of pets that doctors, dentists, and long-term care facilities are setting up programs to have a trained therapy pet (typically a dog) visit on scheduled days.[6][7] Pets also improve your cholesterol according to one study.[8]

However, one might argue that people who own pets tend to be healthier than non-pet owners because they know they can handle the daily routine of taking care of a pet. Or are people who have pets just happier to begin with?

I'm just playing devil's advocate here. I have four cats myself. I know how beneficial having a pet can be. Because of the amount of pain I am in, I often spend much of the night awake despite pain medication. I don't want to wake my husband so I get up and go to another part of the house. The cats keep me company.

Two other benefits of having a dog are for self-protection, and to pull a manual wheelchair if you have a large dog. I will discuss self-defense in a later chapter.

Dogs are "date magnets" according to one article. People will approach a person with a dog much more readily than they will approach someone they do not know without a dog.[9]

I had the opportunity to speak with Glenn McIntyre during a spinal cord conference in Little Rock in the summer of 2007. Mr. McIntyre is a motivational speaker and consultant and is in a wheelchair. He echoed the idea that dogs are "date magnets." He told the conference attendees that pretty girls come up to him all the time to see his service dog.

One question I have never seen asked is if one pet has a certain level of positive effect on your health, does having x times the number of pets have x times the level of positive effect on your health? Is having three dogs three times as beneficial as having one dog?

If you do not have a pet and are considering getting one, you first need to figure out what kind of pet you want. You have many choices, dogs, cats, birds, fish, reptiles, or small mammals like ferrets. Talk to people who have the type of pet you are considering to learn more about taking care of that particular type of pet. Research on the Internet.

The five factors you must consider before getting a pet are:

1. Cost. Can you handle the all the assorted costs of having a pet?
2. Space. Is there enough space where you live to accommodate a pet or will your landlord allow a pet?
3. Time. Do you have the time to take care of a pet?

4. Patience. Do you have the patience to take care of a pet?
5. Physical demands. Are you physically able to take care of a pet? You can't always count on a family member who says he or she will take care of the pet.[10]

If you were not a pet person before your injury, you're probably not going to be a pet person after your injury unless the injury has made some major changes in your personality. You should not consider having a pet. But if you are a pet person, then enjoy the health benefits your pet offers.

It's nice to find something that improves our health after a spinal cord injury.

86

Sports After A Spinal Cord Injury

Get busy living or get busy dying—
Stephen King

In an earlier chapter I discussed sports as a way to acquire a spinal cord injury. In this chapter I will discuss sports as a means to get your life back after a spinal cord injury. I will start with a brief history of wheelchair sports and then talk about the different wheelchair sports and adaptive equipment that exist today.

Only after doctors figured out how to keep a person alive after a spinal cord injury could life after a spinal cord injury be contemplated. Wheelchair Sports, USA has an excellent discussion on the history of wheelchair sports:

> The initial impetus [driving force] to organize Wheelchair Sports, USA grew out of the interests of athletes with disabilities—many of whom were veterans of World War II. They wanted to participate in sports other than basketball, which had seen rapid growth in the early 1950's through teams sponsored by veterans hospitals and other rehabilitation agencies. General Omar N. Bradley was one of the leaders of the early efforts to develop wheelchair sports programs, principally for servicemen injured during the war. In the early days, many wheel-chair basketball players saw participation in individual wheelchair sports as supplementary training for their primary interest in basketball. However, the Wheelchair Sports, USA, program appealed to even greater numbers of athletes with disabilities because it was able to incorporate women and quadriplegics (those with paralysis in upper as well as lower extremities); two populations which basketball could not reasonable accommodate at that time.
>
> Europe's first organized wheelchair sports program was introduced In 1948 by well-known neurosurgeon, Dr. Ludwig Guttman, founder of The Spinal Injury Center in Stoke-Mandeville, England. The first Stoke-Mandeville games included only a handful of participants (26) [*sic*], and few events (shot put, javelin, club throw, and archery), but growth in both the number of events and participants came quickly.[1]

Many people are aware of wheelchair sports because of the popularity of the movie, *Murderball*, a movie documentary that came out in 2005. For those not familiar with the movie, it is about a group of wheelchair athletes with driven personalities, who are preparing to compete in the Paralympic Games in wheelchair rugby. The athletes compete in full contact style. The documentary received both praise and criticism, and increased the general public's awareness of wheelchair sports and the determination that goes into them.

I was quite amazed to learn about the variety of wheelchair sports that exist during the research for this chapter. Not only do "regular" sports exist for the wheelchair athlete, but "extreme" sports also exist.

The Twenty-Seventh National Veterans Wheelchair Games in June 2007 featured the following sports:

1. Air Guns
2. Archery
3. Basketball
4. Bowling
5. Field Events
6. Handcycling
7. Motor Rally
8. Nine Ball
9. Power Chair Relay
10. Power Soccer
11. Quad Rugby
12. Slalom
13. Softball
14. Swimming
15. Table Tennis [ping pong]
16. Track
17. Weightlifting

There were also exhibition events in trapshooting and wheelchair curling.[2]

The Paralympic Games feature the following sports:

1. Archery
2. Basketball
3. Boccia
4. Curling
5. Cycling
6. Equestrian [horses]
7. Fencing
8. Goalball
9. Judo
10. Powerlifting
11. Rowing
12. Rugby
13. Sailing
14. Skiing—Alpine
15. Skiing—Nordic
16. Sled Hockey
17. Soccer
18. Swimming
19. Table Tennis
20. Tennis
21. Track & Field
22. Volleyball[3]

If you're not familiar with boccia, it is a sport specifically for athletes with a disability. The non-disabled version of the sport is called bocce. Boccia is played by disabled athletes with locomotor disabilities affecting motor skills. Individuals, pairs, or teams of three can play it. There are different classes for competition, depending upon the degree of an athlete's disability.[4]

Curling is another sport you may not be familiar with. It is a complex sport played on a rectangular sheet of ice with granite stones. It is similar to hockey is some ways. There are two teams of four players each. The idea is to steer a heavy, polished granite stone toward a goal. Players sweep the ice in front of it as it moves.[5]

Goalball is a game for blind athletes. In teams of three, players throw a ball with bells embedded in it toward a goal, again like hockey. Players with partial sight and those with normal vision can compete in the sport by wearing blindfolds.[6]

The Paralyzed Veterans of America (PVA) sponsors two wheelchair events: The PVA Bass Tour for people who enjoy fishing. The wheelchair fisherman is teamed up with an able-bodied person who operates the boat.[7]

The Paralyzed Veterans Association also sponsors the PVA Trapshoot Circuit for all trapshooters.[8]

As for extreme wheelchair sports, Apparalyzed.com, a spinal cord injury peer support organization, has a section on extreme wheelchair sports on its website. This section lists the extreme sports:

1. UK Four Cross Downhill Mountain Biking
2. TankChair—Extreme Off Road Wheelchair [you've got to see this to believe it]
3. Extreme Wheelchair Racing and Jumping
4. Wheelchair Jousting with Cattle Prods
5. SitSki (adaptive skiing with one ski done in a sitting position)
6. Amped Riders (skateboarding, surfing, and snowboarding)
7. No Limits (climbing)
8. Wheelchair Junkie (various extreme sports)
9. Team Tyler (all extreme sports)
10. Extreme Chairing (for people who enjoy watching or participating in extreme wheelchair sports)[9]

For those interested in shooting, the National Rifle Association offers information on disabled shooting services free of charge. See the Resources chapter for more information.[10]

If you or a family member wishes to participate in a wheelchair sport, please make yourself or your family member aware of the benefits and the risks involved before you or he/she plays. Any sport carries the risk of additional injury.

87

Driving and Transportation After a Spinal Cord Injury

They are just getting on transportation and taken some place they have never lived before.... That has to be hard in itself, going to the unknown.—
Salvation Army

I want to briefly discuss transportation options after a spinal cord injury for individuals in a manual or electric wheelchair. What options are available to you or your family member will depend upon where you live.

I am going to discuss driving a car, truck, or van first. The degree of injury determines what driving options a person has. A paraplegic with a complete injury obviously can no longer use his or her legs. Driving in a pre-injury manner is no longer possible. A complete quadriplegic will not have use of his or her arms and driving in a pre-injury manner is also out of the question.

The level of injury also determines what driving options a person has. An incomplete quadriplegic may be unable to drive in a pre-injury manner. An incomplete paraplegic may also be unable to drive in a pre-injury manner.

If an injured individual has sufficient use of his or her hands, then adaptive hand driving controls are an option. Many different companies make these. The basic idea behind hand controls is to use the hand-operated controls instead of the legs to push the pedals down. Hand controls come in either permanently installed systems or portable systems for use in rental cars or similar situations. Computer assisted hand controls are also available.[1]

Three categories of basic vehicle adaptations exist:

1. People with disabilities ride as passengers in a private vehicle
2. People with disabilities drive with adaptive equipment

3. People with disabilities use devices to assist in loading an unoccupied wheelchair or scooter into a vehicle.[2]

People who use hand controls to drive and use manual wheelchairs can often continue to use their cars, SUVs, station wagons, or trucks especially if their wheelchairs will fold or are very light.[3] Manual wheelchairs can be carried on top of some cars with the right equipment.[4] Power wheelchairs can weigh as much as three hundred pounds and are more difficult to transport.[5]

Three types of vans exist for the transport of wheelchairs and their occupants: full-size vans, mid-size vans, and minivans. There are pros and cons to each. Most vans need to have lifts installed and need to have raised roofs to allow sufficient headroom for the person in the wheelchair.

Van conversion can be very expensive. Most financial assistance programs will only pay for modifications of used vehicles and not the purchase of new vehicles with adaptive equipment installed.

Full-size vans have the advantage of being able to hold passengers as well as the wheelchair occupant. They also can transport sporting equipment, groceries, or whatever else you may need to carry. Some people believe full-size vans are more durable than smaller vans. The downside of full-size vans is they are very expensive to modify, sometimes costing as much as the van itself to modify. They are also large vehicles and more difficult to park and drive. A larger garage may be necessary as well. The cost of gasoline is also becoming more of an issue as time passes.[6]

I don't have any information on mid-size vans. I do have some on minivans. There are two different types of mini-vans available for wheelchair users. The first is a side-entry, lowered-floor minivan. The second is a rear-entry minivan. Some rear-entry minivans can lower to the ground.

The advantages to both of these types of minivans are they will fit in most garages or assigned parking spaces such as in an apartment complex. In a rear-entry minivan, other vehicles to the side do not block the ramp. There are two possible positions for a wheelchair. In a side-entry minivan, a wheelchair can be secured in the passenger position. Side-entry minivans convert well for disabled drivers. Many different wheelchair positions are possible.

The disadvantages to both the side-entry and the rear-entry minivan is they are complicated to modify and very expensive to do so. It may cost as much or more to modify a minivan as it would to buy a full-size van. A disadvantage of the rear-entry minivan the wheelchair cannot be secured in the front passenger or driver position.[7]

There are many ways to purchase a used vehicle for use with or by a wheelchair driver. Some of these include car dealers, adaptive equipment companies, classified ads in your local newspaper, the Internet, and eBay. However, purchasing vehicles on the Internet or eBay is not without risk. Adaptive equipment may have been improperly installed. The vehicle may have been wrecked and not repaired. It is advisable to purchase a vehicle from a National Mobility Equipment Dealers Association (NMEDA) member. This organization has a strict Quality Assurance audit program (QAP) for all its dealers. Ideally, you should find a qualified QAP dealership.[8]

If you have enough control over your movements that you can drive with hand controls, you will need to be certified to be able to drive with them. Check with your local Department of Motor Vehicles to learn where you can find a certified trainer. If you have a Veterans' Affairs agency near you, it may offer hand control certified training. You might also contact your state chapter of the Paralyzed Veterans of America, even if you are not a veteran.

Public ground transportation may be available for wheelchair users in larger metropolitan areas. Public buses and dedicated Para transit vehicles may be in use in larger cities. Some large cities may have light rail systems. I do not know if these are typically accessible by individuals using wheelchairs.

I want to mention one little detail in this chapter. For those who have a spinal cord injury in the neck or chest, you may find yourself more subject to centrifugal force riding in a car than you were before your accident. In English, your chest, stomach, and abdominal muscles are weaker than they used to be. You may find yourself getting pushed to the side when you go around curves in a car.

Whatever method of transportation you choose, be prepared for getting from one place to another to take longer than it did before your (or your family member's) accident.

88

Travel and Accessibility After a Spinal Cord Injury

Certainly, travel is more than the seeing of sights;
it is a change that goes on, deep and permanent,
in the ideas of living.—
Miriam Beard

You may be wondering what the difference is between travel after a spinal cord injury and transportation after a spinal cord injury. In this chapter I intend to talk about vacation-type and business travel instead of local ground travel.

Vacation or business travel after a spinal cord injury is also going to contain its share of challenges. Airlines are going to vary in their degree of accessibility. Hotels that claim to be accessible may or may not be. Bed and breakfast inns may or may not be accessible.

I have read mixed results from wheelchair users flying on airplanes. Some people report horrible experiences. Others found the airline they flew with very willing to accommodate them and their wheelchairs. I have heard that if you fly and are a wheelchair user, be prepared for your wheelchair to be damaged during the flight.

You are going to have to do your homework planning your travel before you leave.

You will need to check with the airlines if you are flying regarding their degree of accessibility and their policies. You will need to check with hotels, motels, and bed and breakfast inns on their degree of accessibility. Some hotels and motels claim to be accessible, when in reality they are not. It is common to read letters to the editor in *New Mobility* and *PN* magazines about bad experiences people have had with hotels or motels that claimed to be accessible and were not. There may be issues of doorway width, bathroom accessibility, and bed height accessibility.

In years past it used to be nearly impossible to travel if you were in a wheelchair. Nowadays, there are travel agencies that specialize in disabled travel for all types of disabilities. There are even package tours for the disabled.

There are some issues in worldwide travel that are the same for non-disabled and disabled people. You may need a passport. Electricity voltages may be different and adapters may be needed for laptop computers, hairdryers, electric razors, etc.

Some countries have laws that may seem unusual to people in other countries. For example, for years chewing gum was outlawed in Singapore. Now the partial ban has been lifted. Chewing gum can be purchased through licensed dealers. Customers must supply identity information and register to purchase chewing gum.

See the Resources chapter for more information on travel.

89

Parking After a Spinal Cord Injury

Going to church does not make you a Christian
anymore than going to the garage makes you a car—
Lawrence J. Peter

I couldn't find a good quotation on parking so I used one of my favorites on cars.

There isn't much in life that a spinal cord injury doesn't affect. Down to the most trivial things. Like parking your vehicle. Your ability to get out of your vehicle and the distance you are able to travel from a parking place to your desired destination changes after a spinal cord injury. If you are using a cane, crutches, or walker, you cannot tolerate the type of distances from your parked vehicle to a store the way you used to. If you are using a manual or electric wheelchair, it is also better to be able to park closer to the store.

A similar system of placards is used worldwide to signify a permit to park in disabled parking places. It is the familiar blue background with a white side view of a person in a wheelchair. Very generic. But understood worldwide.

And who wouldn't want a disability parking permit? It allows you to park much closer to a business. I don't think there is a car in Arkansas without one. Arkansas has become a retirement state because of its warm winters. It is pretty much impossible to find an open disabled parking space in Arkansas unless the store that you want to go to is closed. Arkansas has recently strengthened its accessible parking laws.

Forgery of disability parking permits became so widespread in Illinois that the state had to start using a punch card system with the driver's birth date. This was too easy to fake so the state became the first in the country to use a hologram sticker on its permits. Illinois also instituted a $500 fine and possible driver's license suspension for disabled parking permit forgery.[1]

Another recent development in disability parking permits is the settlement of a lawsuit by the United Spinal Association and The Equal Rights Center against Washington, D.C. It seems the District of Columbia would not recognize disabled parking permits from other jurisdictions and was fining drivers accordingly.[2]

You get a disabled parking permit from the governmental agency in your state or country that issues driver's licenses and license plates. There is usually a standard form to complete that must be signed by your doctor stating your reason for needing a disabled parking permit. Your doctor will also need to state whether or not the disability is temporary or permanent. Some states have both disability parking hangtags that hang from the rear view mirror and disability license plates.

90

Selecting a Wheelchair After a Spinal Cord Injury

We may take Fancy for a companion, but must follow Reason as a guide.—
Samuel Johnson

If you thought buying a new vehicle pre-injury was difficult, wait until you start shopping for a wheelchair (or wheeled chair as they can be called). It can be an overwhelming task. It is a purchase you need to research before you buy, consult with experts (your doctor, your occupational therapist, your physical therapist), talk with other people already in wheelchairs, talk with wheelchair retailers and rehab centers, and take into consideration what you can afford.

I am going to do my best to assist you with your choices, but what you select is ultimately up to you. For those of you who are thinking "what kind of chair are you using, Carolyn," I am a "walking quad" so at the moment I do not own a wheelchair. I do not know if that will continue forever, but for the moment I can walk with walking crutches or a walker on level surfaces. I cannot handle unlevel surfaces, like grass. I lose my balance and fall.

You are going to have to make your decision for your primary chair by process of elimination in some ways. You may acquire additional specialty wheelchairs over time for different purposes. I have provided a rough guideline below:

Need for wheelchair: Permanent or Temporary?

Amount of upper body strength: Paraplegic or Quadriplegic?

Weight and size restrictions: Under 250/300 pounds or Over 250/300 pounds?

Wheelchair condition: New or Used?

Most people buy totally the wrong thing for them on their first wheelchair, so I have been told. This is especially true if you are younger when choosing your first wheelchair. Keep in mind that this is a very expensive purchase that must last you for many years. Your needs in wheelchairs will change over time. Most wheelchairs, like everything else, have a limited lifespan.

Wheelchairs are so expensive because they must be custom manufactured from specialty materials such as titanium. Each individual requiring a wheelchair needs to be measured and it is very important to be sure to purchase a wheelchair that fits you.

One accessory you must purchase when you purchase a wheelchair is a wheelchair cushion. Many different types and styles are available. Each different type of cushion has its advantages and disadvantages. You will have to figure out what works best for you. Wheelchair cushions increase sitting comfort and help prevent pressure sores. It is also possible to purchase additional optional accessories for wheelchairs like bags, backpacks, trays, cup holders, etc.

Wheelchairs manufactured in the United States must conform to strict manufacturing standards. The American National Standards Institute (ANSI), which regulates many different types of standards in the U.S., sets the standards to which all manufacturers must conform.[1]

You can purchase a brand new wheelchair or you can purchase a used chair. If you purchase a new chair, you will most likely be purchasing it through a medical supply store or similar retail store. It is possible to purchase new wheelchairs on the Internet or off eBay.

The disadvantages to purchasing a wheelchair you cannot see before you buy are that it may not fit you, it may have something wrong with it you could not tell because you could not personally inspect it before purchase. You may not get exactly what you paid for. You may not get your purchase at all. If you purchase a new wheelchair off the Internet, make sure you have a guarantee with it.

Purchasing used chairs can be done at yard or tag sales, estate sales, consignment shops, through word of mouth at support groups, or off the Internet or eBay. If you purchase an expensive used chair off the Internet or eBay, make sure you have a guarantee with it.

Although this chapter is mainly concerned with helping you (or your family member) choose your primary wheelchair, I am going to provide a little bit of information on different types of wheelchairs and specialty wheelchairs as well. When I use the word "wheelchair" I am using it to mean all different types of devices that individuals use for mobility including manual wheelchairs, powered wheelchairs, and scooters.

There are several different types of wheelchairs:

1. Standard manual wheelchairs: for use less than four hours a day

2. Lightweight wheelchairs: for use with air, cruise, train, or ground transportation
3. Transport wheelchairs: for use to transport someone to and from the house or around the mall.
4. Extra Wide/Heavy Duty wheelchairs: for use with large or obese individuals
5. Shower wheelchairs: for use during personal hygiene care and made of rust-free materials
6. Reclining wheelchairs: for use as a more comfortable chair or for more specialized needs such as for individuals who cannot pressure release manually
7. Pediatric wheelchairs: for use by children, young adults, or very small adults
8. Power wheelchairs: specialized wheelchairs operated by battery power with some form of controller operated by the wheelchair occupant
9. Standing wheelchairs: very specialized wheelchairs that allow the occupant to stand up
10. Scooters: small specialized powered transport devices used best inside and around the home
11. Dedicated Specialty Sports wheelchairs: specialized lightweight manual wheelchairs for individuals to participate in wheelchair sports such as basketball
12. Specialized Outdoor Sports wheelchairs: specialized manual wheelchairs for individuals to use on all terrains for sports such as hunting or fishing[2 3 4]

I want to make another point about wheelchairs before I continue. They are like cars in one way. They require routine maintenance and they do break down.

I found a general set of issues to consider in the selection of a wheelchair by Gary Karp, who has written many books on spinal cord injury and related issues:

1. How wide are your doors—main entry, kitchen, bedrooms, bathrooms, etc.?
2. Are there tight angles to negotiate, such as a hallway that turns sharply at the bedroom door?
3. How large is the bathroom? Will it be possible to wheel your chair alongside the bathtub, or must you face it directly? Is the door smaller than the others in your house? Will you be able to close the door once inside with your wheelchair?
4. What is the knee clearance of the tables and desks you will deal with at home and at work if you work?
5. How high are cabinets and shelves you might need to reach?
6. Is the terrain around your home paved? If not, what kind of surface is it? Is it level?
7. What are the surfaces where you will do most of your wheeling? Carpet, tile, concrete, packed soil?
8. If you drive, do you have a car, or a van? Two or four doors?

9. What is the size of the trunk in the family car?
10. What kind of public transportation might you use?
11. What kind of hobbies or activities do you participate in that might affect the type of chair you use?
12. If you like to "hang out" at your best friend's house, can you fit through those doors?
13. Is the appearance of your chair important to you or are you only interested in functionality? Do you want something sporty? Eye-catching?
14. What is your preferred level of exercise? Do you get lots of exercise or are you a "couch potato?"[5]

Next, I want to discuss manual wheelchairs. One consideration in the selection of a manual wheelchair is who will be propelling the chair. Is the injured person going to be propelling the chair or is the person going to have someone pushing the chair all the time? This is a major factor in the choice of a manual chair. Chairs that the injured person will propel have very large wheels in the back of the wheelchair and small wheels in the front. Chairs that another person typically propels have four small wheels.

The information I am going to provide you on manual wheelchairs comes from a fact sheet that is more than ten years old, but the basic information is still good. A lot changed in the wheelchair market between the 1960s and the 1990s, but the basics between the 1990s and the early twenty-first century are still the same.

Here are the considerations for manual wheelchairs:

1. Frame type: Rigid or folding frame. Rigid frames cannot be folded. Folding frames can obviously be folded.
2. Upholstery: You must consider the type of upholstery you want on the wheelchair. Bear in mind you may be dealing with extreme heat, extreme cold, rain, snow, and everything in-between.
3. Braking Systems: Braking systems on manual wheelchairs consist of stopping the back wheels with your hands. However, there are different types of parking brakes.
4. There are different types of wheelchair tires now: sold tires, semi-pneumatic tires, and radial tires. There are also mag wheels and off road wheels. All wheels other than what is standard with a particular chair come with extra cost.
5. Casters: Casters in front vary in size and composition (pneumatic, sold rubber, plastic, or a combination).
6. Footrests: Footrests can be incorporated into the frame of the chair as part of the design or they can swivel, flip up, or be removed.

7. Armrests: Some wheelchairs have no armrests. Armrests are helpful if the person has difficulty with upper body balance while seated. Armrests are an important consideration when dealing with the height of counters, desks, and tables.[6]

Let's talking briefly about steering and pushing your manual wheelchair. The strength in your upper body is something you will have to build up over time. It is important to use proper pushing techniques because using a manual wheelchair puts abnormal stress on your wrists, arms, and shoulders. This can lead to carpal tunnel syndrome in the wrists and elbow and shoulder joints wearing out.

To learn the proper technique for pushing a manual wheelchair, talk to your rehabilitation hospital or consult the article in the March 2007 issue of *PN* magazine that discusses the topic thoroughly and even provides pictures and diagrams of proper procedures.[7]

Several companies on the market have introduced a "power assist" manual wheelchair. These wheelchairs still have to be moved by hand. The power assist feature is controlled by a joystick and is used for going up a hill and for additional braking down a hill. The drawback to these wheelchairs is the batteries are even more expensive than batteries for power chairs and have about half the charge range, meaning they need to be recharged more often.[8]

Powered wheelchairs are the way to go for the spinal cord injury survivor who does not have sufficient control or strength in the upper body for a manual chair. Many advances have been made in powered wheelchairs in recent years.

Here is a quick list of the some of the variety of choices available in powered wheelchairs:

1. Rear wheel drive: power is behind the person so the person feels as if he or she is being pushed from behind.

2. Front wheel drive: power is in front of the person so the person feels as if he or she is being pulled from the front.

3. Mid wheel drive: power is under the person. This option has the smallest turning radius. I have also had front wheel drive recommended to me for small turning radius.

4. Retracting or stationary armrests

5. Foot plate options

6. Front casters

7. Tires
8. Manual or power lift, recline, or both
9. Manual or power elevating leg rests[9]

The controller on a powered wheelchair is an important consideration. A joystick is the typical method of operating a powered wheelchair. If the spinal cord injury survivor does not have sufficient use of his or her arms then another form of controller must be used. Swing away joystick controllers are also available and are better for some situations. Wheelchairs can be controlled through a sipping or puffing breathing system, a system of switches built into the headrest, or by means of a switch and scanner so that a finger tap or toe tap can be used to control movement.[10]

For information on powered wheelchair batteries I am going to refer you to two different articles that explain range and charge considerations and the different types of batteries available. The information is fairly complex so I am not going to reproduce it here.[11] [12]

There are several general considerations in the purchase of a powered wheelchair:

> 1. Where will I be using the wheelchair? Will it be used indoors or outdoors? If the wheelchair will be used outdoors, will there be rough or uneven ground?
> 2. What is the turning radius of the wheelchair? Will this work in my home?
> 3. Does the wheelchair have a weight limit?
> 4. Does the chair accommodate a tilt system?
> 5. Can I operate the joystick and turn the wheelchair on and off?
> 6. Will the chair accommodate other types of controls (head control or single switch)?
> 7. Can I mount a seating system on the wheelchair?
> 8. If you are buying a used wheelchair, check with the manufacturer to learn if you can modify the chair at a later date. (The electronics may not be current to be able to install alternative controllers).[13]
> 9. If the wheelchair will be used by a child or a person with a condition that will deteriorate, make sure to ask if the chair can be modified accordingly with different controllers or other options.[14]

Now I want to talk more about sports wheelchairs. Many sports wheelchairs are more expensive than standard manual wheelchairs. There are basically four types of sports wheelchairs:

1. Handcycles: These are basically bicycles with a wheelchair seat built in.

2. Court Chairs: These are for use in wheelchair basketball.

3. Racers: These are manually propelled with the rear wheels for racing.

4. Miscellaneous Sports Chairs: These are the fat tire all-terrain chairs.[15]

I believe it is safe to say that if you are a paraplegic or a quadriplegic with a good amount of upper body strength you will be able to operate a Sports Wheelchair.

I have heard and read that many people are very frustrated because they have found "the perfect chair" for their needs and they cannot get their insurance, Medicare, or Medicaid to pay for it. Many states have grant programs to assist with paying for wheelchairs. Check with your local Department of Health or equivalent state agency to see if there are any programs. If you can find a local spinal cord injury support group, someone there may also know of any programs. Also check with local rehabilitation hospitals. The only person I know of who was able to get exactly the "right chair" and a very expensive chair at that (which he really does need), was a person who was injured on the job. His expenses are being paid by the state Workers' Compensation agency.

Wheelchairs are one of the most common frustrations I have heard discussed in support group meetings. People complain they cannot get their chairs properly repaired or parts of the chair wore out before they thought was a reasonable time.

For any wheelchair you purchase new, the quality and availability of customer service is very important. Talk with retailers, people who have been in chairs for many years, and anyone else you can find to learn about the customer service of the company's product(s) you are interested in.

I found a wheelchair checklist to help a person get a proper fit in a wheelchair:

1. Your feet are flat on the footrests.
2. Your elbows are comfortably bent on the armrests.
3. Your thighs are parallel with your seat or slightly higher.
4. Your knees are comfortably bent at the edge of the seat.
5. You have a half-inch breathing room between your hips and the sides of the wheelchair.
6. Your bottom is flush with the seat angle of your chair.
7. You are sitting in a balanced position. This doesn't mean heads up and stomach in, but rather a position where your knees are slightly high and bent and your head is slightly down. This provides better trunk control, reaching ability, and coordination. But make sure you keep up your strengthening exercises, particularly the muscles of the shoulders, girth, neck, and legs. And keep on pressure relieving.

8. Your brakes, control panel, and on/off switches [if you have the latter two] are easy to reach.
9. You can maneuver easily in your chair and can stop when you have to.
10. You feel comfortable.[16]

The history of wheelchair development is very interesting, but I am not going to discuss it in this chapter. It is not immediately relevant to the early stages of recovering from a spinal cord injury. It is something you can research on your own later on if you are interested.

You sometimes see antique metal or wooden wheelchairs on eBay with photographs. I'll bet someplace out there someone actually collects antique wheelchairs.

91

Accessible Living, Home Modifications and Universal Design

A good home must be made, not bought.—
Joyce Maynard in *Domestic Affairs*

There is so much information available on the subjects of accessibility, home modifications, and universal design that I could write for days and still not cover everything.

I am going to discuss some basics in this chapter. I have provided references for you to do future research in the Resources chapter. This is an area where you or your family members are doing to have to do a lot of research, and learn the information yourselves. I cannot teach you everything you need to know in a short little chapter.

It is a given that almost every spinal cord injured person will require some kind of modification to their "living space" after their injury. I use the phrase "living space" because there are so many different types of dwellings people can occupy. People live in condominiums, apartments, single family homes, nursing homes, duplexes, and probably some other type of arrangement I am forgetting about.

Required modifications may be minimal, such as installing grab bars in the bathroom, or they may involve a complete remodeling of the inside and outside of a home. Some homeowners are forced to sell their existing homes and buy more accessible homes. Another option is to buy a home that is still inaccessible, but more easily modified than their existing home. Other people sell their homes and have a new home custom built that is accessible.

There are some other "givens" in accessible living. First, the kitchen and bathroom are the most difficult rooms to make accessible. Second, the type of flooring in the house is very important for a wheelchair user. Wheelchairs require a nice smooth floor. Wheelchair wheels will destroy carpet or hardwood floors very quickly. Linoleum is also not recommended because it can tear easily.

New laminate floors that look like wood may or may not work. I know people in power chairs who swear by them, but I have also seen information that says the floating laminate floors tend to spread and separate from the weight of a power chair. Tile also works well. It is best to find a flooring professional who has experience installing flooring for wheelchair users.

Other areas that can be problematic for wheelchair users are small bathrooms and stairs. A variety of different lifts exist for staircases, but the cost can be very high. In some houses, elevators are installed. I shudder to think of the cost, but having never investigated it, it may be more reasonable than I think. As for small bathrooms, it may be difficult or impossible to renovate a very small bathroom because the room itself is too small for the wheelchair user to turn the chair. I have heard that it is easier to add an accessible bathroom onto a house than to try to modify an existing bathroom.

One subject I do want to address is wheelchair ramps on the exterior of the house. Wheelchair ramps are required to be built to specific building code specifications to be safe. There are formulas for the maximum angle of slope to the ramps for them to comply with code. Ramps are made from metal or wood.

It is advisable to have handrails on the sides of the ramps to keep the wheelchair from rolling off the ramp. Ramps can be temporary or permanently installed. If you are having ramps custom installed, don't skimp on code regulations to save a few dollars. You are setting yourself up for an accident later on.

I strongly recommend that you have smoke detectors and carbon monoxide detectors in your "living space" and that you test them on a regular basis. Make sure their batteries are good. Long life nine-volt batteries can be purchased at Radio Shack or on the Internet. If you can afford a whole house alarm system that is monitored by a commercial alarm service, this is also advisable.

Take action to reduce mold in your "living space." Make sure ventilation in your "living space" is good. It is also important that your "living space" be as quiet as possible to allow you to rest.[1]

One quick thought. If you are building a home and you or a family member uses a wheelchair, make sure the fuse box and main breaker are inside and are installed at an accessible height.

One final thing I want to mention is the concept of "Universal Design." This is a phrase you may have heard on TV or read about. The definition of Universal Design I found is "Universal Design is the design of products and environments to be usable by all people, to the greatest extent possible, without need for adaptation or specialized design."[2]

Ok, so that was written in "architectese." How about a more simple explanation? It means someplace that anybody with any disability can live comfortably and function. Universal Design seems to be the newest rage among architects at universities. Model houses are being built all over the country.

When it comes to Universal Design and the typical architect who actually designs houses for people, I'm going to bet that most of them have never been exposed to the concept of Universal Design. It has been my experience that something that is supposed to be suitable for all is rarely suitable for anybody.

Over time, more and more architects will become familiar with home design for people with disabilities. I believe that college architecture degrees have started training new architects along these lines.

Who knows, someday every new home may be required to be wheelchair accessible.

92

Equipment You May Need After a Spinal Cord Injury

I didn't want to be encumbered by
what anyone else's abilities were,
their equipment or environment or
their ability to get certain products—
Thomas Keller

This is a difficult chapter to write. It's like fortune-telling. There is no way I can tell an individual person exactly what equipment he or she will need after a spinal cord injury. It depends on the injury, the person's abilities, their living environment after the injury, their doctor's opinions, and other factors.

One thing is certain when it comes to equipment. It is all expensive. It can be challenging to find the financial resources to obtain the equipment you need.

There are basics when it comes to spinal cord injury equipment. You may not need or want everything in the list. Here is the list:

1. Wheelchairs (see the chapter on Selecting a Wheelchair for more details)
2. Cushions and positioning equipment
3. Hospital bed and mattress
4. Bathroom safety equipment (grab bars etc.)
5. Transfer equipment (mechanical lifts and transfer boards)
6. Upper and lower extremity splints and braces
7. Devices for walking (canes, crutches, walkers, shoe inserts etc.)
8. Exercise equipment.
9. Driver training and adaptive equipment

10. Computer access (specialized keyboard, mouse, or dictation software)
11. Environmental control units (garage door openers, etc.)
12. Respiratory equipment[1]

Your doctors, therapists, and caseworker should be able to provide you with a list of specifically what equipment you will need.

93

Self-Defense After a Spinal Cord Injury

Self-defense is the clearest of all laws, and for this reason lawyers didn't make it.—
Douglas William Jerrold

One of the sad truths after a spinal cord injury is that we are no longer able to defend ourselves in the same ways we could before the injury because our bodies no longer work the way they used to.

This emphasizes the fact that each of us, as spinal cord injury survivors, must take full responsibility for our own safety. We are more vulnerable to attack now that we are disabled.

Spinal cord injury and being the victim of a crime have one thing in common. In both situations, most people think it will never happen to them. We've already been wrong once. *Let's not be wrong again.*

Self-defense is defined as actions taken by a person to prevent another person from causing harm to oneself, one's property, or one's home.[1] In this chapter I will be concerned with preventing harm to oneself.

I found an appropriate quotation on self-defense and disability on the Internet: "As a person with a disability, you want to be able to go anywhere like everybody else, and not feel you're easy prey. You want to be as confident and secure as possible when you get on the street, whether or not you are a wheelchair user.... Nonetheless, people with disabilities are vulnerable to attack and often are seen as easy targets."[2]

Here are some tips to help you stay safe:

1. Your ability to recognize a dangerous person or situation makes you safer.
2. Awareness involves knowing what to look for and disciplining yourself to pay attention.

3. The ultimate success is self-defense is when nothing happens!
4. The earlier you detect and recognize a potential problem, the more options you have to resolve it.
5. Detecting and recognizing danger is based on accurate mental maps.
6. Attention involves adjusting your conscious focus toward what is relevant to a particular situation.
7. Accept full responsibility for your safety.
8. Identify situations in your own life requiring a higher level of vigilance.
9. Build and refine your self-defense maps by continuous learning.
10. Analyze the news. Familiarize yourself with criminal patterns and factors which contribute to violent crime. Apply the questions who, what, when, where, why and how to these incidents and use your acquired knowledge to stay out of the news yourself!
11. Practice observations skills.
12. Establish self-defense habits.[3]

You have two basic options for defending yourself: using some form of martial arts as self-defense or using a firearm. If you have a complete injury, the odds are that you will have someone with you. That person needs to be practicing the above tips, and be prepared to defend you and him- or herself as well. There is additional information in the Resources chapter on self-defense training for the disabled.

If you are comfortable using firearms (or wish to become comfortable and are capable of doing so), many states allow for citizens to obtain a concealed carry permit. This will allow you to carry a licensed firearm with you. Federal, state and local governments and some places of business such as hospitals strictly forbid firearms even if you have a concealed carry permit.

Check with a local gun shop, your local state police office, or the National Rifle Association (http://www.nra.org) for more information on concealed carry permits. You will have to take a short class under a certified instructor and take a shooting test to obtain a concealed carry permit. You will need to have a clean criminal record to get your permit.

94

In Case of Emergency

Be prepared.—
Boy Scout Motto

If anything can go wrong, it will go wrong says the famous Murphy's Law of western culture.

The bad thing about having a spinal cord injury is that things do go wrong with our bodies, sometimes unexpectedly. And some of those things can be life threatening. This chapter is written for friends and family members of spinal cord injury survivors so you have a better idea of what to do to prepare for an emergency.

If the injured person in question has enough use of his arms and hands to use a cell phone, then make sure he or she has a cell phone with him or her at all times. Make sure to keep the battery well charged. Don't depend on a pre-paid cell phone in this situation.

The injured person should program (or have a family member) program contact names and phone numbers into his or her cell phone. The contact names should be preceded with the letters "ICE." This is a common abbreviation for In Case of Emergency. This way hospital staff knows who to call if the person is rushed to the emergency room by ambulance.

The injured person should obtain an autonomic dysreflexia card to put in his/her wallet if he/she has this condition. A printable card can be obtained from http://www.sci-info-pages.com/ad_card.html. Omit the final period from the web address. These cards can be obtained from other sources. Check with your local spinal cord injury support group or rehabilitation hospital. Medical alert necklaces and/or bracelets can also be worn.

Another tip is for the injured person to carry a medical ID card listing medical conditions other than autonomic dysreflexia. If the person wears contact lenses, this should be noted on the card. State Farm Insurance offers a free service where you can create and print a medical ID card online. You do not have to have State

Farm Insurance to use this service. The web address is https://online.statefarm.com/apps/MedicalCard/Medical_Card.asp. Omit the final period. If you search for "medical ID card" on a search engine, this site will come up.

There are companies that will print and laminate these cards for you for a nominal charge. I prefer to create and laminate my own card. I don't want anyone else having access to my medical information.

Another tip for in the home is to have a baby monitor in the room where the injured person sleeps if you are responsible for caring for the person, and you sleep in another room. The sending unit is in the injured person's room and the receiving units are in the rooms of the other occupants of the house.

Commercial alarm companies have services where a person can press a button on a device and this will signal the alarm company in the event of a medical emergency. This, of course, is only useful for the injured person if he or she does not have a complete quadriplegic injury. If you already have an alarm system, this may be an option you want to consider. This service is available for a modest additional fee.

I have been told by a reliable source that it is a good idea to visit your local police substation. Bring a box of donuts with you. Don't buy cheap donuts when you do this. Go to a real donut shop. You or a family member can do this.

You want to talk to the dispatcher and make sure there is information stored in the computer your medical conditions (or the medical conditions of the person in question). Make sure to include that the person is a spinal cord injury survivor, and either a paraplegic or quadriplegic if it is not obvious (like me). This way the first responders and paramedics will have the appropriate information if there is an emergency. This is a good idea for anyone who has medical problems.

Be prepared in advance for natural disasters as well. Have a plan in case of a tornado. Decide where all the family members will go before there is a storm. Designate one room in the house if the tornado sirens sound. Make sure everyone in the house knows how to transport the injured person to the destination room.

The Red Cross advises families to have an evacuation plan in case of natural disaster. Specific instructions are available at http://www.redcross.org. It is advisable to have extra prescription medication on hand in case of a natural disaster if at all possible. Also having an extra two weeks' worth of food is recommended. Have a spare pair of prescription glasses may be a good idea.

If the injured person is ventilator dependent, make sure battery backups are ready if severe weather is approaching. If possible, have a generator to back up the household electricity. Having a good quality surge suppressor on critical equipment is also advisable. Don't depend on cheap, poor quality equipment to save equipment that someone's life depends on.

Don't forget about pets in an emergency. You should create a "pet emergency supply kit." This kit needs to contain: food (at least three days), water (at least three days), medicines and medical records, first aid kit (talk to your vet), collar with ID, harness, or leash, a crate or pet carrier, pet litter or a reasonable substitute such as newspaper, and a picture of you and your pet together.[1]

Next, plan what you will do in case of emergency. Where will you go? Make sure you know in advance of a place that will take you and your pet(s). If you are unable to evacuate your pets yourself, make arrangements with family, friends, or neighbors to do so.[2]

Finally, stay informed about the different types of emergencies. Planning ahead will save regrets later.

People Don't Treat Me the Same Way After the Accident

95

Spinal Cord Syndromes as an Invisible Disability

Everyone needs a strong sense of self.
It is our base of operations for everything
that we do in life.—
Julia T. Alvarez

I have lost count of how many times I have been stopped by someone, usually a female in her 50s, who says to me "you're too young to be using a walker." I always respond with "you're never too young for a spinal cord injury."

In our society, people assume if you walk with a limp or are having difficulty walking (and you don't have crutches or a cane or a walker), that you are drunk. If you are using crutches or a walker, they assume you have a lifelong disability. Or have an acquired disability such as multiple sclerosis.

I'm not alone with the problem of having an invisible disability. If you're reading this book and have a spinal cord syndrome or have a family member with a spinal cord syndrome, you're may already be quite familiar with the problem of an invisible disability. There are many different kinds of invisible disabilities.

I saw a posting on the National Spinal Cord Injury Association (NSCIA) forum from a lady with Brown-Sequard Syndrome who posted:

> My biggest problem other than dealing with the disabilities (and I would love to hear how you deal with this) is that I look normal other than my right hand, which never completely came back, and a limp. I feel like no one understands when I can't keep up. My doctor gave me the most relief last month when he told me that just sitting in a chair I am doing more work than he is. I feel like I need to justify when I can't do anymore.[1]

I found a website that was created by people who understand the problem that I and others with spinal cord syndromes have. It is called the Invisible Disabilities Advocate.

The website sells a booklet called "But You LOOK Good!" [*sic*] for people with invisible disabilities to help their friends and family members understand. The website explains:

> Society tells us that we can measure a person's character by what they drive, the size of the house they live in and the labels on their clothing.... American society puts extreme value of image.... We get so wrapped up in "who we are" being defined by "what we do" that it is no wonder why so many who become disabled also become insecure and feel like their lives no longer have importance.... The truth is, there are millions of people in this world who suffer from what I call "invisible disabilities." They may have a ruptured disk in their back, a spinal injury, brain injury or a disease that is attacking their cells, muscles and/or nervous system. They may have heart problems, lung problems, neurological disorders, severe pain and/or weakness. In other words, their debilitation is just as real, even though the damage lies under the skin.[2]

Another website devoted to invisible disabilities is The Invisible Disabilities Page.[3] Wikipedia defines an invisible disability as "a disability that is not (always) immediately apparent to casual observers; that is, it is not visible to the naked eye."[4]

An observation I want to make about invisible disabilities is that people are always going to make judgments about you and your disability. There is not much you can do to stop it. Don't let it bother you.

For those of us with an acquired disability, in some ways it is a badge of honor, if you will. We earned it. We endured some traumatic event, and have the disability to show for it. If the disability isn't visible, then people don't give us the respect we deserve for enduring the disability.

96

Disability Rights and Discrimination

You are the embodiment of the information you choose to accept and act upon. To change your circumstances you need to change your thinking and subsequent actions.—
Anonymous

Discrimination against the disabled has become such a concern than many countries have taken action to reduce and/or eliminate discrimination against people with disabilities. In the United States, The Americans with Disabilities Act (ADA) was passed in 1990 in the hope of preventing or at least reducing the amount of discrimination experienced by the disabled in the workplace.[1]

The Disability Discrimination Act (DDA) was passed in 1995 in the U.K., and supplemented by the Disability Discrimination Act of 2005 (DDA 2005).[2] Europe has the European Network on Independent Living (ENIL) whose purpose is to promote independent living among persons with disabilities and the general public.[3] Australia's Human Rights & Equal Opportunity Commission oversees the rights of disabled individuals in Australia.[4] Canada has similar legislation to what I have mentioned above.

Private organizations also exist in the United States to protect the rights of disabled individuals. The National Disability Rights Network is a group dedicated to the protection and advocacy of individuals with disabilities.[5] The National Council for Support of Disability Issues is another advocacy group.[6]

The Equal Employment Opportunity Commission (EEOC) is the government agency in the United States charged with elimination of illegal discrimination from the workplace. The Americans with Disabilities Act describes what a disability is (you certainly have one after having a spinal cord injury), what a prospective employer may or may not ask you about your disability during a job interview, and what an employer is required to do by law to make it possible for you to do to your job. There must be a record of your disability for you to be covered under the ADA (your medical records are proof).

Employers covered under the ADA are: private employers, state and local governments, employment agencies, labor organizations, and labor-management committees. The ADA applies to all employers with at least fifteen employees.

You must be qualified for the job you are in to be covered by the ADA. If you are in the United States, and you believe you have been discriminated against based on your disability; contact the nearest Equal Employment Opportunity Commission office. Look in your telephone book under the government pages. If you are in one of the countries or regions I discussed at the beginning of this chapter, then contact the appropriate governmental agency.

97

"My Introduction to Disabled People"

Few things are harder to put up with than the annoyance of a good example—
Mark Twain

When I first found out I had a spinal cord injury, I started thinking back through my life. I thought about the people I knew who had been disabled and how they dealt with their situations. This chapter is intended as a tribute to those individuals.

I remember hearing about one of our neighbors, who fell out of a tree in his yard while trimming it and broke his neck. We lived on a u-shaped street so everybody who lived on the street were "our neighbors," no matter how far away their house was because we knew every family. I remember seeing him from a distance in his powered wheelchair after his accident.

One of the first people I remember meeting who used a wheelchair was my student teacher in fourth grade. His name was Silas Singh. He was from Fiji. He was unable to walk because he had contracted polio while on Fiji. He was always in excellent spirits and cheerful.

I went to junior high school with a Chinese girl named Dorothy Chu. She was from Taiwan. She, like Mr. Singh, was also always happy and always smiling. She shared another similarity with Mr. Singh. She had also contracted polio. She did not use a wheelchair, but walked with leg braces and a cane. I remember her saying that she wanted to be a neurologist when she grew up so she could help others with neurological problems. Her family moved to Hawaii and she is now a neurologist there. I contacted her recently and it was nice to do some catching up.

Another person that had a positive influence on me was Chris Smith. Chris has cerebral palsy. Chris was in a wheelchair during high school and college years and had a personal attendant. I never actually met him, but I knew who he was.

He was in the class ahead of me in high school. He was an incredible painter. I had the opportunity to chat with Chris via e-mail during the planning for our two classes' thirtieth reunion. It was the first time he and I have actually communicated in all these years. His ability to paint always impressed me.

One of the most influential spinal-cord-injury people to come into my life was Barry Vuletich, although I didn't know it at the time I first met him. Barry has been a well-known figure in Arkansas Rehabilitation Services for many years in many different capacities. I'll bring this story full circle after I give you a little bit of background.

Shortly before my accident I was working for a temporary service in Little Rock in 1994 while I was looking for full-time employment with my MBA. I was assigned as a "temp" for Barry for a week. He was the first quadriplegic I had ever had the opportunity to get to know fairly well. While working for Barry I learned that spinal-cord-injured people are still people. They are just people with limitations. I never had any idea that I would be joining the quadriplegic ranks shortly thereafter.

In an unusual twist of fate and to show you how small a world it can be, I had the opportunity to meet Barry again in the Fall of 2006. I had attended a disabilities conference where I met Barry's assistant, Sharon Wofford (a truly delightful lady). I spoke with her about an issue at the conference, but our conversation turned to adaptive typing software. She offered to demonstrate the software to me.

She mentioned that she worked for Barry, and I filled her in on my previous history with Barry. She insisted I come talk to him when I was through with the demonstration. I spent the next hour and a half in Barry's office filling him in on what had happened since I temped for him in 1994. Then they asked me if I wanted to serve on the Arkansas Increasing Capabilities Access Network (ICAN) advisory council.

I have typed this manuscript, rather than using adaptive software. The adaptive software is pricier than my budget can afford, at close to $1,000. I hope someday to be able to afford the software (Tell your friends about this book. Just kidding. I truly hope they never need it.)

I figured if all these people could deal with their disabilities and be cheerful and functional, then so could I. If you think back through your life, I am sure you can think of people who can be similar examples for you.

The Questions Nobody Wants to Ask After a Spinal Cord Injury

98

Sexuality After a Spinal Cord Injury

I've always felt that sexuality is a really slippery thing.
In this day and age, it tends to get categorized
and labeled, and I think labels are for food.
Canned food.—
Michael Stipe

Sexuality/sex after a spinal cord injury is something that everybody wants to know about, but nobody wants to talk about.

In this chapter I am going to discuss sexuality in general after a spinal cord injury. In the following chapter, I will discuss sex for males after a spinal cord injury. I will discuss sex for females after a spinal cord injury in the chapter after the chapter for men.

Dr. Marca Sipski has observed that "maintaining a healthy sex life after a spinal cord injury is an important priority to many people."[1] Really? No kidding.

I found another study on sexual function related to spinal cord injury I thought was very interesting. Studies of the spinal cord injury population have shown that walking is not the most important function to recover to improve quality of life after a spinal cord injury. According to the article, "regaining sexual function is the combined number one or number two priority to a significant proportion of all individuals living with SCI, regardless of injury level." The other functions important to quality of life were regaining bladder and bowel function, eliminating autonomic dysreflexia, and improving arm/hand function.[2]

I want to make a clarification regarding the above quotation. The quotation uses the word references "all individuals" living with a spinal cord injury. The article I read cites an earlier article by the same author. In the current article the study on sexual health of spinal cord injury population was of adults eighteen years and older. I have not read the original article, but I am going to assume that the study group was also of an adult population eighteen years and older. I want to make it clear that the researchers are not surveying teenagers, pre-teens, and children when it comes to sexual issues.

The book *The Ultimate Guide to Sex and Disability* lists several myths about disability and sexuality:

1. People living with disabilities and chronic illnesses are not sexual.
2. People living with disabilities and chronic illnesses are not desirable.
3. Sex must be spontaneous.
4. People who live with disabilities and chronic illnesses can't have "real" sex.
5. People living with disabilities and chronic illnesses are pathetic choices for partners.
6. People living with disabilities and chronic illnesses have more important things than sex to worry about.
7. People living with disabilities and chronic illnesses are not sexually adventurous.
8. People living with disabilities and chronic illnesses who have sex are perverts.
9. We are get what we deserve, and we can always do more to help ourselves.
10. People living in institutions shouldn't have sex.
11. Sex is private.
12. People living with disabilities and chronic illnesses don't get sexually assaulted.
13. People living with disabilities and chronic illnesses don't need sex education.
14. People living with disabilities and chronic illnesses are unnatural.[3]

Do any of these myths interfere with your life? This is not a question to be answered immediately and quickly. Really think about it for a period of time. And if they do, do you want to take action to stop them from interfering with your life?

Sexuality is all about self-esteem. People do many things to make themselves more attractive. To have high self-esteem, you need to feel good about yourself. If you feel good about yourself, then you can "market" yourself. (Well, not in *that* sense. I don't mean you should become a "streetwalker." Even if you can still walk.) to men or women (or both, I suppose). I am getting *old*.

Spinal cord injuries don't generally make us feel better about ourselves. For a variety of reasons. We may no longer have normal control of our bodily functions. We may no longer have normal control of our arms and legs. We may rely upon canes, crutches, walkers, manual or electric wheelchairs for mobility. We may have lost or gained weight as a result of our injuries. We may have removed ourselves from our normal social activities as a result of our accident and loss of functionality, where we would meet people.

You are not alone if your injury has made your self-esteem not what it used to be.

"How do I get that self-esteem back? How do I become where I feel attractive again?" There are many resources available. The book I mentioned earlier in this chapter is a very thorough self-help (I hate that phrase but I don't know what else to call it) guide. There are other books on sex and disability. Support groups and counseling come to mind as other options.

But whatever route you take to recover your self-esteem and your sexuality, take it at your own pace. Don't let anyone force you to recover at a speed faster than you are ready for.

And don't let anyone make you feel you are unattractive.

99

Sex After a Spinal Cord Injury—Men

So many men, so little time—
Mae West

This is one of the most important topics to discuss after a spinal cord injury. I am not going to go into a great deal of detail because the information and scientific advances are changing so fast that whatever I say will be out of date immediately. It's like buying a computer and the computer becomes obsolete six months after you buy it. I just want to cover some basics.

Gentlemen, I am going to assume that you are familiar with the construction of your genitalia ("private parts") so that I don't have to explain how you are built. If you don't know, ask someone you are comfortable discussing the subject, do some research on the Internet, or ask your doctor.

I am going to state one universal fact when it comes to spinal cord injury and sex. As Dr. Marca Sipski states in doctorese:

> The effect of a spinal cord injury on sexual response is generally discussed based upon the degree of completeness or incompleteness of the patient's injury[,] and whether the neurologic damage affecting the individual's sacral spinal segments is an upper or lower motor neuron injury."[1]

Whew! Take a deep breath after that quotation. Let's talk in English. What still works and how well depends on if your injury is complete or incomplete and whether the damage to your spinal cord prevents information getting from your brain to your "private parts" or if the damage prevents information getting from your "private parts" to your brain. Why was that so difficult for a doctor to say? It's a great quotation, but unfortunately the article is already ten years old.

I've already discussed how you know if your injury is complete or incomplete so there is no need to explain that part of the quotation again.

I am going to talk about how your sex organs react before a spinal cord injury and after a spinal cord injury. Bear in mind that every injury is different. Every person's functionality is different after a spinal cord injury.

Doctors say that "nothing will work downstairs" after a spinal cord injury for you men. I know of one fellow with a T-level injury who cannot feel or move his legs who doesn't even have pain, but whose "everything else" still works fine. So much for what doctors say.

Let's talk about how things work before a spinal cord injury. Guys, you see a pretty girl. Your brain reacts. You are programmed that way automatically. Your brain sends a signal downstairs. The nerves between levels T10 and L2 in your spinal cord receive the signal from your brain. The T10 to L2 nerves order a "wake up call" to certain parts that are near and dear to you. You know what happens, or should happen next.[2]

I'm going to throw in some humor before I go on to the next paragraph. Say you are staying in a motel or hotel. Assume there is no alarm clock in your room. You need to wake up at a certain time to start your day. In the United States you call the front desk and ask for a wake up call. In the United Kingdom you call the front desk and ask for a knock up call. In American English slang, knocking someone up means to get them pregnant.

Back to my discussion. Guys, let's assume that someone makes contact with your near and dear parts, your ears, your nipples, your neck, etc. Let's assume that the someone making contact is making contact with your permission. Your near and dear parts react. They send a signal to the S2 to S4 levels of your spinal cord in your very low back.[2]

In both situations, a signal must travel through part of your spinal cord. Depending on where and how badly your spinal cord has been damaged determines how much signal can get through to its destination.

Will your soldier still stand at attention after a spinal cord injury? Quite possibly. Oral medications now exist to assist with such problems. I don't have to name them. Constant commercials for these drugs blare out of your TV. More of them are being developed as we speak. Local injections are also available. Local medications are available. Vacuum pumps exist. As a last resort, surgical implants are also available.[2] Your best bet is going to be to talk with your urologist on the subject. If you don't have a good urologist, ask around in your community. Get one.

Ok, let's assume your "flagpole" is ok. Will everything else go "swimmingly?" If you'll pardon the pun, here is the hard part. Fertility can be a real problem after a spinal cord injury. Doctors don't know why at this point, but you're not making as many of the "little swimmers" as you should be. My own hypothesis is because you are not getting as much blood flow to that area of your body. Your body can no longer produce what it should be producing.

From what I've read, the "little swimmer" population remains normal for about two weeks after your injury. Might want to have some of them frozen for future use if the option is available.[2] Lack of population density is a problem that also plagues men who have not had spinal cord injuries.

Why don't the "little swimmers" swim as well after a spinal cord injury? A recent article says that the "little swimmers" have been joined by white blood cells which destroy foreign bodies and cells that promote inflammatory reactions.[3] I guess the presence of those additional cells is kind of like the alligators in the old video game "Frogger" where you try and get the frog across the stream by jumping from log to log.

Let's talk about a related problem after a spinal cord injury. What about "The Big T?" Testosterone. The production of this hormone makes you look and act like a guy.

We all know that as you age, you don't make as much of "The Big T." Bad news. Some medical conditions like diabetes can also cause problems with 'T" production. So can a spinal cord injury. Replacement therapy is available by prescription in the form of oral medication, creams, or patches.[4]

There is some good news. According to one study:

> A significant amount of adaptation occurs regarding sexual stimulation and arousal in men living with 'complete' spinal cord injury. There was an inverse relationship between developing new areas of sexual arousal above the level of lesion and not having genital sensation, anal sensation, or the ability to lift legs against gravity. The most commonly reported sexual stimulation leading to the best arousal involved touching the genitalia, followed by stimulation of the head/neck and torso areas."[5] If the men with complete injuries can adapt, so can the men with incomplete injuries.

If you do find yourself in a situation where having sex is an option, don't forget about the risk of sexually transmitted diseases. You have enough problems without getting one of those.

If you decide you want to have children after your injury, research your options. Have your situation evaluated by a physician. See what options are available.

If a doctor determines you are still fertile after your accident, and you don't want to have children; please take appropriate precautions. Unless your religion prevents doing so.

100

Sex After a Spinal Cord Injury—Women

Women are meant to be loved, not to be understood.—
Oscar Wilde

Women are also going to issues with sex after a spinal cord injury, but these functionality issues are different from those men face.

Ladies, as I said to the men in the previous chapter, I am going to assume that you are familiar with the construction of your genitalia ("private parts") so that I don't have to explain how you are built. If you don't know, ask someone you are comfortable discussing the subject with, do some research on the Internet, or ask your doctor.

I presented a quotation in the chapter on sex after a spinal cord injury for men (which I am assuming you did not read) and I am going to repeat it here. As Dr. Marca Sipski states in doctorese:

> The effect of a spinal cord injury on sexual response is generally discussed based upon the degree of completeness or incompleteness of the patient's injury and whether the neurologic damage affecting the individual's sacral spinal segments is an upper or lower motor neuron injury.[1]

In English, level and degree of injury determine functionality. Again, every injury is different. Your degree of functionality and feeling will be different from other women.

I read a quotation some years back and I cannot find the article, but I want to mention the idea here. The article discussed the differences between how men's bodies are "wired" for sexual function and how women's bodies are "wired" for sexual function. The article discussed that men's bodies require the spinal cord to be intact because the signals are "hardwired" in men for sexual function (pardon the pun). The article went on to say that women's bodies are not "hardwired" for sexual function, but that women's bodies depend more on the brain.

It is fairly common knowledge that as men age, their "boingers" don't "boing" the way the they used to. Women also experience a problem with aging that their WD-40 doesn't work the way it used to (please *don't* try using WD-40 in bed, unless your bed squeaks when you have sex and you live in an apartment). For those who don't know what WD-40 is, it's a general purpose household, automotive, and marine lubricant in a spray can. Spinal cord injury also intensifies this problem.[2] Not the squeaky bed in an apartment problem, although I suppose it could.

Women, as you know, you may also experience problems if you have no sensation below the waist. Or even if you have partial sensation. Or your muscles "down there" may no longer function properly. The "Big O" may become simply a memory.

Let me go back to the subject of lubrication briefly. There are many dedicated products on the market for this purpose. Use a water-based lubricant. Do not use an oil-based lubricant, especially if your partner is using a condom. You can buy lubricants in discount stores, drug stores, on eBay, or on the Internet. Experiment until you find one that works for you.

Even assuming you have partial or no feeling below the shoulders, earlobes, necks, and the lips on your face still work nicely as erogenous zones.

Women with spinal cord injuries seem to be more concerned than men with spinal cord injuries about the problem of bladder incontinence sexual activity and bowel incontinence during sexual activity.[3]

The most common sources of difficulty in sexual activity in women are "injury level (greater difficulties for cervical injuries), having severe spasticity (during typical daily life), having pain, spasticity, or autonomic dysreflexia during sexual activity, or autonomic dysreflexia in general," according to one article.[4]

As with men, according to the article cited in the previous paragraph, "there was an inverse relationship between developing new areas of arousal above the level of lesion and not having anal sensation or the ability to lift legs against gravity."[5] If the men can adapt, so can you, ladies!

As for menopause after a spinal cord injury, one study reported that the age at which women with spinal cord injuries go through menopause does not differ greatly from the age at which women without spinal cord injuries go through menopause. The SCI women seem to start menopause just slightly earlier than their counterparts without a spinal cord injury. A few women did go through menopause within one year after their injury.[6]

Women who did go through menopause after their injuries reported more mood disorders, and symptoms directly related to spinal cord injury such as spasticity, autonomic dysreflexia, and bladder spasms.[7]

One thing I want to discuss that is not directly related to spinal cord injury is the new vaccine for Human Papilloma Virus (HPV). Almost all strains of this virus can cause cervical cancers. It is recommended that a woman be vaccinated at about ages eleven to twelve, before she becomes sexually active. The vaccination requires three doses in one year. It is also recommended that women ages nineteen through twenty six be vaccinated since they could not be vaccinated at ages eleven or twelve. The vaccine is still being studied to determine its effectiveness in preventing genital cancer in males.[8]

Don't forget that sexually transmitted diseases are still an issue. Protect yourself accordingly. If you don't want to get pregnant, use birth control, if your religion allows it. Yes, you may still be able to become pregnant with a spinal cord injury.

Also don't forget to have a yearly visit to the gynecologist, and have a Pap Smear done. Even if you have the HPV vaccine. You don't need to deal with cancer in addition to everything else.

Women with spinal cord injuries, even complete spinal cord injuries, can still get pregnant and bear children. This is assuming other injuries were not sustained in the accident to prevent it. If you are within childbearing age, and want to get pregnant, it would be advisable to find an OB/GYN who is experienced with spinal cord injury pregnancies.

Getting Help and Quality of Life Improvement

101

"How Do I Find a Doctor Who is Familiar with Spinal Cord Injuries After I'm Recovered?"

Sometimes attaining the deepest familiarity with a question is our best substitute for actually having the answer.—
Brian Greene

Let's assume you have done the hospital phase and the rehabilitation phase. You are living with family, friends, or on your own.

You realize that spinal cord injury survivors have different medical needs than the general population. How do you find doctors who are familiar with treating the medical conditions unique to spinal cord injury survivors? And why do you need to?

The ultimate goal for every one of us with a spinal cord injury is the same: to minimize the effects of the injury and to optimize the quality of life.[1] As I have mentioned several times in the book, the expertise of medical science dealing with long-time spinal cord injury survival is relatively limited. Not every doctor is going to have experience treating a single spinal cord injury survivor, much less many of them.

There is both an up side and a down side to the increasing rate of spinal cord injury in the United States. The bad part is that more people have spinal cord injuries. The good part is that more doctors will become experienced treating people with spinal cord injuries because there are more spinal cord injuries (and the survivors are living longer).

Why aren't all doctors familiar with treating spinal cord injury survivors? When I say "doctor" I am referring to a general practitioner ("GP" as they are often called). I supposed the same discussion could be used with particular types of specialists such as urologists or cardiologists. Not having been to medical school, I don't know how much emphasis is placed on the ongoing treatment of spinal cord injury survivors. But I can take a stab at another way to approach the question.

If a doctor sees a lot of strep throat cases, he or she is going to be very familiar with how to treat strep throat. If he or she does not see that many cases, the doctor may be unfamiliar with all the ins and outs of treatment. So let's do some calculations. Oh no, you say, not math! I will do the calculations for you.

There are approximately 3,000,000 people in the United States.[2] There are about 300,000 spinal cord injury survivors in the United States.[3] So about ten percent of the population in the United States has a spinal cord injury. But just because one out of every ten people has a spinal cord injury doesn't mean a doctor will have a spinal cord injury survivor in his or her patient group.

I could not find any information on geographic distribution of spinal cord injury survivors in the United States. If any of you medical professionals out there do this kind of research, maybe you could do a study sometime. Let me know if you have any such information.

If spinal cord injury survivors were spread among the general population in an even distribution, the odds would be greater than each doctor would have a spinal cord injury survivor in his or her patient group.

I am guessing that spinal cord injury survivors in each community tend to go to the same doctor(s) because they talk to other survivors. This is how they find out who has experience with this type of medicine. I know my spinal cord injury support group has had this discussion.

A quotation I found in a book on spinal cord injury and aging that fits this chapter very well is "There is no adequate way to describe the many different healthcare needs of persons with SCI."[4] The authors of this source continue by saying:

> While the healthcare needs of persons with SCI are similar to those in the general population, they are different in six major ways:
> 1. Persons with SCI generally have a "thinner margin of health" that must be scrupulously guarded if serious medical problems are to be averted … SCI people are highly vulnerable to a variety of acute conditions.
> 2. Once an acute condition sets in, the recovery and recuperation period is likely to be longer for persons with SCI than for persons in the general population. The mobility limitations of a person with SCI may also limit participation in selected therapies.
> 3. People with SCI may be at greater risk of acquiring new chronic health conditions that often accompany the aging process—we do know they are not always able to participate in some of the prevention strategies available to the non disabled population.…

> 4. Unlike most in the general population, persons with SCI may need intermittent rehabilitative services and assistive technologies. An example is going from crutches and braces to a wheelchair.
> 5. Unlike most of the general population, about half of all persons with SCI need some assistance with their daily personal care. The assistance is not only essential to their ability to lead active and productive lives but is also essential to health maintenance.…
> 6. A small but growing minority of persons with SCI need mechanical ventilation.[5]

Another excellent point that the authors of the book on spinal cord injury and aging make is that spinal cord injury survivors make an average of eighteen doctor visits a year. That is approximately four times the rate of visits for people without spinal cord injuries. They also mention that spinal cord injury survivors have an average of forty eight contacts per year with other medical professionals such as nurses, physical therapists, or psychologists. Finally they add that spinal cord injury survivors are "among the highest users of hospital inpatient care during their post-rehabilitation life."[6]

The authors of the above also make three more excellent points regarding spinal cord injury survivors and the medical community:

> 1. Persons with SCI are far more likely to be using prescription drugs than the general population. They are usually long-time users of prescription drugs.…[7]
> 2.… [T]he "work" of living with disability continues to tax the coping abilities of the individual on a much more immediate and personal level—throughout the course of his or her life.[8]
> 3. In addition, there is the additive effect of aging and disability, which magnifies the impact of typical and expected stresses into even larger, more unmanageable crisis [*sic*][9]

Now you know why a spinal cord injury survivors needs doctors who are familiar with treating medical issues that may arise after a spinal cord injury. Now comes the more difficult question. How do you find them?

Ask other spinal cord injury survivors. Find support groups and ask. Ask rehabilitation and occupational therapists. Ask medical vendors. Ask anybody you think might know.

If you are not happy with the treatment you receive or the doctor's level of familiarity with treating issues that arise after a spinal cord injury, then find another doctor.

It is *your* health and *your* life.

102

"Should I Go To a Chiropractor After a Spinal Cord Injury?"

The treatments themselves do not 'cure' the condition, they simply restore the body's self-healing ability.—
Leon Chaitow

"Should I go to a chiropractor?" is one of those questions that is very difficult to answer. It depends on what your situation is.

It is my understanding that reputable chiropractors will generally not work on self-referred people with disc fusions. You certainly don't want to go to a chiropractor until your fusion is fully healed and completely fused. This generally takes about a year. Your fusion may take more time to heal, depending on your circumstances. Do be sure to follow your surgeon's instructions. If you don't, you run the risk of your recovery being less than expected. Also make sure you read the last chapter of the book before the Endnotes.

There are instances where an individual may be referred to a chiropractor by his or her primary care physician after having a spinal fusion. This is to increase the range of motion in the neck.

I did see improvement in range of motion after going to a chiropractor. But I was very careful as to how much I would let him adjust my neck. When the adjustment started causing pain, I stopped going to the chiropractor.

If you have not had a confirmed spinal cord injury, then the decision will have to be yours. You will need to research your decision carefully and consider all the pros and cons.

If you are considering a particular chiropractor, research and find out if any complaints have been filed against the particular doctor with your appropriate state agency. See if you can find other people in your community who have used that particular doctor. The doctor him- or herself will likely be happy to give you references of patients who are happy with his or her services (imagine that!) with the patient's consent, of course.

There are many people who are very happy with the services of their chiropractor as opposed to their family doctor in relieving their symptoms. There are also people who have suffered spinal cord injuries as a result of the manipulations of a chiropractor.[1 2]

For those not familiar with what a chiropractor does, a chiropractor is a person who diagnoses and treats patients whose health problems are associated with the body's muscular, nervous, and skeletal systems, especially the spine. They provide natural, drugless, non-surgical treatments and rely on the body's inherent healing powers. Chiropractors are authorized to take x-rays.

Increasingly, states are requiring chiropractors to have a four-year undergraduate degree along with completion of a four-year program at an accredited chiropractic college leading to the Doctor of Chiropractic degree. After completing a degree program, an individual must pass the appropriate licensing procedures in the state(s) he or she wishes to practice in.

This may be all or part of the four-part test administered by the National Board of Chiropractic Examiners and/or a state examination. All states except New Jersey require continuing education hours each year to maintain licensure. A professional with the initials D.C. after his or her name is a chiropractor.[3] In China a chiropractor is called a bonesetter.[4]

Chiropractic care is covered by some insurance plans and by some HMOs, generally with limited coverage. Does Medicare cover chiropractic care? Yes with very severe restrictions.

First, you must have a subluxation (here we go again, more "doctorese") of the spine. [5]A subluxation is where your vertebrae in your spinal column no longer line up properly.[6] Next, you must have an x-ray, CT scan, or MRI image taken by your family doctor. Medicare will not cover the imaging if it is performed by your chiropractor. The benefit paid will be determined by your medical need.[7]

Does Medicaid cover chiropractic care? This is an easy question with a very complication answer. Yes and no. Chiropractic services are technically allowed under Medicaid. But the individual states regulate the benefits. So the coverage is extremely variable from state to state.[8]

State mandates do exist for coverage for group health insurance plans. There are two types of mandated benefits for chiropractic. The first consists of a minimum coverage standard for all group polices sold in a state. As of 1999, this was in effect in forty-four of the fifty states. There may be a specified number of chiropractic visits covered in a group health insurance policy. The second mandate, effective only in Washington state as of 1999, requires insurance companies to offer specified chiropractic coverage for sale.[9]

If you decide to go to a chiropractor, make sure the chiropractor you select is reputable. Check with your state (regional or national) chiropractic regulating agency, depending on what country you are in. You want to know in advance if there have been any complaints against the person. Also ask around in your community who is good.

103

"Should I Go To a Massage Therapist After a Spinal Cord Injury?"

So no tennis for the moment,
but lots of treatment and massage.—
Kim Clijsters

You may also be curious about massage therapy after a spinal cord injury. As with a chiropractor, you need to wait until your fusion has completely healed.

I found an article that discusses massage therapy for spinal cord injury patients. The author of the article states that very few massage therapists actually have experience with spinal cord injury patients. The purpose of the article was to educate therapists how massage can be useful for spinal cord injury patients.

The same massage therapy that is used for normal people can be used on spinal cord injurees. If a person is in a wheelchair and cannot get to the massage table, the therapist can use stretching techniques to help his or her client to improve spasticity.[1]

Depending on your degree of injury, going to a massage therapist may not be possible because of the lack of a lift to get you from your wheelchair to the massage table. Hydraulic massage tables do exist which would make it easier to transfer a person from a wheelchair to the massage table.[2] The massage therapist's place of business may not be accessible.

Other benefits that spinal cord injurees may see from massage are to limit the process of postural distortions. In plain English this is not being able to sit up straight. Massage therapists are as bad as doctors with their jargon. Getting regular massages can help reduce the process and the pain that comes with it.[3]

People who are in manual wheelchairs are going to have problems with overuse of their shoulders, arms, and hands. Massage can also help with the chronic tendonitis associated with overuse.[4]

"Massage has no risk of injury or further injury," according to a posting I found on the Internet. [Everything has some risk to it, even if it is a small one. There is always the risk of being injured by an incompetent professional.] Massage can help with circulation, keeping joints loose, and relieving minor aches and pains.[5] It can also help with spasticity, from my own experience.

Does Medicare cover massage therapy? Not as of July 2005.[6] What about Medicaid? I was unable to find a clear answer to this question. Some states, such as Florida, are experimenting with offering massage therapy under Medicaid for treatment of chronic pain.[7]

My answer to the question of "should I go to a massage therapist?" is if you are interested in having a massage, you should investigate the possibility. Make sure the person you go to is properly certified by the state you live in.

104

"Should I Participate in a Clinical Trial?"

All life is an experiment.—
Ralph Waldo Emerson

"Carolyn, I'm desperate. I can't go through the rest of my life like this. I've got to find a clinical trial and get into it! I've got to be cured."

I know exactly how you feel. I've been living with a spinal cord injury going on thirteen years. Spinal cord injuries get old very quickly.

If you decide you are interested in participating in a clinical trial, here are some things you need to know. New treatments move from the laboratory environmental to a clinical environment. They must undergo clinical trials before being released on the market.[1]

Clinical trials are necessary because pharmaceutical companies need to find out if their new drugs really do have beneficial effects. They also need to make sure their new drugs do not cause harm to the patients.

If you are considering joining a clinical trial, there are two things you need to avoid: 1) experimental treatments offered without having completed a trial, and 2) treatments offered for material gain. You should not have to pay for any procedure specifically related to a clinical trial program.[2]

Don't join any clinical program that offers to pay you for participating. This is different from being paid to complete a survey related to your disability.

There are three steps in legitimate clinical trials. The first (Phase One) is to find out if the treatment is safe. The second (Phase Two) is to determine if there is a positive effect from the treatment being tested. The third (Phase Three) is to make sure there is a positive effect from the treatment being tested and to determine there are no serious side effects. If the treatment passes two separate Phase Three trials, then it will be approved for clinical use.[3]

Just because you have applied to join a clinical trial does not mean you will be accepted. All clinical trials have very specific criteria (specifics for being included). An example of a clinical trial criteria might be: males between the ages of thirty and thirty five with blue eyes and brown hair who rode bicycles as children. These are not serious clinical trial criteria, but you get the idea.

You will be required to give what is called informed consent to participate in a clinical trial. I will repeat the definition of informed consent in case you have forgotten from the chapter on Transitional Syndrome. Informed consent is a legal condition whereby a person can be said to have given consent based upon an appreciation and understanding of the facts and implications of an action.[4]

Let's not talk like lawyers. Let's talk like real people. What informed consent means is that you (or your family) must understand all the pros and cons of what is about to be done to you. You have to be given all the relevant information. You (or your family) also have to be capable of giving informed consent.

You cannot give informed consent if you are mentally retarded or mentally ill, drunk, seriously ill in some situations, are not coherent due to lack of sleep, stoned, medically partially sedated, or have any other condition which would cause you to be unable to understand the pros and cons of the situation.[5] A head injury might be another example of a situation why you would not be able to give proper informed consent.

If you have been accepted to a clinical trial, you will have to undergo various medical tests first. Examples of these tests are a full physical exam, blood tests, and tests of the ability to perform daily living tasks to test your spinal cord function. You should not have to pay for these tests.[6]

If you have participated in previous clinical trials or have been given experimental treatment, you may be excluded from a clinical trial.[7]

Assuming you have been accepted into a clinical trial, you now have to make a decision. Do you participate or do you decline? There are some factors that will help you make your decision.

You need to find out before you agree to participate what experimental evidence there is that the treatment works. You also need to find out the evidence that the treatment is safe. After all, if you receive an unsafe treatment, your condition could worsen or you could die. There is a lot at stake here. Finally, you need to find out if you have been invited to participate in Phase One, Phase Two, or Phase Three of the clinical trial. You should know what follow-up studies there will be after the clinical trial is over. If you are asked to pay for the follow-up studies, then the clinical trial is not legitimate.[8]

If you are really serious about participating in a clinical trial, then the following organizations can be contacted for more information:

Christopher and Dana Reeve Foundation: http://www.christopherreeve.org
Institut pour la Recherche sur la Moelle épinière et l'Enéphale: http://www.irme.org
International Spinal Research Trust: http://www.spinal-research.org
Fondation Internationale pour la recherche en paraplèie: http://www.irp.ch
Japan Spinal Cord Foundation: http://www.jscf.org
Miami Project to Cure Paralysis: http://www.themiamiproject.org
Neil Sachse Foundation: http://www.nsf.org.au
Paralyzed Veterans of America: http://wwww.pva.org
Rick Hansen Foundation: http://www.rickhansen.com
Spinal Cure Australia: http://www.spinalcure.org.au
Wings for Life: http://www.wingsforlife.com[9]

You can also contact spinal cord injury researchers. The foundations listed above can give you more information on this. It is best to contact the researchers by e-mail. [10]

I recommend that anyone who is serious about participating in clinical trials go to http://www.campaignforcure.org. Read the full document I have referenced in this chapter. It goes into much more detail about the phases of a clinical trial.

Final Thoughts

105

"Final Thoughts"

It is now September 2007. Nearly thirteen years have passed since my accident. Where am I emotionally and physically at this point?

Raymond and I, like everybody else, take life one day at a time. We don't try to plan beyond the current day. We just take life as it comes. This is something we have had to learn. Plans change. Spinal cord injuries happen.

I was going to say in the previous paragraph that we "put one foot in front of the other like everybody else." I realized this phrase carried with it an inherent humor, because I don't walk normally.

Raymond, of course, worries about me more than he did before my accident.

Each day brings with it new challenges. I never know from one minute to the next how my body is going to function. How my neurons are going to misfire. What strange and new difficulty the attempt to move is going to bring.

Do I still carry anger about my accident? No. Not after this many years. I have accepted that it was meant to be for some reason. I am grateful to still be alive.

I do feel frustration, of course. Not being able to do the things I used to be able to do. I miss working in the yard like I used to. I miss being able to write by hand. I miss being able to walk normally. And a host of other things. Little things like looking up at the stars. Or watching an airshow. I miss being able to be employed full-time in traditional work. I miss the camaraderie of having fellow employees.

I will always have physical challenges to contend with, as a result of the accident.

I still I feel alienated from others in two different ways. I feel alienated from "normal," non-spinal-cord-injured people. This will probably never change. I also feel alienated from people in wheelchairs. I don't want to join the ranks of those in wheelchairs, of course. Nothing personal. I want to be able to continue walking with assistance. But the nature of my injury makes it difficult sometimes for me to be able to relate to others with spinal cord injuries. And for them to be able to relate to me. I hope, given more time, I will be able to resolve these feelings of alienation.

I have benefited in many ways since my accident as well.

I have met many wonderful people I would not have met otherwise, but for my spinal cord injury. I would not have had the opportunity to write this book, if not for my spinal cord injury. And I have recently started a new career, as a freelance writer, because of my spinal cord injury. I have also become more involved with religion since my injury. I depend upon daily prayer more now than at any time in my life.

My life certainly has not turned out the way I planned. Or the way I could ever have foreseen. This does not make it bad.

Just different.

106

"A Word of Warning"

If you have an incomplete spinal cord injury and have a relative degree of independence, you may be tempted to resume some of your pre-injury activities. This is especially true if you have Central Cord Syndrome.

If you want to engage in any of the following activities, check with your physician first:

1. Snow skiing
2. Water skiing
3. Any carnival or theme park rides (especially a roller coaster)
4. Skydiving
5. Ice skating
6. Roller skating
7. Skateboarding
8. Using a trampoline
9. Any extreme sports

You certainly do not want to engage in any of these activities while your fusion is still healing.

Your fusion(s) may not be able to withstand the physical forces put on them by some of these activities. Especially by activities such as riding a roller coaster. I have read reports of people suffering closed head injuries and spinal cord injuries from riding roller coasters. For activities where there is a high risk of falling, you run the risk of damaging your fusion or even your spinal cord further.

If you live in an area where ice develops on hard surfaces in the winter, be very, very careful. As I have mentioned previously, my first neurosurgeon warned me before I had my first surgery if I slipped and fell on the ice, I could completely tear my spinal cord. Then I would be a complete quadriplegic from the shoulders down.

Remember, having a spinal cord injury doesn't mean your life is over. It just means you have to live the rest of your life more carefully and more cautiously. This can be a good thing, though.

Living your life with excessive caution leads to old age.

Endnotes

Abbreviations

Preface

1. *Wikipedia*, s.v. "Quadriplegia," http://en.wikipedia.org/wiki/Quadriplegia (Accessed June 23, 2007).

2. *Wikipedia*, s.v. "Paraplegia," http://en.wikipedia.org/wiki/Paraplegia (Accessed June 23, 2007).

Chapter 1 "Thoughts Immediately After a Spinal Cord Injury"

Chapter 2 "A Little Bit About Me"

Chapter 3 "My Accident"

Chapter 4 "My First Surgery"

Chapter 5 "My Complications One"

Chapter 6 My Complications Two

Chapter 7 "Good Days, Bad Days Even Still"

Chapter 8 "What If?…."

1. "What is Posttraumatic Stress Disorder (PTSD)?" National Center for Post-traumatic Stress Disorder (undated): 1 http://www.ncptsd.va.gov/ncmain/index.jsp (Accessed May 2, 2007).

2. *Urban Dictionary*, s.v. "T-bone," http://www.urbandictionary.com (Accessed May 2, 2007).

3. "Cars," an episode of *Crash Test Human.*

4. Lindsay Carswell. "Paralysis Push" *ScienCentralNews* (undated): 1 http://www.Sciencentral.com/articles/view.php3?article_id=21839251 (Accessed May 2, 2007).

5. S. Laurance Johnston. "Methylprednisone Revisited" *PN* (December 2006): 35-6.

Chapter 9 "Carolyn, What Syndrome and Symptoms Do You Have?"

Chapter 10 Ways The Spinal Cord Can Be Injured

1. Joseph S. Torg, James T. Guille, and Suzanne Jaffe. "Injuries to the Cervical Spine in American Football Players" *J Bone Joint Surg Am* 84 (2002): 121.

Chapter 11 The Neck Bone is Connected to the Hip Bone....?

1. Wise Young, "Spinal Cord Injury Levels & Classification" Sci-Info-Pages.com (June 25, 2006): 4 http://www.sci-info-pages.com/levels.html (Accessed January 29, 2007).

Chapter 12 "You Are Not Alone"

Chapter 13 A Brief History of Spinal Cord Injury and Treatment

1. Ben Hollis, "A History of Spinal Cord Injury" (lecture, Arkansas Spinal Cord Commission monthly support group meeting, Sherwood, AR, February 16, 2006).

2. Albert Bosch, E. Shannon Stauffer, and Vernon L. Nickel, "Incomplete Traumatic Quadriplegia: A Ten Year Review" *JAMA* 216 no. 3 (April 19, 1971): 473.

3. *Wikipedia*, s.v. "Teddy Pendergrass," http://en.wikipedia.org/wiki/Teddy_Pendergrass (Accessed May 9, 2007).

4. *Wikipedia,* s.v. "Vic Chesnutt," http://en.wikipedia.org/wiki/Vic_Chesnutt (Accessed May 9, 2007).

5. *Wikipedia,* "Chuck Graham," http://en.wikipedia.org/wiki/Chuck_Graham (Accessed May 9, 2007).

6. William C. Hanigan and Chris Sloffer, "Nelson's Wound: Treatment of Spinal Cord Injury in the 19th and Early 20th Century Military Conflicts" *Neurosurg Focus* 16 (March 2004): 1-12 http://www.medscape.com (Accessed January 31, 2007).

7. Lee Goldstein, *So Far So Good!* (Palm Coast, Florida: Paraplegia Press, 2005): vi, ix.

Chapter 14 Why You Need a Sense of Humor After a Spinal Cord Injury

1. *Wikipedia,* s.v. "Sense of humor," http://en.wikipedia.org/wiki/Sense_of_humor (Accessed July 10, 2007).

2. Richard Hollicky, *Roll Models: People Who Live Successfully Following Spinal Cord Injury and How They Do It* (Victoria, British Columbia: Trafford Publishing, 2004): 9.

Chapter 15 Know Your Surgeon and Anesthesiologist

1. "Know Your Anesthesiologist" American Society of Anesthesiologists (1999): 1-3 http://www.asahq.org/patient/Education/know.htm (Accessed May 24, 2007).

Chapter 16 Surgery for Spinal Cord Injuries

1. "Evaluating spinal fusion surgery" Spine-health.com (2007): 1 http://www.spine-health.com/topics/surg/discorfusion/discorfusion02.html (Accessed January 26, 2007).

2. "Cervical Artificial Disc Preserves Neck Mobility An Interview with Richard Guyer, MD" Spineuniverse.com (August 18, 2006): 2 http://www.spineuniverse.com/displayarticle.php/article2522.html (Accessed January 26, 2007).

3. Thomas Morrow, "Spinal Disc Technology Seeks To Replace Body's Engineering Marvel" *Managed Care Magazine* (June 2005): 1 http://www.managedcaremagazine.com/archives/0506/0506.biotech.com (Accessed January 26, 2007).

4. "Cervical Artificial Disc Preserves Neck Mobility: Part 2 An Interview with Richard Guyer, MD" Spineuniverse.com (August 16, 2006): 1 http://www.spineuniverse.com/displayarticle.php/article2525.html (Accessed January 26, 2007).

5. "Low Back Artificial Disc Device Approved! PRODISC-L® Total Disc Replacement" Spineuniverse.com (August 16, 2006): 1 http://www.spineuniverse.com/displayarticle.php/article1987.html (Accessed January 26, 2007).

6. David DeWitt, "Bone graft site pain and morbidity after spinal fusion" Spine-health.com (June 20, 2007): 1 http://www.spine-health.com/topics/surg/graftpain/graftpain.html (Accessed July 7, 2007).

7. See Note 6.

8. See Note 6.

9. *Wikipedia,* s.v. "Anterior superior iliac spine," http://en.wikipedia.org/wiki/Anterior_Superior _Iliac_Spine (Accessed July 7, 2007).

10. See Note 1.

Chapter 17 Communicating With Your Doctor

1. Gemmy Allen, "Communicating" Modern Management BMGT-1301 (1998): 1-5 http://www.telecollege.dcccd.edu/mgmt1374/book_contents/3organizing/commun/communic. htm+communication+process&hl=en&ct=clnk&cd=1&gl=us (Accessed May 27, 2007).

2. "Communicating with Your Doctor" Ohio State University Medical Center (2007): 1 http://medicalcenter.osu.edu/patientcare/findadoctor/choosing/communication (Accessed May 24, 2007).

3. "How to Help Your Doctor—Easy Steps To Improve Your Medical Care" MedicineNet.com (September 16, 2004): 6 http://www.MedicineNet.com/pdf/howtohelpyourdoctor.pdf (Accessed May 24, 2007).

Chapter 18 The Importance of Peer Support After a Spinal Cord Injury

1. Richard Hollicky, *Roll Models: People Who Live Successfully Following Spinal Cord Injury and How They Do It* (Victoria, British Columbia: Trafford Publishing, 2004): 43.

2. Roxanne Furlong, "Pay It Forward" *New Mobility* (June 2007): 48-49.

3. Steve Fiffer, *Three Quarters, Two Dimes, and A Nickel: A Memoir of Becoming Whole* (New York: The Free Press, 1999), 245.

Chapter 19 Family and Friends Adjustment to a Spinal Cord Injury

1. Theresa Jaworski and J. Scott Richards, "Family Adjustment to Spinal Cord Injury" Spain Rehabilitation Center Department of Rehabilitation Medicine University of Alabama, Birmingham (1998): 4 http://images.main.uab.edu/spinalcord/pdffiles/FamilyAdjustment.pdf (Accessed July 10, 2007).

2. Theresa Jaworski and J. Scott Richards, "Family Adjustment to Spinal Cord Injury" Spain Rehabilitation Center Department of Rehabilitation Medicine University of Alabama, Birmingham (1998): 5-6 http://images.main.uab.edu/spinalcord/pdffiles/FamilyAdjustment.pdf (Accessed July 10, 2007).

3. Theresa Jaworski and J. Scott Richards, "Family Adjustment to Spinal Cord Injury" Spain Rehabilitation Center Department of Rehabilitation Medicine University of Alabama, Birmingham (1998): 7 http://images.main.uab.edu/spinalcord/pdffiles/FamilyAdjustment.pdf (Accessed July 10, 2007).

4. Theresa Jaworski and J. Scott Richards, "Family Adjustment to Spinal Cord Injury" Spain Rehabilitation Center Department of Rehabilitation Medicine University of Alabama, Birmingham (1998): 10 http://images.main.uab.edu/spinalcord/pdffiles/FamilyAdjustment.pdf (Accessed July 10, 2007).

5. Richard C. Senelick and Karla Dougherty, *beyond* [*sic*] *please and thank you: The Disability Awareness Handbook for Families, Co-Workers, and Friends* (Birmingham: HealthSouth Press, 2001), 4-5.

Chapter 20 Trauma Centers

1. *Wikipedia*, s.v. "Trauma center," http://en.wikipedia.org/wiki/Trauma_center (Accessed May 19, 2007).

2. "Verified Trauma Centers" American College of Surgeons Trauma Programs (May 10, 2007): 1-8 http://www.facs.org/trauma/verified.html (Accessed May 19, 2007).

Chapter 21 How an Incomplete Spinal Cord Injury is Diagnosed

1. "Spinal Cord Trauma" *WebMD InteliHealth®* (2007): 2 http://www.intelihealth.com/IH/ihtIH/WSIHW000/9339/28083.html (Accessed July 9, 2007).

2. See Note 1.

3. Karim Brohi, "Indications for spinal immobilisation" trauma.org 7 no. 4 (April 2002): 1 http://www.trauma.org/archive/spine/cspine-stab.html (Accessed July 9, 2007).

4. Karim Brohi, "Indications for spinal immobilisation" trauma.org 7 no. 4 (April 2002): 2 http://www.trauma.org/archive/spine/cspine-stab.html (Accessed July 9, 2007).

5. See Note 1.

6. *Wikipedia*, s.v. "Computed tomography," http://en.wikipedia.org/wiki/Ct-scan (Accessed July 9, 2007).

7. *Wikipedia*, s.v. "Magnetic resonance imaging," http://en.wikipedia.org/wiki/MRI (Accessed July 9, 2007).

8. Charles H. Tator and Edward C. Benzel, "Clinical Manifestations of Acute Spinal Cord Injury" in *Contemporary Management of Spinal Cord Injury From Impact to Rehabilitation.* 2nd ed. American Association of Neurological Surgery (2000): 21-22.

9. Merriam, W.F., T.K. Taylor, S.J. Ruff, and M.J. McPhail, "A reappraisal of acute traumatic central cord syndrome" *J Bone Joint Surg Br* 68 no. 5 (November 1986): 709.

10. Tator, Charles H. and Edward C. Benzel, "Clinical Manifestations of Acute Spinal Cord Injury" in *Contemporary Management of Spinal Cord Injury From Impact to Rehabilitation.* 2nd ed. American Association of Neurological Surgery (2000): 23.

11. Wise Young, "Spinal Cord Injury Levels & Classification" Sci-Info-Pages.com (June 25, 2006): 9-10 http://www.sci-info-pages.com/levels.html (Accessed January 29, 2007).

Chapter 22 Hoffman's and Babinski's Signs

1. *Wikipedia*, s.v. "Central nervous system," http://en.wikipedia.org/wiki/Central_nervous _system (Accessed June 29, 2007).

2. *Wikipedia*, s.v. "Peripheral nervous system," http://en.wikipedia.org/wiki/Peripheral_nervous _system (Accessed June 29, 2007).

3. *Wikipedia*, s.v. "Neuron," http://en.wikipedia.org/wiki/Neuron (Accessed June 29, 2007).

4. *Wikipedia*, s.v. "Motor neuron" http://en.wikipedia.org/wiki/Motor_neuron (Accessed June 29, 2007).

5. *Wikipedia*, s.v. "Upper motor neuron," http://en.wikipedia.org/wiki/Upper_motor_neuron (Accessed June 29, 2007).

6. *Wikipedia*, "Lower motor neuron," http://en.wikipedia.org/wiki/Lower_Motor_neuron (Accessed June 29, 2007).

7. "Finger Flexors" neuroexam.com (undated): 1 http://www.neuroexam.com/content.php?p=33 (Accessed April 30, 2007).

8. "Hoffmann's reflex (Johann Hoffmann)" Whonamedit.com (undated): 1 http://www.whonamedit.com/synd.cfm/1560.html (Accessed April 30, 2007).

9. *Wikipedia*, s.v. "Plantar reflex," http://en.wikipedia.org/wiki/Plantar_reflex (Accessed June 29, 2007).

Chapter 23 "What Does Paralysis After a Spinal Cord Injury Feel Like?"

1. *Wikipedia*, s.v. "Paralysis," http://en.wikipedia.org/wiki/Paralysis (Accessed June 10, 2007).

Chapter 24 An Introduction to Spinal Cord Injuries and Syndromes

1. Charles H. Tator and Edward C. Benzel, "Clinical Manifestations of Acute Spinal Cord Injury" in *Contemporary Management of Spinal Cord Injury From Impact to Rehabilitation.* 2nd ed. American Association of Neurological Surgery (2000): 26.

2. Valerie Rich and Elizabeth McCaslin, "Central Cord Syndrome in a High School Wrestler: A Case Report" *J Athletic Training* 41 no. 3 (2006): 2 http://www.pubmedcentral.nih.gov/ articlerender.fcgi?artid=1569555 (Accessed July 11, 2007). [note: my copy of this article was obtained on the Internet. The pages of my copy do not show the original page numbers so the citation within the chapter must be based on the page numbers from my copy which run 1 through 7.]

3. "Injury Complications" Paraplegic-Online.com (February 2, 2007): 6 http://www.paraplegic-online.com/einjuricomplic01.html (Accessed August 2, 2007).

Chapter 25 Anterior Cord Syndrome

1. "Anterior Cord Syndrome" Apparelyzed.com (2005): 1 http://www.apparelyzed.com/spinal-cord-injury/anterior-cord-syndrome.html (Accessed July 15, 2007).

2. *Wheeless' Textbook of Orthopedics Online*, s.v. "Anterior Cord Syndrome," http://www.wheelessonline.com/ortho/anterior_cord_syndrome (Accessed July 15, 2007).

3. See Note 2.

4. See Note 1.

5. Albert Bosch, E. Shannon Stauffer, and Vernon L. Nickel, "Incomplete Traumatic Quadriplegia: A Ten Year Review" *JAMA* 216 no. 3 (April 19, 1971): 477.

Chapter 26 Brown-Sequard Syndrome

1. Michael S. Beeson and Scott T. Wilber, "Brown-Sequard Syndrome" *eMedicine* (February 1, 2007): 1 http://www.emedicine.com/emerg/topic70.htm (Accessed July 15, 2007).

2. "Brown Sequard" PeaceHealth.org (July 5, 2005): 1 http://www.peacehealth.org/kbase/nord/nord950.htm (Accessed July 15, 2007).

3. Michael S. Beeson and Scott T. Wilber, "Brown-Sequard Syndrome" *eMedicine* (February 1, 2007): 2-3 http://www.emedicine.com/emerg/topic70.htm (Accessed July 15, 2007).

4. Michael S. Beeson and Scott T. Wilber, "Brown-Sequard Syndrome" *eMedicine* (February 1, 2007): 2 http://www.emedicine.com/emerg/topic70.htm (Accessed July 15, 2007).

5. "Incomplete C1 Quad" The National Spinal Cord Injury Association Discussion Forum (August 20, 2005): 2 http://www.spinalcord.ord/forum/viewtopic.php/?t=416&highlight =brown+sequard (Accessed January 23, 2007).

6. "Living With Brown Sequard" The National Spinal Cord Injury Association Discussion Forum (February 8, 2006): 1-4 http://www.spinalcord.ord/forum/viewtopic.php/?t=416 &highlight=brown+sequard (Accessed January 23, 2007).

7. "Nice To Know I'm Not Alone With Brown Sequard" The National Spinal Cord Injury Association Discussion Forum (November 6, 2006): 1 http://

www.spinalcord.org/forum/viewtopic.php/?t=416&highlight=brown+sequard (Accessed January 23, 2007).

Chapter 27 Central Cord Syndrome

1. Albert Bosch, E. Shannon Stauffer, and Vernon L. Nickel, "Incomplete Traumatic Quadriplegia: A Ten Year Review" *JAMA* 216 no. 3 (April 19, 1971): 476.

2. Jim Pointer, "The Case of the Mysterious Motorist" Alameda County EMS (undated): 7-8 http://www.acgov.org/ems/Presentations/25_The_Case_of_The_mysterious_motorist.ppt (Accessed May 22, 2007).

3. R.C. Schneider, Glenn Cherry, and Henry Pantek, "The Syndrome of Acute Central Cervical Spinal Cord Injury with Special Reference to the Mechanisms Involved in Hyperextension Injuries of Cervical Spine" *J Neurosurg* 11 (July 26, 1954): 546.

4. R.C. Schneider, Glenn Cherry, and Henry Pantek, "The Syndrome of Acute Central Cervical Spinal Cord Injury with Special Reference to the Mechanisms Involved in Hyperextension Injuries of Cervical Spine" *J Neurosurg* 11 (July 26, 1954): 568.

5. R.C. Schneider, Glenn Cherry, and Henry Pantek, "The Syndrome of Acute Central Cervical Spinal Cord Injury with Special Reference to the Mechanisms Involved in Hyperextension Injuries of Cervical Spine" *J Neurosurg* 11 (July 26, 1954): 576.

6. See Note 3.

7. R.C. Schneider, Glenn Cherry, and Henry Pantek, "The Syndrome of Acute Central Cervical Spinal Cord Injury with Special Reference to the Mechanisms Involved in Hyperextension Injuries of Cervical Spine" *J Neurosurg* 11 (July 26, 1954): 547.

8. "Central Cord Syndrome" American Association of Neurological Surgeons (2007): 1 http://www.neurosurgerytoday.org/what/patient_e/central_cord_syndrome (Accessed July 11, 2007).

9. Valerie Rich and Elizabeth McCaslin, "Central Cord Syndrome in a High School Wrestler: A Case Report" *J Athletic Training* 41 no. 3 (2006): 2 http://www.pubmedcentral.nih.gov/ articlerender.fcgi?artid=1569555 (Accessed July 11, 2007). [note: my copy of this article was obtained on the Internet. The pages of my copy do not show the original page numbers so the citation within the chapter must be based on the page numbers from my copy which run 1 through 7.]

10. "Central Cord Syndrome" The National Spinal Cord Injury Association Discussion Forum (February 3, 2005): 1-8 http://www.spinalcord.ord/forum/viewtopic.php/?t=261&highlight =central+cord+syndrome (Accessed January 30, 2007).

Chapter 28 Posterior Cord Syndrome

1. Charles H. Tator and Edward C. Benzel, "Clinical Manifestations of Acute Spinal Cord Injury" in *Contemporary Management of Spinal Cord Injury From Impact to Rehabilitation.* 2nd ed. American Association of Neurological Surgery (2000): 28.

2. "Types of Paralysis" Apparelyzed.com (2005): 2 http://www.aparelyzed.com/quadriplegia.htm (Accessed July 15, 2007).

3. Jim Pointer, "The Case of the Mysterious Motorist" Alameda County EMS (undated): 23-24 http://www.acgov.org/ems/Presentations/25_The_Case_of_The_mysterious_motorist.ppt (Accessed May 22, 2007).

Chapter 29 Cauda Equina Syndrome

1. Charles H. Tator and Edward C. Benzel, "Clinical Manifestations of Acute Spinal Cord Injury" in *Contemporary Management of Spinal Cord Injury From Impact to Rehabilitation.* 2nd ed. American Association of Neurological Surgery (2000): 26.

2. Sarah Smith, "The Tale of the Horse's Tail: Cauda Equina Syndrome" Cauda Equina Support Group (August 2000): 1-10 http://www.caudaequina.org/definition.html (Accessed January 24, 2007).

Chapter 30 Arachnoiditis

1. *Wikipedia,* s.v. "Arachnoid," http://en.wikipedia.org/wiki/Arachnoid (Accessed June 27, 2007).

2. "Arachnoiditis Information & Support" Circle of Friends With Arachnoiditis (COFWA) (September 15, 2006): 1 http://www.cofwa.org (Accessed January 24, 2007).

3. Mary Claire Walsh, "Arachnoiditis" SpineUniverse.com (September 20, 2006): 1-2 http://www.spineuniverse.com/displayarticle/php/article180.html (Accessed January 24, 2007).

4. "National Institute of Neurological Disorders and Stroke Arachnoiditis Information Page" National Institute of Neurological Disorders and Stroke (August 4, 2006): 1 http://www.ninds.nih.gov/disorders/arachnoiditis/arachnoiditis.htm (Accessed January 24, 2007).

5. See Note 1.

Chapter 31 Conus Medullaris

1. *Wikipedia,* s.v. "Conus Medullaris," http://en.wikipedia.org/wiki/Conus_medullaris (Accessed July 10, 2007).

2. Segun T. Dawodu and Nicholas Lorenzo, "Cauda Equina and Conus Medullaris Syndromes" *emedicine* (January 16, 2007): 1-20 http://www.emedicine.com/neuro/topic667.htm (Accessed July 15, 2007).

Chapter 32 Cervicomedullary Syndrome

1. Robert A. Minns and Anthony Busuttil, "Letter Patterns of Presentation of the shaken baby syndrome Four types of inflicted brain injury predominate" *BMJ* 328 (2004): 766 http://www.bjm.com/cgi/content/full/328/7442/766 (Accessed July 15, 2007).

Chapter 33 Anterior Spinal Artery Syndrome

1. Kensuke Suzuki, Kotoo Megure, Mitsuyoshi Wada, Kei Nakai, and Tadao Nose, "Anterior Spinal Artery Syndrome Associated with Severe Stenosis of the Vertebral Artery" *AJNR Am N Neuroradiol* 19 (August 1998): 1353 http://www.ajnr.org/cgi/reprint/19/7/1353 (Accessed July 1, 2007).

2. William F. Zuber, Max R. Gaspar, and Philip D. Rothschild, "The Anterior Spinal Artery Syndrome—A Complication of Abdominal Aortic Surgery" *Ann Surg* 172 no. 5 (November 1970): 909 http://www.pubmedcentral.nih.gov/picrender.fcgi?artid=1397362&blobtype=pdf (Accessed July 2, 2007).

3. William F. Zuber, Max R. Gaspar, and Philip D. Rothschild, "The Anterior Spinal Artery Syndrome—A Complication of Abdominal Aortic Surgery" *Ann Surg* 172 no. 5 (November 1970): 913 http://www.pubmedcentral.nih.gov/picrender.fcgi?artid=1397362&blobtype=pdf (Accessed July 2, 2007).

4. See Note 3.

5. See Note 3.

6. *Wikipedia,* s.v. "Angiogram," http://en.wikipedia.org/wiki/Angiogram (Accessed July 2, 2007).

7. See Note 1.

8. *Wikipedia,* s.v. "Arteriosclerosis," http://en.wikipedia.org/wiki/Arteriosclerosis (Accessed July 2, 2007).

9. See Note 1.

10. See Note 1.

11. *Wikipedia,* s.v. "Vasculitis," http://en.wikipedia.org/wiki/Vasculitis (Accessed July 2, 2007).

12. See Note 1.

13. See Note 1.

14. *Wikipedia,*s.v. "Sickle-cell disease," http://en.wikipedia.org/wiki/Sickle_cell_anemia (Accessed July 2, 2007).

15. See Note 1.

16. See Note 1.

17. William F. Zuber, Max R. Gaspar, and Philip D. Rothschild, "The Anterior Spinal Artery Syndrome—A Complication of Abdominal Aortic Surgery" *Ann Surg* 172 no. 5 (November 1970): 911-913 http://www.pubmedcentral.nih.gov/picrender.fcgi?artid=1397362&blobtype=pdf (Accessed July 2, 2007).

18. *Wikipedia*, s.v. "Aorta," http://en.wikipedia.org/wiki/Aorta (Accessed July 2, 2007).

19. See Note 1.

Chapter 34 Spinal Cord Concussion aka Spinal Cord Shock aka Spinal Shock

1. *Wikipedia*, s.v. "Hypotonia," http://en.wikipedia.org/wiki/Hypotonia (Accessed July 6, 2007).

2. *Wikipedia,* s.v. "Spinal shock," http://en.wikipedia.org/wiki/Hypotonia (Accessed May 18, 2007).

3. Thomas J. Zwimpfer and Mark Bernstein, "Spinal Cord Concussion" *J Neurosurg* 72 no. 6 (June 1990): 894-5.

4. Charles H. Tator and Edward C. Benzel, "Clinical Manifestations of Acute Spinal Cord Injury" in *Contemporary Management of Spinal Cord Injury From Impact to Rehabilitation.* 2nd ed. American Association of Neurological Surgery (2000): 24.

5. "Spinal Cord Injury—Early Days" multikulti.org.uk (undated): 1-2 http://www.multikulti.org.uk/en/health/spinal-cord-injury-early-days/(Accessed April 18, 2007).

6. "What are the symptoms of an acute spinal cord injury?" Ohio State University Medical Center (2007): 2 http://medicalcenter.osu.edu/patientcare/healthcare_services/nervous_system/acutespinal/(Accessed July 6, 2007).

7. Donald Schreiber, "Spinal Cord Injuries" *emedicine* (August 8, 2006): 3 http://www.emedicine.com/emerg/topic553.htm (Accessed January 31, 2007).

8. Ryan Grove, John Norwig, and Joseph Maroon, "Management of a Cerebral and Spinal Cord Concussion in a Professional Football Player" *Pro Football Athletic Trainer* 21 no. 1 (Summer 2003): 1.

9. Marc R. Del Bigio and Garth E. Johnson, "Clinical Presentation of Spinal Cord Concussion" *Spine* 14 no. 1 (January 1989): 37.

10. Marc R. Del Bigio and Garth E. Johnson, "Clinical Presentation of Spinal Cord Concussion" *Spine* 14 no. 1 (January 1989): 40.

Chapter 35 SCIWORA (Spinal Cord Injury Without Radiographic Abnormality)

1. J.R. Ruge and others [not listed], "Spinal Cord Injury Without Radiographic Abnormality (SCIWORA) Recommendations" SpineUniverse.com (May 14, 2001): 2 http://www.spineuniverse.com/pdf/traumaguide/13.pdf (Accessed July 1, 2007).

2. Jeffrey S. Schiff, Brian Moore, and Jeff Louie, "Pediatric Trauma—Unique Considerations in Evaluating and Treating Children" *Minnesota Medicine* Minnesota Medical Association 88 (January 2005): 2-3.

3. Anonymous, "Spinal cord injury without radiographic abnormality (SCIWORA) in the adult: A case presentation and literature review." *J Neurol Sciences* Turkey 21 (2004): 1 http://med.ege.edu.tr/~norolbil/2004/NBD31604.htm (Accessed February 11, 2005).

4. David A. Wald, "Spinal Cord Injuries" AHC Media freecme.com (undated): 8 http://www.thrombosis-consult.com/ articles/Textbook/42_spinalcordinjuries (Accessed February 11, 2005).

5. H.S. Bhatoe, "Cervical spinal cord injury without radiographic abnormality in adults" *Neurol India* 48 no. 3 (2000): 245 http://www.neurologyindia.com/article.asp?issn=0028-3886; year=2000;volume=48;issue=3;spage=243;epage=8;aulast=Bhatoe (Accessed February 11, 2005).

6. See Note 3.

7. Gregory W. Hendey, Allan B. Wolfson, William R. Mower, and Jerome R. Hoffman, "SCIWORA—It's Not Just Child's Play Analysis of the NEXUS Data." *Acad Emer Med* 9 no. 5. (2002): 1.

8. Izumi Koyanagi, Yoshinobu Iwasaki, Kazutoshi Hida, Minoru Akino, Hiroyuki Imamura, Hiroshi Abe, "Acute cervical cord injury without fracture or dislocation of the spinal column" *J Neurosurg Online* 93 no. 1 (July 2000 Suppl): 4 http://www.thejns-net.org/spine/issues/v93n1/ pdf/s0930015.pdf (Accessed February 6, 2007).

Chapter 36 SCIWORET (Spinal Cord Injury Without Radiographic Evidence of Trauma)

1. Charles H. Tator and Edward C. Benzel, "Clinical Manifestations of Acute Spinal Cord Injury" in *Contemporary Management of Spinal Cord Injury From Impact to Rehabilitation.* 2nd ed. American Association of Neurological Surgery (2000): 31.

2. Izumi Koyanagi, Yoshinobu Iwasaki, Kazutoshi Hida, Minoru Akino, Hiroyuki Imamura, Hiroshi Abe, "Acute cervical cord injury without fracture or dislocation of the spinal column" *J Neurosurg Online* 93 no. 1 (July 2000 Suppl): 4 http://www.thejns-net.org/spine/issues/v93n1/pdf/s0930015.pdf (Accessed February 6, 2007).

Chapter 37 Burning Hands Syndrome aka "Stingers" or "Burners"

1. J.C. Maroon, "'Burning Hands' in football spinal cord injuries" *JAMA* 238 no. 19 (November 7, 1977): 1049.

2. Kurt E. Jacobson, "Stingers and Burners" *Hughston Health Alert* Hughston Sports Medicine Foundation (December 2, 2001): 1 http://www.hughston.com/hha/a_12_2_1.htm (Accessed May 3, 2007).

3. "NCAA® Guideline 2n 'Burners' (Brachial Plexus Injuries)" (2003): 1 http://www.ncaa.org/ library/sports_sciences/sports_med_handbook/2003-04/2n.pdf (Accessed July 10, 2007).

4. Charles H. Tator and Edward C. Benzel, "Clinical Manifestations of Acute Spinal Cord Injury" in *Contemporary Management of Spinal Cord Injury From Impact to Rehabilitation.* 2nd ed. American Association of Neurological Surgery (2000): 26.

5. "Burners and Stingers" American Academy of Orthopaedic Surgeons (January 2006): 1 http://orthoinfo.aaos.org/fact/hr_report.cfm?Thread_ID=226&topcategory=Shoulder (Accessed July 10, 2007).

6. "Physical Therapy Corner: Burner Syndrome" Nicholas Institute of Sports Medicine and Athletic Trauma (2007): 1 http://www.nismat.org/ptcor/burners (Accessed July 10, 1007).

7. See Note 5.

8. See Note 6.

9. See Note 6.

10. "Burners and Stingers" American Academy of Orthopaedic Surgeons (January 2006): 2 http://orthoinfo.aaos.org/fact/hr_report.cfm?Thread_ID=226&topcategory=Shoulder (Accessed July 10, 2007).

11. See Note 6.

12. See Note 6.

13. Ilian Elias, Michael A. Pahl, Adam C. Zoga, Maurice L. Goins, and Alexander R. Vaccaro, "Recurrent burner syndrome due to presumed cervical spine osteoblastoma in a collision sport athlete—a case report" *J Brachial Plexus and*

Periph Nerve Inj (June 6, 2007): 3-4 http://www.jbppni.com/content/2/1/13 (Accessed July 10, 2007).

14. "Physical Therapy Corner: Burner Syndrome" Nicholas Institute of Sports Medicine and Athletic Trauma (2007): 2 http://www.nismat.org/ptcor/burners (Accessed July 10, 1007).

15. See Note 14.

Chapter 38 Bruising of the Spinal Cord (Contusio Cervicalis)

1. Charles H. Tator and Edward C. Benzel, "Clinical Manifestations of Acute Spinal Cord Injury" in *Contemporary Management of Spinal Cord Injury From Impact to Rehabilitation.* 2nd ed. American Association of Neurological Surgery (2000): 26.

2. "Spinal Cord Injury" U*X*L Complete Health Resource: Sick! 4 (2007): 2 http://www.faqs.org/health/Sick-V4/Spinal-Cord-Injury.html (Accessed April 18, 2007).

3. "Spinal Cord Trauma" *WebMD InteliHealth*® (2007): 1 http://www.intelihealth.com/IH/ihtIH/WSIHW000/9339/28083.html (Accessed July 9, 2007).

Chapter 39 The Hangman's Fracture

1. Igor Boyarsky and Gary Godorov, "C2 Fractures" *emedicine* (March 15, 2006): 4 http://www.emedicine.com/orthoped/topic597.htm (Accessed July 15, 2007).

2. See Note 1.

3. Safwan Halabi, "Hangman's Fracture" MyPACS.net Radiology Teaching Files Case 1775820 MyPACS.net (June 22, 2005): 1 http://www.mypacs.net/cases/HANGMANS-FRACTURE-1775820.html (Accessed July 15, 2007).

4. "Definition of Hangman's fracture" MedicineNet.com (2007): 1 http://www.medterms.com/script/main/art.asp?articlekey=25212 (Accessed July 15, 2007).

5. "Hangman Fracture of the Cervical Spine" SpineUniverse.com (undated): 1 http://www.spineuniverse.com/Ip/ejournal/ag_030400danek_hangman.html (Accessed July 14, 2007).

6. Abhay Sanan and Setti S. Rengachary, "The History of Spinal Biomechanics" *Neurosurgery* 39 (1996): 1-17 http://www.c3.hu/~mavideg/ns/Sananetal.html (Accessed July 15, 2007).

Chapter 40 Hysterical Paralysis (Ganser Syndrome)

1. Charles H. Tator and Edward C. Benzel, "Clinical Manifestations of Acute Spinal Cord Injury" in *Contemporary Management of Spinal Cord Injury From Impact to Rehabilitation.* 2nd ed. American Association of Neurological Surgery (2000): 26.

2. P. Roy-Byrne, "The Neuroanatomy of Hysterical Paralysis" *J Watch Psych* (July 26, 2001): 1 http://psychiatry.jwatch.org/cgi/content/full/2001/26/7 (Accessed July 10, 2007).

3. "Mental Health: Ganser Syndrome" *WebMD®* (July 1, 2005): 1 http://www.webmd.com/mental-health/ganser-syndrome (Accessed July 10, 2007).

4. Daniel Schneider and Brian R. Szetela, "Ganser Syndrome" *emedicine* (August 30, 2006): 1 http://www.emedicine.com/med/topic840.htm (Accessed July 10, 2007).

5. See Note 2.

6. See Note 3.

7. Daniel Schneider and Brian R. Szetela, "Ganser Syndrome" *emedicine* (August 30, 2006): 2 http://www.emedicine.com/med/topic840.htm (Accessed July 10, 2007).

8. See Note 2.

9. Maria Ron, "Explaining the unexplained: understanding hysteria" *Brain* 124 no. 6 (June 2001): 1066 http://brain.oxfordjournals.org/cgi/content/full/124/6/1065 (Accessed July 10, 2007).

10. Daniel Schneider and Brian R. Szetela, "Ganser Syndrome" *emedicine* (August 30, 2006): 3-4 http://www.emedicine.com/med/topic840.htm (Accessed July 10, 2007).

11. Eric J. Letonoff, Troy R.K. Williams, and Kanwaldeep S. Sidhu, "Hysterical paralysis: a report of three cases and a review of the literature" *Spine* 27 no. 15 (October 2002): E446.

12. "Mad Dogs and Servicemen," an episode of *M*A*S*H.*

Chapter 41 Closed Head Injury aka Traumatic Brain Injury

1. "Closed head injury" Providence Health & Services Alaska (2007): 1 http://www.providence.org/alaska/tchap/glossary/C.htm (Accessed June 10, 2007).

2. Patrick McCaffrey, "The Neuroscience on the Web Series: CMSD 636, Neuropathologies of Language and Cognition Unit 12 Traumatic Brain Injury: Recovery and Remediation" California State University, Chico (2001): 1 http://www.scuchico.edu/~pmccaffrey//syllabi/SPPA336/336unit12.html (Accessed May 1, 2007).

3. Glen Johnson, "How The Brain Is Hurt" *Traumatic Brain Injury Survival Guide* (1998): 1 http://www.tbiguide.com/howbrainhurt.html (Accessed May 1, 2007).

4. Glen Johnson, "Common Indicators of a Head Injury" *Traumatic Brain Injury Survival Guide* (1998): 1-2 http://www.tbiguide.com/indicators.html (Accessed May 1, 2007).

5. "What is a Neuropsychologist?" *A Neuropsychology Homepage* (1997): 1 http://www.tbidoc. com/Appel2.html (Accessed June 10, 2007).

6. "Psychologist" *Medical Terminology & Drug Database* St. Jude Children's Research Hospital Memphis, Tennessee (2007): 1 http://www.stjude.org/glossary (Accessed June 10, 2007).

7. Orly Avitzur, "Avoid Insult to Brain Injury" *Neurology Now* (March/April 2007): 44-45.

Chapter 42 Spina Bifida

1. *Wikipedia*, s.v. "Spina Bifida," http://en.wikipedia.org/wiki/Spina-bifida (Accessed June 23, 2007).

2. "Genetics and Spina Bifida" Spina Bifida Association (2007): 1 http://www.sbaa.org/site/c.liKWL7PLLrF/b.2700269/k.5527/Genetics_and_Spina_Bifida.htm (Accessed June 23, 2007).

3. See note 2.

Chapter 43 Prognosis After a Complete Spinal Cord Injury

1. *Wikipedia*, s.v. "Spinal Cord Injury," http://en.wikipedia.org/wiki/Spinal_cord_injury (Accessed May 25, 2007).

Chapter 44 Prognosis After an Incomplete Spinal Cord Injury

1. Shirley McCluer, "Predicting Outcome (Prognosis) in Spinal Cord Injury—Fact Sheet #12" Spinalcord [*sic*] Injury Information Network (June 2003): 2-3 http://www.spinalcord.uab.edu/show.asp?durki=21502 (Accessed July 1, 2007).

2. Janis Kelly, "Late Recovery After Major Spinal Cord Injury—Is It Possible? The Christopher Reeve 'N of One' Study" *Neurology Reviews* 10 no. 11 (November 2002): 1-2 http://www.neurologyreviews.com/nov02/nr_nov02_superman.html (Accessed July 1, 2007).

3. Janis Kelly, "Late Recovery After Major Spinal Cord Injury—Is It Possible? The Christopher Reeve 'N of One' Study" *Neurology Reviews* 10 no. 11 (Novem-

ber 2002): 2-3 http://www.neurologyreviews.com/nov02/nr_nov02_superman.html (Accessed July 1, 2007).

4. *Wikipedia*, s.v. "Functional Electrical Stimulation," http://en.wikipedia.org/wiki/Functional_electrical_stimulation (Accessed July 1, 2007).

5. "The Body Electric," an episode of *Discover Magazine*.

Chapter 45 Prognosis After a Central Cord Syndrome Spinal Cord Injury

1. W.F. Merriam, T.K. Taylor, S.J. Ruff, and M.J. McPhail, "A reappraisal of acute traumatic central cord syndrome" *J Bone Joint Surg Br* 68 no. 5 (November 1986): 709.

2. Albert Bosch, E. Shannon Stauffer, and Vernon L. Nickel, "Incomplete Traumatic Quadriplegia: A Ten Year Review" *JAMA* 216 no. 3 (April 19, 1971): 477.

3. Martyn L. Newey, Pradeep K. Sen, and Robert D. Fraser, "The long-term outcome after central cord syndrome A study of the Natural History." *J Bone Joint Surg Br* 82-B no. 6 (August 2000): 855.

Chapter 46 Rehabilitation After a Spinal Cord Injury

Chapter 47 Aging with a Spinal Cord Injury

1. Phil Klebine and Daniel Lammertse, "Summary Transcript from Aging with Spinal Cord Injury Teleconference for Consumers & Families." Aging with SCI. Department of Physical Medicine & Rehabilitation University of Alabama, Birmingham (October 26, 1999): 1 http://www.spinalcord.uab.edu/show.asp?durki=25829 (Accessed January 7, 2006).

2. Gale G. Whiteneck, Susan W. Charlifue, Kenneth A. Gerhart, Daniel P. Lammertse, Scott Manley, Robert R. Menter, and Kathie R. Seedroff, *Aging With Spinal Cord Injury* (New York: Demos Publishing Company, 1993), 4.

3. See Note 2.

4. See Note 2.

5. Gale G. Whiteneck, Susan W. Charlifue, Kenneth A. Gerhart, Daniel P. Lammertse, Scott Manley, Robert R. Menter, and Kathie R. Seedroff, *Aging With Spinal Cord Injury* (New York: Demos Publishing Company, 1993), 10.

6. Gale G. Whiteneck, Susan W. Charlifue, Kenneth A. Gerhart, Daniel P. Lammertse, Scott Manley, Robert R. Menter, and Kathie R. Seedroff, *Aging With Spinal Cord Injury* (New York: Demos Publishing Company, 1993), 183.

7. Joseph Surkin, Melissa Smith, Alan Penman, Mary Currier, H. Louis Harkey III, and Yue-Fang Chang, "Spinal Cord Injury Incidence in Mississippi: A Capture-Recapture Approach." *J Trauma-Injury Infection & Critical Care* 45 no. 3 (September 1998): 502-4.

8. Gale G. Whiteneck, Susan W. Charlifue, Kenneth A. Gerhart, Daniel P. Lammertse, Scott Manley, Robert R. Menter, and Kathie R. Seedroff, *Aging With Spinal Cord Injury* (New York: Demos Publishing Company, 1993), 199.

9. Gale G. Whiteneck, Susan W. Charlifue, Kenneth A. Gerhart, Daniel P. Lammertse, Scott Manley, Robert R. Menter, and Kathie R. Seedroff, *Aging With Spinal Cord Injury* (New York: Demos Publishing Company, 1993), 239.

10. Gale G. Whiteneck, Susan W. Charlifue, Kenneth A. Gerhart, Daniel P. Lammertse, Scott Manley, Robert R. Menter, and Kathie R. Seedroff, *Aging With Spinal Cord Injury* (New York: Demos Publishing Company, 1993), 275.

11. "Understanding Damage in Human Injury" *The Miami Project E-News* The Miami Project to Cure Paralysis. (January 13, 2006): 1-2.

12. M.A. McColl, "A house of cards: women, aging and spinal cord injury" *Spinal Cord* 40 no. 8 (August 2002): 371-3 http://www.nature.com/sc/journal/v40/n8/full/31013321.html (Accessed May 9, 2007).

13. Josie Byzek, Tim Gilmer, and Roxanne Furlong, "Active Aging" *New Mobility* (May 2007): 34.

Chapter 48 Life Expectancy After a Spinal Cord Injury

1. "Life Expectancy Hits Record High" Center for Disease Control National Center for Health Statistics (February 28, 2005): 1-3 http://www.cdc.gov/nchs/pressroom/05facts/lifeexpectancy.htm (Accessed June 2, 2007).

2. "Spinal Cord Injury Statistical Information" Spinal Cord Injury Association of Illinois (undated): 1-3 http://www.sci-illinois.org/Pages/factsheets/literature/stats.htm (Accessed June 2, 2007).

3. David J. Strauss, Michael J. DeVivo, David R. Paculdo, and Robert M. Shavelle, "Trends in Life Expectancy After Spinal Cord Injury" *Arch Phys Med Rehab* 87 (August 2006): 1081.

4. See Note 2.

5. "Facts and Figures at a Glance Spinal Cord Injury" Spinalcord [*sic*] Injury Information Network University of Alabama, Birmingham (June 2006): 3-4 http://www.spinalcord.uab.edu/show.asp?durki=21446 (Accessed May 2, 2007).

Chapter 49 Quality of Life After a Spinal Cord Injury

1. S. Wood-Dauphinée, G. Exner, and the SCI Consensus Group, "Quality of life in patients with spinal cord injury—basic issues, assessment, and recommendations" (Quality of Life after Multiple Trauma Conference Wermelskirchen, Germany September 29-October 2, 1999): 137.

2. "Quality of Life: What's Important" Craig Hospital (undated): 1 http://www.craighospital.org/SCI/METS/quality.asp (Accessed June 1, 2007).

3. "Quality of Life: What's Important" Craig Hospital (undated): 1-2 http://www.craighospital.org/SCI/METS/quality.asp (Accessed June 1, 2007).

4. "Quality of Life: What's Important" Craig Hospital (undated): 2-3 http://www.craighospital.org/SCI/METS/quality.asp (Accessed June 1, 2007).

5. "Quality of Life: What's Important" Craig Hospital (undated): 3 http://www.craighospital.org/SCI/METS/quality.asp (Accessed June 1, 2007).

Chapter 50 The Importance of Hope After a Spinal Cord Injury

1. *Wikipedia*, s.v. "Hope," http://en/wikipedia.org/wiki/Hope (Accessed June 10, 2007).

2. Jerome Groopman, *The Anatomy of Hope* (New York: Random House, 2004), 193.

Chapter 51 Religion and Faith After a Spinal Cord Injury

1. Esther Isabelle Wilder, *Wheeling and Dealing: Living with Spinal Cord Injury* (Nashville: Vanderbilt University Press, 2006), 105.

2. Esther Isabelle Wilder, *Wheeling and Dealing: Living with Spinal Cord Injury* (Nashville: Vanderbilt University Press, 2006), 106.

3. Esther Isabelle Wilder, *Wheeling and Dealing: Living with Spinal Cord Injury* (Nashville: Vanderbilt University Press, 2006), 111.

4. Esther Isabelle Wilder, *Wheeling and Dealing: Living with Spinal Cord Injury* (Nashville: Vanderbilt University Press, 2006), 113.

5. Esther Isabelle Wilder, *Wheeling and Dealing: Living with Spinal Cord Injury* (Nashville: Vanderbilt University Press, 2006), 118.

6. Christopher Reeve, *Nothing is Impossible: Reflections on a New Life* (New York: Random House, 2002), 67, 81.

Chapter 52 Survivor Guilt I—"What Did I Do To Deserve This?"

1. *Wikipedia*, s.v. "Survivor guilt," http://en.wikipedia.org/wiki/Survivor_guilt (Accessed May 11, 2007).

2. *Wikipedia*, "Survivor syndrome," http://en.wikipedia.org/wiki/Survivor_syndrome (Accessed May 11, 2007).

3. See Note 1.

4. *Wikipedia*, "Post traumatic stress disorder" http://en.wikipedia.org/wiki/Post-traumatic_stress _disorder (Accessed May 11, 2007).

5. Donna Marzo, "Why Not Me? Dealing with Survivor Guilt in the Aftermath of a Disaster" *SelfhelpMagazine* (September 24, 2001): 1-2 http://www.self-helpmagazine.com/articles/trauma/guilt.html (Accessed May 11, 2007).

6. "Device Liberates Quadriplegic From Ventilator" *ScienceDaily* (May 15, 2001): 2 http://www.sciencedaily.com/releases/2001/05/010515075604.htm (Accessed May 11, 2007).

7. See Note 5.

Chapter 53 Survivor Guilt II—"I Did Something Stupid To Get Hurt"

Chapter 54 Survivor Guilt III—"My Actions Unintentionally Killed or Seriously Injured Another Person"

Chapter 55 Survivor Guilt IV—"Why Wasn't I Hurt Worse or as Badly as So-and-So?"

1. "Central Cord Syndrome" The National Spinal Cord Injury Discussion Forum (August 22, 2005): 2 http://www.spinalcord.org/forum/view-topic.php?t=261 (Accessed January 30, 2007).

Chapter 56 Depression After a Spinal Cord Injury

1. "Depression After Spinal Cord Injury" Drugs.com (undated): 1 http://www.drugs.com/cg/depression-after-spinal-cord-injury.html (Accessed June 28, 2007)

2. "Depression and Spinal Cord Injury" Research: Spinal Cord Injury Update. University of Washington Rehabilitation Medicine 10 no. 2 (Summer 2001): 1 http://depts.washington.edu/rehab/sci/updates/01sum_depression.html (Accessed May 9, 2007).

3. Donna M. Dryden, L. Duncan Saunders, Brian H. Rowe, Laura A. May, Niko Yiannakoulias, Lawrence W. Svenson, Donald P. Schopflocher, and Donald C.

Voaklander, “Depression following Traumatic Spinal Cord Injury” *Neuroepidemiology* 25 no. 2 (2005): 55.

4. Y. Kishi, R.G. Robinson, and A.W. Forrester, “Comparison between acute and delayed onset major depression after spinal cord injury” *J. Nerv Ment Dis* 183 no. 5 (May 1995): 290, 292.

5. “Depression and Spinal Cord Injury” Research: Spinal Cord Injury Update University of Washington Rehabilitation Medicine 10 no. 2 (Summer 2001): 1-2 http://depts.washington.edu/rehab/sci/updates/01sum_depression.html (Accessed May 9, 2007).

6. Phil Ullrich, Marylou Guihan, and Frances M. Weaver, “Feature Article: Psychological Treatments for Pain and Depression After Spinal Cord Injury: Rationale and Challenges to Implementation” United Spinal Association (March 8, 2007): 1 http://www.unitedspinal.org/publications/process/2007/03/08/feature-article-psychological-treatments-for-pain-and-depression-after-spinal-cord-injury-rationale-and-challenges-to-implementation/(Accessed May 10, 2007).

7. Phil Klebine and Linda Lindsey, “Pain After Spinal Cord Injury” University of Alabama, Birmingham (May 2001): 5 http://www.spinalcord.uab.edu/show.asp?durki=41119 (Accessed May 9, 2007).

8. Elisabeth Kübler-Ross and David Kessler, “An excerpt from *On Grief and Grieving*” Davidkessler.org (January 2007): 1 http://www.davidkessler.org (Accessed May 10, 2007).

Chapter 57 Addiction After a Spinal Cord Injury

1. “Uncontrollable Trauma, PTSD and Alcohol Addiction” eNotAlone.com (2006): 1 http://www.enotalone.com/article/11325.html (Accessed July 9, 2007).

2. *Wikipedia*, s.v. “Endorphin,” http://en.wikipedia.org/wiki/Endorphin (Accessed July 9, 2007).

3. “United States Prescribing Information Lyrica” Pfizer (June 2007): 1, 7 http://www.pfizer.com/pfizer/download/uspi_lyrica.pdf (Accessed July 19, 2007).

4. "Drug Rehab & Treatment The Disease of Addiction" Casa Palmera Treatment Center (undated): 1 http://www.casapalmera.com/treatments/drug-rehab-treatment.php (Accessed July 9, 2007).

Chapter 58 Spinal Cord Injury Statistics

1. Cindy Mervis (Maine Department of Health & Human Services Public Health), e-mail message to author, October 18, 2005.

2. "Spinal Cord Injury (SCI): Fact Sheet" Center for Disease Control National Center for Injury Prevention and Control (September 7, 2006): 1-3 http://www.cdc.gov/ncipc/factsheets/scifacts. htm (Accessed June 15, 2007).

3. Alabama: Phil Klebine (Assistant Director of Research Services University of Alabama Birmingham Department of Physical Medicine & Rehabilitation), e-mail message to author, August 22, 2005; state population from http://www.50states.com/alabama.html (Access date unknown): 1.

Alaska: Sam Warren, Martha Moore, and Mark S. Johnson. "Traumatic head and spinal cord injuries in Alaska (1991-1993)" *Alaska Med* 37 no. 1 (Jan-Mar 1995): 14.

Arizona: "Facts & Figures" Arizona Governor's Council on Spinal and Head Injuries (May 2003): 1 http://www.azheadspine.org/spinal_facts.htm (Accessed August 2, 2005); state population from http://www.50states.com/arizona.html (Accessed August 2, 2005).

Arkansas: "Spinal Cord Injury Statistics Arkansas" Arkansas Spinal Cord Commission (June 2004): 1 http://www.spinalcord.ar.gov/General/stats.html (Accessed September 23, 2005).

California: Roger B. Trent (Chief, Injury Surveillance and Epidemiology Section, California Department of Health Services, Sacramento), e-mail message to author August 3, 2005.

Colorado: Susan Charlifue (Research Supervisor, Craig Hospital, Englewood), e-mail message to the author, September 26, 2005.

Connecticut: Marica Matika (Reference Librarian Government Information Services Connecticut State Library), e-mail message to the author, February 9, 2006.

Delaware: MarySue Jones (Trauma System Coordinator, Delaware Office of Emergency Medical Services, Delaware Trauma System Registry, Division of Public Health, Office of Emergency Medical Services), e-mail message to the author, October 5, 2005.

District of Columbia: Steven A. Towle (Spinal Cord Injury Network), e-mail to the author, September 5, 2005.

Florida: "Brain & Spinal Cord Injury Program" *The Florida Department of Health Facility Designation Standards* (April 18, 2005): 5 (Accessed July 4, 2007); "July 2005 estimated Florida population" FactMonster http://www.factmonster.com/ipka/A0004986.html (Accessed July 4, 2007).

Georgia: Kristen E. Vincent (Executive Director Brain & Spinal Injury Trust Fund Commission, Atlanta), e-mail message to the author, February 9, 2006; estimated Georgia 2004 population from http://quickfacts.census.gov (Accessed September 26, 2005).

Hawaii: "Hawaii health status indicators and baseline data (1990)" Hawaii State Department of Health (undated): 1 http://www.hawaii.gov/health/healthy-lifestyles/healthy_hawaii/opd-2ex.htm (Accessed September 23, 2005).

Idaho: estimated 2005 population from "Population by State" infoplease.com (2007): 1 http://www.infoplease.com/ipa/A0004986.html (Accessed July 4, 2007).

Illinois: "Hospital Discharge Database Inpatient Interactive Query Results" Illinois Department of Public Health Health Statistics 2nd Quarter 1998, 3rd Quarter 1998, 4th Quarter 1998 (2004): 1-6 http://app.idph.state.il.us/hospitaldischarge/IPResults.asp (Accessed July 4, 2007); Illinois estimate 2004 population "Illinois Estimated Population 2000-2004" Illinois Department of Public Health Health Statistics (undated): 1 http://www.idph.state.il.us/health/estpop2000_2009.htm (Accessed July 4, 2007).

Indiana: Linda Stemnock (Data Analyst Indiana State Department of Health Epidemiology Resource Center, Data Analysis Team), e-mail message to the author, February 17, 2006; estimated 2004 Indiana population from Vincent Thompson. "Population Estimates for 2004: Indiana Barely Maintains Its Rank" *incontext* 6 no. 1 (January-February 2005): 1.

Iowa: estimated 2005 population from "Population by State" infoplease.com (2007): 1 http://www.infoplease.com/ipa/A0004986.html (Accessed July 4, 2007).

Kansas: estimated 2005 population from "Population by State" infoplease.com (2007): 1 http://www.infoplease.com/ipa/A0004986.html (Accessed July 4, 2007).

Kentucky: W. Jay Christian, "Traumatic Brain & Spinal Cord Injury Surveillance Project Fiscal Year 2003 Final Report" Kentucky Injury Prevention and Research Center University of Kentucky (July 1, 2003): 6 http://www.kiprc.uky.edu/projects/tbi/tbi_FY03.doc (Accessed July 13, 2007).

Lousiana: "Injury Research and Prevention Program," Louisiana Office of Public Health (undated): 1 http://www.oph.dhh.louisiana.gov/injuryprevention/page5316.htm?php (Accessed September 23, 2005).

Maine: estimated 2005 population from "Population by State" infoplease.com (2007): 1 http://wwwinfoplease.com/ipa/A0004986.htm (Accessed July 4, 2007).

Maryland: Audrey S. Regan, "Maryland State Board of Spinal Cord Injury Research 2003 Research Grant Competition Announcement" Maryland Department of Health & Mental Hygiene (March 1, 2004): 1-4 http://www.fha.state.md.us/oipha/html/spinal.html (Accessed February 7, 2006); estimated Maryland 1998 population from "ST-99-1 State Population Estimates and Demographic Components of Population Change: July 1, 1998 to July 1, 1999" U.S. Census Bureau (December 29, 1999): 1-3 http://www.census.gov/population/estimates/state/st-99-1.txt (Accessed July 4, 2007).

Massachusetts: Beth C. Hume (Injury Surveillance Project Director Massachusetts Department of Public Health), e-mail message to the author, February 13, 2006.

Montana: estimated 2005 population from "Population by State" infoplease (2007): 1 http://www.infoplease.com/ipa/A0004986.html (Accessed July 4, 2007).

Minnesota: Anna Gaichas (state of Minnesota), e-mail message to the author, October 1, 2005.

Mississippi: Joseph Surkin, Melissa Smith, Alan Penman, Mary Currier, H. Louis Harkey III, and Yue-Fang Chang, "Spinal Cord Injury Incidence in Mississippi: A Capture-Recapture Approach." *J Trauma-Injury Infection & Critical Care* 45 no. 3 (September 1998): 502.

Missouri: "Health Snapshot Spinal Cord Injury and SCI personal assistant services in Missouri (1995-2000)" Missouri Department of Health and Senior Services and contained in the Missouri Department of Health and Senior Services Missouri Information for Community Assessment database (April 2004): 1-2 http://www.muhealth-org/~momscis/snaps/sciinmoa.htm (Accessed February 7, 2006).

Montana: estimated 2005 population from "Population by State" infoplease.com (2007): 1 http://www.infoplease.com/ipa/A0004986.html (Accessed July 4, 2007).

Nebraska: Victor Filos (Nebraska Department of Health and Human Services), e-mail message to the author, October 5, 2005.

Nevada: "Nevada's Injury Data Surveillance Project" Bureau of Family Health Services Nevada State Health Division Department of Human Resources (October 2002): 28 http://health2k.state.nv.us/BFHS/injury/NevadaInjuryReportFinal.pdf (Accessed July 13, 2007).

New Hampshire: Lisa M. Thompson (President, New Hampshire Chapter of the National Spinal Cord Injury Association), e-mail message to the author, October 5, 2006.

New Jersey: Darryl R. Brown (Registry Manager—Central Nervous System Injuries, Center for Health Statistics, New Jersey State Commissions on Spinal Cord Research and Brain Injury Research, New Jersey Department of Health and Senior Services), e-mail message to the author, October 1, 2005.

New Mexico: Ajoy Kumar (Injury Epidemiologist Epidemiology & Response Division New Mexico Department of Health), e-mail message to the author, March 16, 2006.

New York: "Current Trends Trends [*sic*] in Traumatic Spinal Cord Injury—New York, 1982-1988" *Morbidity and Mortality Weekly Report* 40 no. 31 (August 09, 1991): 535-7, 543; Centers for Disease Control and Prevention http://www.cdc.gov/mmwr/preview/mmwrhtml/00014953.html (Accessed August 2, 2005).

North Carolina: Catherine P. Sanford, Katrina R. Baggett, and J. Michael Bowling, "Hospitalizations from Injuries: A Report on the Completeness of External-Cause-of-Injury Coding in the State's Hospital Discharge Data North Carolina, 1997-1999) *NCPH SCHS* no. 128 (December 2001): 4 http://www.schs.state.nc.us/SCHS/(Accessed July 4, 2007); estimated 2005 state population from ST-99-3 "State Population Estimates: Annual Time Series July 1, 1990 to July 1, 1999" U.S. Census Bureau (December 29, 1999): 1 (Accessed July 4, 2007).

North Dakota: estimated 2005 population from "Population by State" infoplease.com (2007): 1 http://www.infoplease.com/ipa/A0004986.html (Accessed July 4, 2007).

Ohio: estimated 2005 population from "Population by State" infoplease.com (2007): 1 http://www.infoplease.com/ipa/A0004986.html (Accessed July 4, 2007).

Oklahoma: "Number of hospitalized spinal cord injuries by year of injury and survival status, Oklahoma, 1988-1994" OSDH surveillance data (fatal and nonfatal injuries) *Oklahoma Injury Facts* (undated): 1 http://www.health.state.ok.us/program/injury/okfacts/fig78.html (Accessed September 25, 2005); 1990 population of Oklahoma from ST-99-3 "State Population Estimates: Annual Time

Series July 1, 1990 to July 1, 1999" U.S. Census Bureau (December 29, 1999): 1 (Accessed July 4, 2007).

Oregon: estimated 2005 population from "Population by State" infoplease.com (2007): 1 http://www.infoplease.com/ipa/A0004986.html (Accessed July 4, 2007).

Pennsylvania: "Facts & Prevention Strategies Head & Spinal Cord Injuries in Pennsylvania 1995" Injury Prevention Program Pennsylvania Department of Health (1998): 4 http://www.dsf.health.state.pa.us/health/cwp/view.asp?a=174&Q=197963 (Accessed July 13, 2007).

Rhode Island: Jay S. Buechner, Mary C. Speare, and Janice Fontes, "Hospitalizations for Spinal Cord Injuries, 1994-1998," Web Edition *Health by Numbers* 2 no. 3 (March 2000): 1 Rhode Island Department of Health; 2000 state population from http://quickfacts.census.gov (Access date unknown).

South Carolina: "Department of Disabilities and Special Needs Annual Accountability Report Fiscal Year 1995-1996" (May 24, 2005): 3 http://www.scstatehouse.net/reports (Accessed September 26, 2005); estimated state population from http://quickfacts.census.gov (Access date unknown).

South Dakota: estimated 2005 population from "Population by State" infoplease.com (2007): 1 http://www.infoplease.com/ipa/A0004986.html (Accessed July 4, 2007).

Tennessee: estimated 2005 population from "Population by State" infoplease.com (2007): 1 http://www.infoplease.com/ipa/A0004986.html (Accessed July 4, 2007).

Texas: Nancy Hudgins, "Neurosurgeon Named Head of TIRR's Mission Connect" *Texas Medical Center News* 24 no. 5 (March 15, 2002): 1 http://www.tmc.edu/tmcnews/03_15_02/page_05.html (Accessed September 25, 2005).

Utah: Cyndi L. Bemis (Media & Education Coordinator, Utah Department of Health, Violence and Injury Prevention Program), e-mail message to the author, September 26, 2005.

Virginia: Patricia (Patti) A. Goodall (Department of Rehabilitation Services), to the author, February 9, 2006.

Vermont: Caroline Dawson (Public Health Analyst, Public Health Statistics, Health Surveillance, Vermont Department of Health), e-mail message to the author, February 7, 2006.

Virginia: ST-99-3 "State Population Estimates: Annual Time Series July 1, 1990 to July 1, 1999" U.S. Census Bureau (December 29, 1999): 1 (Accessed July 4, 2007).

Washington: estimated 2005 population from "Population by State" infoplease.com (2007): 1 http://www.infoplease.com/ipa/A0004986.html (Accessed July 4, 2007).

West Virginia: Bradley A. Woodruff and Roy C. Baron. "A description of nonfatal spinal cord injury using a hospital-based registry" *Am J Prev Med* 10 no. 1 (Jan-Feb 1994): 11.

Wisconsin: "Spinal Cord Injury in Wisconsin 2000" (December 2002): 17 http://dhfs.wisconsin.gov/Disabilities/physical/SCI.HTM (Accessed September 25, 2005).

Wyoming: estimated 2005 population from "Population by State" infoplease.com (2007): 1 http://www.infoplease.com/ipa/A0004986.html (Accessed July 4, 2007).

4. "Spinal Cord Injury—Incidence and Prevalence—US and Europe" Google Answers.com (June 21, 2004): 1-6 http://answers.google.com/answers/threadview?id=364371 (Accessed July 4, 2007).

5. "Census 2001 at a glance" *Statistics South Africa Census 2001* (undated): 1 http://www.statssa.gov.za/census01/html/default.asp (Accessed July 4, 2007).

Chapter 59 Spinal Cord Injury Prevention

1. The Foundation for Spinal Cord Injury Prevention, Care & Cure (1999): 1-2 http://www.fscip.org (Accessed May 28, 2007).

2. "Preventing Spinal Cord Injury" The Foundation for Spinal Cord Injury Prevention, Care & Cure (1999): 1-3 http://www.fscip.org/prevention.htm (Accessed May 28, 2007).

3. "Trampoline Injuries" The Foundation for Spinal Cord Injury Prevention, Care & Cure (1999): 1-2 http://www.fscip.org/tramp.html (Accessed May 28, 2007).

4. Barth A. Green, M. Alexander Gabrielsen, Wiley J. Hall, and James O'Heir. "Analysis of swimming pool accidents resulting in spinal cord injury" *Paraplegia* 18 no. 2 (April 1980): 100.

5. Michael DeVivo. "Prevention of Spinal Cord Injuries that Occur in Swimming Pools" *Pushin' On Newsletter* 15 no. 1 (Winter 1997): 2-3 http://www.spinalcord.uab.edu/show.asp?durki=21422 (Accessed May 28, 2007).

6. "Healthy People 2010 Chapter 15 Injury and Violence Prevention" Safetypolicy.org (August 19, 2001): 1-2 http://www.safetypolicy.org/hp2010/15-2.htm (Accessed May 28, 2007).

7. "Spinal Cord Injury (SCI): Prevention Tips" Center for Disease Control. National Center for Injury Prevention and Control (September 7, 2006): 2 http://www.cdc.gov/ncipc/factsheets/scipvention.htm (Accessed May 28, 2007).

8. Michael DeVivo. "Prevention of Spinal Cord Injuries that Occur in Swimming Pools" *Pushin' On Newsletter* 15 no. 1 (Winter 1997): 3 http://www.spinalcord.uab.edu/show.asp?durki=21422 (Accessed May 28, 2007).

9. "NRA Gun Safety Rules" The National Rifle Association (2007): 1-3 http://www.nrahq.org/education/guide.asp (Accessed May 28, 2007).

10. "Section 3: Being A Hunter Chapter 6: Hunter Safety" The Ohio Department of Natural Resources (2005): 34-35 http://www.dnr.state.oh.us/wildlife/PDF/chapter6.pdf (Accessed May 28, 2007).

11. "Before You Ride" ATV Safety Institute (undated):1 http://www.atvsafety.org/asi.cfm?spl=2&action=display&pagename=Before%20You%20Ride (Accessed May 28, 2007).

12. "Winter Season Prompts Concern on Snowmobile Safety" United Spinal Association (January 16, 2007): 1 http://www.unitedspinal.org/2007/01/16/339/#more-339/(Accessed January 19, 2007).

13. Pat O'Hare and Karyl M. Hall. "Preventing Spinal Cord Injuries Through Safety Education Programs" *American Rehabilitation* (Spring 1997): 1 http://www.ed.gov/pubs/AmericanRehab/spring97/sp9705.html (Accessed August 2, 2005).

14. See Note 12.

15. See Note 12.

16. Pat O'Hare and Karyl M. Hall. "Preventing Spinal Cord Injuries Through Safety Education Programs" *American Rehabilitation* (Spring 1997): 1-2 http://www.ed.gov/pubs/AmericanRehab/spring97/sp9705.html (Accessed August 2, 2005).

17. Pat O'Hare and Karyl M. Hall. "Preventing Spinal Cord Injuries Through Safety Education Programs" *American Rehabilitation* (Spring 1997): 2 http://www.ed.gov/pubs/AmericanRehab/spring97/sp9705.html (Accessed August 2, 2005).

Chapter 60 Sports as a Cause of Spinal Cord Injury

1. "Factsheet #2: Spinal Cord Injury Statistics" National Spinal Cord Injury Association Resource Center (May 1996): 2 http://www.makoa.org/nscia/fact02.html (Accessed May 2, 2007).

2. "Spinal Cord Injury" Mayo Clinic Rochester, Minnesota (August 22, 2005): 4 http://www.mayoclinic.com/health/spinal-cord-injury/D00460/DSECTION=3 (Accessed May 2, 2007).

3. "Spinal Cord Injury (SCI): Fact Sheet" National Center for Injury Prevention and Control Center for Disease Control (undated): 1 http://www.cdc.gov/nipc/factsheets/scifacts.htm (Accessed May 2, 2007).

4. "Spinal Cord Injury" U*X*L Complete Health Resource: Sick! 4 (2007): 1 http://www.faqs.org/health/Sick-V4/Spinal-Cord-Injury.html (Accessed April 18, 2007).

5. "Facts and Figures at a Glance Spinal Cord Injury" Spinalcord [*sic*] Injury Information Network University of Alabama, Birmingham (June 2006): 2 http://www.spinalcord.uab.edu/show.asp?durki=21446 (Accessed May 2, 2007).

6. See Note 1.

7. "Spinal Cord Injury" American Association of Neurological Surgeons (November 2005): 2 http://www.neurosurgerytoday.org/what/patient_e/spinal.asp (Accessed May 2, 2007).

8. See Note 2.

9. David W. Lawrence, Gregory W. Stewart, Dena M. Christy, Lynn I. Gibbs, and Marcy Ouellete, "High School Football-Related Cervical Spinal Cord Injuries in Louisiana: The Athlete's Perspective" (1996): 4 http://www.injuryprevention.org/states/la/football/football.htm (Accessed May 2, 2007).

10. J.S. Torg, R.J. Naranja Jr., H. Pavlov, B.J. Galinat, R. Warren, and R.A. Stine, "The relationship of developmental narrowing of the cervical spinal canal to reversible and irreversible injury of the cervical spinal cord in football players" *J Bone Jnt Surg Am* 80 no. 10 (October 1998): 1554-5.

11. Robert C. Cantu, "Stingers, transient quadriplegia, and cervical spinal stenosis: return to play criteria" *Medicine & Science in Sports & Exercise* 29 no. 7 (Supplement July 1997): 234.

12. "Heads Up, Don't Duck! A Player & Coaches Guide to Help Decrease the Risk of Spinal Cord Injuries in Hockey" Michigan Amateur Hockey Association (November 30, 2006): 1-3 http://www.maha.org/coaches/headsup (Accessed May 3, 2007).

13. Barry P. Boden, Robin Tachetti, and Fred O. Mueller. "Catastrophic Injuries in High School and College Baseball Players" *Am J Sports Med* 32 no. 5 (July 1, 2004): 1195.

Chapter 61 Breathing Problems After a Spinal Cord Injury

1. Phil Klebine and Linda Lindsey, "Understanding and Managing Respiratory Complications after SCI" Spinal Cord Injury—InfoSheet #19 University of Alabama, Birmingham (September 2001): 1 http://www.spinalcord.uab.edu/show.asp?durki=44544 (Accessed May 29, 2007).

2. Phil Klebine and Linda Lindsey, "Understanding and Managing Respiratory Complications after SCI" Spinal Cord Injury—InfoSheet #19 University of Alabama, Birmingham (September 2001): 1-2 http://www.spinalcord.uab.edu/show.asp?durki=44544 (Accessed May 29, 2007).

3. Phil Klebine and Linda Lindsey, "Understanding and Managing Respiratory Complications after SCI" Spinal Cord Injury—InfoSheet #19 University of Alabama, Birmingham (September 2001): 2 http://www.spinalcord.uab.edu/show.asp?durki=44544 (Accessed May 29, 2007).

4. Phil Klebine and Linda Lindsey, "Understanding and Managing Respiratory Complications after SCI" Spinal Cord Injury—InfoSheet #19 University of Alabama, Birmingham (September 2001): 3 http://www.spinalcord.uab.edu/show.asp?durki=44544 (Accessed May 29, 2007).

5. See Note 4.

6. See Note 4.

7. Phil Klebine and Linda Lindsey, "Understanding and Managing Respiratory Complications after SCI" Spinal Cord Injury—InfoSheet #19 University of Alabama, Birmingham (September 2001): 4 http://www.spinalcord.uab.edu/show.asp?durki=44544 (Accessed May 29, 2007).

8. Phil Klebine and Linda Lindsey, "Understanding and Managing Respiratory Complications after SCI" Spinal Cord Injury—InfoSheet #19 University of Ala-

bama, Birmingham (September 2001): 6 http://www.spinalcord.uab.edu/show.asp?durki=44544 (Accessed May 29, 2007).

9. Phil Klebine and Linda Lindsey, "Understanding and Managing Respiratory Complications after SCI" Spinal Cord Injury—InfoSheet #19 University of Alabama, Birmingham (September 2001): 5 http://www.spinalcord.uab.edu/show.asp?durki=44544 (Accessed May 29, 2007).

10. See Note 8.

11. *Wikipedia*, s.v. "Spirometer," http://en.wikipedia.org/wiki/Spirometer (Accessed July 1, 2007).

Chapter 62 Blood Flow Problems After a Spinal Cord Injury

1. "Heart and Circulatory System" KidsHealth® (February 2004): 1 http://www.kidshealth.org/parent/general/body_basics/heart.html (Accessed May 29, 2007).

2. *Wikipedia*, s.v. "Artery," http://en.wikipedia.org/wiki/Artery (Accessed May 29, 2007).

3. William McKinley, Susan V. Garstang, and Houman Danesh, "Cardiovascular Concerns in Spinal Cord Injury" *emedicine* (December 12, 2006): 2 http://www.emedicine.com/pmr/topic20.htm (Accessed May 29, 2007).

4. See Note 3.

5. See Note 3.

6. George Deitrick, Joseph Charalel, William Bauman, and John Tuckman, "Reduced Arterial Circulation to the Legs in Spinal Cord Injury as a Cause of Skin Breakdown Lesions" *Angiology* 58 no. 2 (2007): 176.

7. "Complications" Mayo Clinic Rochester, Minnesota (August 22, 2005): 7 http://www.mayoclinic.com/health/spinal-cord-injury/DS00460/DSECTION=7 (Accessed May 29, 2007).

8. "Leg Blood Clot Symptoms" *eMedicineHealth* (September 12, 2005): 1 http://www.emedicinehealth.com/blood_clot_in_the_legs/page3_em.htm#Leg%20Blood%20Clot%20Symptoms (Accessed May 29, 2007).

9. "Injury Complications" Paraplegic-Online.com (February 2, 2007): 6 http://www.paraplegic-online.com/einjuricomplic01.html (Accessed August 2, 2007).

Chapter 63 Digestive System Problems After a Spinal Cord Injury

1. Linda Lindsey, "Bowel Management" Spinal Cord Injury—InfoSheet #9 Department of Physical Medicine & Rehabilitation University of Alabama, Birmingham (September 1999): 1-2 http://www.spinalcord.uab.edu/show.asp?durki=21482 (Accessed April 30, 2007).

2. See Note 1.

3. See Note 1.

4. See Note 1.

5. See Note 1.

6. "Spinal Cord Injury Bowel Management" Sci-Info-Pages.com (June 7, 2006)): 6-7 http://www.sci-info-pages.com/bowel.html (Accessed June 27, 2007).

7. "Fecal impaction" *MedlinePlus* (October 13, 2006): 1 http://www.nlm.nih.gov/medlineplus/print/ency/article000230.htm (Accessed July 15, 2007).

Chapter 64 Autonomic Dysreflexia (Hyperreflexia): A Life-Threatening Condition After a Spinal Cord Injury

1. Thomas Cody and Veronica (Roni) Zieroff, "Autonomic Dysreflexia?" Northeast Rehabilitation Health Network (September 7, 2005): 1 http://www.northeastrehab.com/Articles/dyreflexia.htm (Accessed April 30, 2007).

2. "Other Complications of Spinal Cord Injury: Autonomic Dysreflexia (Hyperreflexia) Symptoms and Causes" The Louis Calder Memorial Library of the Uni-

versity of Miami/Jackson Memorial Medical Center (1998): 1 http://calder.med/miami/edu/pointis/automatic.html (Accessed April 30, 2007).

3. "Autonomic Dysreflexia" The National Spinal Cord Injury Association (NSCIA) (2006): 1 http://www.spinalcord.org/html/factsheets/aut_dysreflexia.php (Accessed April 30, 2007).

4. See Note 1.

5. "Other Complications of Spinal Cord Injury: Autonomic Dysreflexia (Hyperreflexia) Symptoms and Causes" The Louis Calder Memorial Library of the University of Miami/Jackson Memorial Medical Center (1998): 1 http://calder.med/miami/edu/pointis/automatic.html (Accessed April 30, 2007).

6. Autonomic Dysreflexia" The National Spinal Cord Injury Association (NSCIA) (2006): 1-2 http://www.spinalcord.org/html/factsheets/aut_dysreflexia.php (Accessed April 30, 2007).

7. Samuel L. Stover, "Heterotopic Ossification" Spinal Cord Injury InfoSheet #12 University of Alabama, Birmingham (June 1997): 1 http://www.spinalcord.uab.edu/show.asp?durki=21485 (Accessed April 30, 2007).

8. Thomas Cody and Veronica (Roni) Zieroff, "Autonomic Dysreflexia?" Northeast Rehabilitation Health Network (September 7, 2005): 2 http://www.northeastrehab.com/Articles/dyreflexia.htm (Accessed April 30, 2007).

9. "Autonomic Dysreflexia" The National Spinal Cord Injury Association (NSCIA) (2006): 2 http://www.spinalcord.org/html/factsheets/aut_dysreflexia.php (Accessed April 30, 2007).

Chapter 65 Skin Problems After a Spinal Cord Injury

1. "Dermatology" University of Maryland Medical Center (2007): 1-2 http://www.umm.edu/dermatology~info/anatomy.htm (Accessed May 29, 2007).

2. See Note 1.

3. See Note 1.

4. "Pressure Sores" familydoctor.org (December 2006): 2 http://www.familydoctor.org/online/fandocen/home/seniors/endoflife (Accessed May 24, 2007).

5. "Pressure Ulcer" *Medline Plus* (October 17, 2005): 1 http://www.nlm.nih.gov/medlineplus/ency/article007071.htm (Accessed May 24, 2007).

6. Pressure Sores" familydoctor.org (December 2006): 1 http://www.familydoctor.org/online/fandocen/home/seniors/endoflife (Accessed May 24, 2007).

7. See Note 6.

8. "Pressure Sore Stages" Spinal-Injury.net (2004): 1-2 http://www.spinal-injury.net/pressure-sore-stages-sci.htm (Accessed June 17, 2007).

9. "Pressure Sores" familydoctor.org (December 2006): 3 http://www.familydoctor.org/online/fandocen/home/seniors/endoflife (Accessed May 24, 2007).

10. "Pressure Sores" familydoctor.org (December 2006): 2-33 http://www.familydoctor.org/online/fandocen/home/seniors/endoflife (Accessed May 24, 2007).

11. See Note 9.

12. See Note 4.

13. See Note 4.

14. Lenette Barker, letter to the editor, *New Mobility* (September 2005): 6.

15. Miracle Mist Plus. http://www.healthylifeandtimes.com (Accessed May 29, 2007).

16. "Spinal Cord Injury Skin Management" Sci-Info-Pages.com (June 25, 2006): 3 http://www.sci-info-pages.com/skin_man.html (Accessed May 29, 2007).

17. "Spinal Cord Injury Skin Management" Sci-Info-Pages.com (June 25, 2006): 4 http://www.sci-info-pages.com/skin_man.html (Accessed May 29, 2007).

18. "Incomplete c5 injury/spastic walking" The National Spinal Cord Injury Association Discussion Forum (January 24, 2005): 3 http://www.spinalcord.org/forum/viewtopic.php?t=256 (Accessed May 24, 2007).

Chapter 66 Fatigue After a Spinal Cord Injury

1. "Fatigue" Craig Hospital (undated): 1-2 http://www.craighospital.org/SCI/METS/fatigue.asp (Accessed June 3, 2007).

2. "Women and Asthma" Women's Health Zone.net (2004): 1 http://www.womenshealthzone.net/zone.net/lung-conditions/asthma/women (Accessed June 3, 2007).

3. See Note 1.

4. "Fatigue" Craig Hospital (undated): 2-3 http://www.craighospital.org/SCI/METS/fatigue.asp (Accessed June 3, 2007).

Chapter 67 Nutrition After a Spinal Cord Injury

1. *Wikipedia*, s.v. "Nutrition," http://en.wikipedia.org/wiki/Nutrition (Accessed June 3, 2007).

2. Vickeri Barton, "Nutrition Guidelines for Individuals with SCI" SCI Forum Reports (from a lecture given June 13, 2006): 1 Northwest Regional Spinal Cord Injury System (NWRSCIS) http://depts.washington.edu/rehab/sci/nutrition.html (Accessed June 3, 2007).

3. Vickeri Barton, "Nutrition Guidelines for Individuals with SCI" SCI Forum Reports (from a lecture given June 13, 2006): 1-2 Northwest Regional Spinal Cord Injury System (NWRSCIS) http://depts.washington.edu/rehab/sci/nutrition.html (Accessed June 3, 2007).

4. Vickeri Barton, "Nutrition Guidelines for Individuals with SCI" SCI Forum Reports (from a lecture given June 13, 2006): 2 Northwest Regional Spinal Cord Injury System (NWRSCIS) http://depts.washington.edu/rehab/sci/nutrition.html (Accessed June 3, 2007).

5. See Note 4.

6. See Note 4.

7. Vickeri Barton, "Nutrition Guidelines for Individuals with SCI" SCI Forum Reports (from a lecture given June 13, 2006): 3 Northwest Regional Spinal Cord Injury System (NWRSCIS) http://depts.washington.edu/rehab/sci/nutrition.html (Accessed June 3, 2007).

Chapter 68 Pain After a Spinal Cord Injury

1. Kenneth McHenry, "Controlling Central Pain: What science can't do, doesn't know and won't learn unless you speak up" *New Mobility* (March 1998): 1 http://www.newmobility.com/review_article.cfm?id=85 (Accessed May 9, 2007).

2. J. Scott Richards and Laura Kezar, "Pain following SCI" *Pushin' On Newsletter* 14 no. 2 (Summer 1996): 1 http//www.spinalcord.uab.edu/show.asp?durki=21428 (Accessed May 9, 2007).

3. Judith Elmore, "Are You in Pain?" *PN* (November 2005): 16.

4. Laskshmi Bangalore, "Rebuilding Circuits" *PN* (February 2007): 29.

5. Kenneth McHenry, "Controlling Central Pain: What science can't do, doesn't know and won't learn unless you speak up" *New Mobility* (March 1998): 2-3 http://www.newmobility.com/review_article.cfm?id=85 (Accessed May 9, 2007).

6. J. Scott and John D. Putzke, "Pain Management following Spinal Cord Injury" Spinal Cord Injury InfoSheet #10 (May 2001): 2 Department of Physical Medicine & Rehabilitation University of Alabama, Birmingham (Accessed May 9, 2007).

7. David Berg, "Introduction to Central Pain" PainOnline.org (2001): 1 http://www.painonline.org/intro.htm (Accessed May 9, 2007).

8. J. Scott Richards and Laura Kezar, "Pain following SCI" *Pushin' On Newsletter* 14 no. 2 (Summer 1996): 2 http://www.spinalcord.uab.edu/show.asp?durki=21428 (Accessed May 9, 2007).

9. Phil Klebine and Linda Lindsey, "Pain After Spinal Cord Injury" University of Alabama, Birmingham (May 2001): 2 http://www.spinalcord.uab.edu/show.asp?durki=41119 (Accessed May 9, 2007).

10. See Note 8.

11. Cynthia Salzman, "Ways to Prevent Pain" *PN* (March 2007): 41.

12. See Note 8.

13. J. Scott Richards and Laura Kezar, "Pain following SCI" *Pushin' On Newsletter* 14 no. 2 (Summer 1996): 3 http://www.spinalcord.uab.edu/show.asp?durki=21428 (Accessed May 9, 2007).

14. *Wikipedia*, s.v. "Referred pain," http://en.wikipedia.org/wiki/Referred_pain (Accessed May 9, 2007).

15. Phil Klebine and Linda Lindsey, "Pain After Spinal Cord Injury" University of Alabama Birmingham (May 2001): 2-3 http://wwwspinalcord.uab.edu/show.asp?durki=41119 (Accessed May 9, 2007).

16. Phil Klebine and Linda Lindsey, "Pain After Spinal Cord Injury" University of Alabama Birmingham (May 2001): 3 http://www.spinalcord.uab.edu/show.asp?durki=41119 (Accessed May 9, 2007).

17. Katie B. Nydam, "SCI Pain: What Makes It Worse" *Pain Research Newsletter* Brigham and Women's Hospital (Fall 2006): 3.

18. Eva G. Widerström-Noga and Dennis C. Turk, "Exacerbation of Chronic Pain following Spinal Cord Injury" *J Neurotrauma* 21 no. 10 (Oct 2004): 1387.

19. Eva G. Widerström-Noga and Dennis C. Turk, "Exacerbation of Chronic Pain following Spinal Cord Injury" *J Neurotrauma* 21 no. 10 (Oct 2004): 1387-8.

20. Jennifer Haupt, "Exercise Rx for Nerve Pain" *Neurology Now* (March/April 2007): 33.

21. Bruce Eimer, "Hypnosis and Pain Management" (undated): 1-2 http://www.hypnosisgroup. com/hypnosis/pain_mgmt.html (Accessed May 9, 2007).

22. *Wikipedia*, s.v. "Transcutaneous Electrical Nerve Stimulator," http://en.wikipedia.org/wiki/Transcutaneous_Electrical_Nerve_Stimulator (Accessed June 30, 2007).

Chapter 69 Kidney and Bladder Problems After a Spinal Cord Injury

1. "Anatomy of the Urinary System" Ohio State University Medical Center (2007): 2 http://medicalcenter.osu.edu/patientcare/healthinformation/otherhealthtopics/Urology/AnatomyoftheUrinarySystem5114/index.cfm (Accessed May 8, 2007).

2. "Bladder Care and Management" SpinalInjury.net (undated): 2-3 http://www.spinalinjury.net/_bladder_care_and_management.html (Accessed May 8, 2007).

3. *Wikipedia*, s.v. "Catheter," http://en.wikipedia.org/wiki/Catheter (Accessed July 7, 2007).

4. "Spinal Cord Injury Bladder Management" Sci-Info-Pages.com (undated): 4 http://www.sci-info-pages.com/bladder.html (Accessed May 8, 2007).

5. "Continence Care FAQs" Hollister—US: Continence Care (undated): 2 http://www.hollister. com/us/continence (Accessed May 8, 2007).

6. "Stadium Pal" and "Stadium Gal" BioRelief (undated): 1 http://www.stadiumpal.com/and www.stadiumgal.com/(Accessed May 8, 2007).

7. "Alpha Blockers" DrugDigest (undated): 1 http://www.drugdigest.org/DD/HC/HCDrugClass/0,4055,5-550236,00.html (Accessed May 8, 2007).

8. "Shadow Buddies" Hollister—US: Continence Care (undated): 1 http//www.hollister.com/us/continence/learning/shadow_buddies.html (Accessed May 8, 2007).

9. Mary Darbey, "Urology Nurses Online: Interview with a Nurse Entrepreneur" (November 1997): 5 *Digital Urol J* http://www.duj.com/Asta.html (Accessed May 8, 2007).

Chapter 70 Spasticity After a Spinal Cord Injury

1. *Wikipedia*, s.v. "Spasticity," http://en.wikipedia.org/wiki/Spasticity (Accessed May 14, 2007).

2. Karen K. Bloom, "Spasticity and Spinal Cord Injury" Spinal Cord Injury Association of Kentucky (February 13, 2004): 1 http://www.sciak.org/articles/5/1/Spasticity-and-Spinal-Cord-Injury (Accessed May 14, 2007).

3. *MedlinePlus Medical Encyclopedia*, s.v. "Spasticity," U.S. National Library of Medicine and the National Institutes of Health (March 5, 2007): 2 http://www.nlm.nih.gov/medlineplus/ency/article/003297.htm (Accessed May 14, 2007).

4. Zeba F. Vanek and John H. Menkes, "Spasticity" *emedicine* (May 23, 2005): 2 http://www.emedicine.com/neuro/topic706.htm (Accessed May 14, 2007).

5. See Note 2.

6. "Spasticity and Spinal Cord Injury" SCI Forum Reports Northwest Regional Spinal Cord Injury System (NWRSCSI) (January 14, 2003): 2 http://depts.washington.edu/rehab/sci/spasticity.html (Accessed May 14, 2007).

7. See Note 1.

8. See Note 6.

9. "Spasticity" Sci-Info-Pages.com (undated): 6 http://www.sci-info-pages.com/other_issues.html (Accessed May 14, 2007).

10. See Note 9.

11. Karen K. Bloom, "Spasticity and Spinal Cord Injury" Spinal Cord Injury Association of Kentucky (February 13, 2004): 1-2 http://www.sciak.org/articles/5/1/Spasticity-and-Spinal-Cord-Injury (Accessed May 14, 2007).

12. "Intrathecal Baclofen Pump System" Cleveland Clinic (2005): 1 http://www.clevelandclinic.org/health/health-info/docs/0300/0369.asp? (Accessed May 14, 2007).

13. "Intrathecal Baclofen Pump System" Cleveland Clinic (2005): 2-3 http://www.clevelandclinic.org/health/health-info/docs/0300/0369.asp? (Accessed May 14, 2007).

14. "Intrathecal Baclofen Pump System" Cleveland Clinic (2005): 2 http://www.clevelandclinic.org/health/health-info/docs/0300/0369.asp? (Accessed May 14, 2007).

15. Loma Cohn. "Mother of son with Baclofen pump warns others: proceed with caution" (undated): 1 http://www.nbiadisorders.org/baclofenpumpcaution.htm (Accessed May 14, 2007).

16. *Wikipedia*, s.v. "Rigidity," http://en.wikipedia.org/wiki/Rigidity (Accessed July 5, 2007).

17. Loma Cohn. "Mother of son with Baclofen pump warns others: proceed with caution" (undated): 1-2 http://www.nbiadisorders.org/baclofenpumpcaution.htm (Accessed May 14, 2007).

18. See Note 6.

19. "BOTOX® Cosmetic" University of Washington Medical Center (2007): 2 http://www.uwmedicine.org/PatientCare/MedicalSpecialties/SpecialtyServices/botox.htm (Accessed May 14, 2007).

20. "Spasticity and Spinal Cord Injury" SCI Forum Reports Northwest Regional Spinal Cord Injury System (NWRSCSI) (January 14, 2003): 3 http://depts.washington.edu/rehab/sci/spasticity.html (Accessed May 14, 2007).

21. See Note 20.

22. Lynn Zimmer and John Morgan, "Marijuana myths facts" Drugpolicy.org (1997): 1 http://www.drugpolicy.org/marijuana/factsmyths/index.cfm? (Accessed July 5, 2007).

23. "Active State Medical Marijuana Programs" The National Organization for the Reform of Marijuana Laws (December 1, 2004): 1 http://www.norml.org/index.cfm?GroupID=3391 (Accessed July 5, 2007).

24. Tom Nordlie, "UF researchers find possible treatment window for spasticity in study of rats with spinal cord injury" *University of Florida News* (November 27, 2002): 1 http://news.ufl.edu/2002/1127/spasticity/(Accessed May 14, 2007).

Chapter 71 Chronic Dizziness After a Spinal Cord Injury

1. Julia Barrett, "Dizziness" Health A to Z.com (August 14, 2006): 1 http://www.healthatoz.com/healthatoz/atoz/common/standard/transform.jsp?requestURI=/heathatoz/Atoz/ency/dizziness.jsp (Accessed May 24, 2007).

2. "Chronic dizziness may have several psychiatric and neurologic causes" *Medical Research News* (February 20, 2007): 1 http://www.news-medical.net/article.asp?id=22022 (Accessed May 24, 2007).

3. Timothy C. Hain, "Vestibular Testing" Timothy C. Hain, MD (November 4, 2004): 1 http://www.tchain.com/otoneurology/testing/engrot.html (Accessed May 24, 2007).

4. Timothy C. Hain, "Benign Paroxysmal Positional Vertigo" Timothy C. Hain, MD (February 27, 2007): 4 http://www.dizziness-and-balance.com/disorders/bppv/bppv.html (Accessed May 24, 2007).

5. "Amitriptyline" *MedlinePlus* (April 1, 2005): 1 http://www.nlm.nih.gov/medlineplus/druginfo/memaster/a682388.html (Accessed May 24, 2007).

Chapter 72 Transitional Syndrome aka Adjacent Segment Disease

1. C.V. Burton, "The Infamous 'Transitional Syndrome'" *The Burton Report®* (undated): 3 http://www.burtonreport.com/infspine/SurgstabilTransitional-Synd.htm (Accessed January 26, 2007).

2. Jeffrey Wood, Michael O'Brien, Thomas Lowe, Paul Alongi, James Eule, and Robert Vraney, "Transition Zone Syndrome: latrogenic Instability or Natural History?" SpineUniverse.com (January 11, 2003): 2 http://www.spineuniverse.com/displayarticle.php/article581.htm (Accessed January 26, 2007).

3. C.V. Burton, "The Infamous 'Transitional Syndrome'" *The Burton Report®* (undated): 2 http://www.burtonreport.com/infspine/SurgstabilTransitional-Synd.htm (Accessed January 26, 2007).

4. Hilibrand, Alan S., Karthik Balasubramanian, Matthew Eichenbaum, John H. Thinnes, Scott Daffner, Scott Berta, Todd J. Albert, Alexander R. Vaccaro, and Sorin Siegler, "The Effect of Anterior Cervical Fusion on Neck Motion" *Spine* 31 no. 15 (July 1, 2006): 2 http://gateway.tx.ovid.com/gw1/ovideweb.cgi (Access date unknown). [note: my copy of this article was obtained from the University of Arkansas for Medical Sciences Interlibrary Loan. The pages of my copy do not show the original page numbers so the citation within the chapter must be based on the page numbers from my ILL copy which run 1 through 9.]

Chapter 73 Range of Motion After Neck Disc Fusion

1. Jill Serbousek, "More on ACDF with Dr. Kenneth Burkus" *InsideSpine* (June 26, 2007):1 http://www.insidespine.com/2007/06/26 (Accessed June 28, 2007).

2. See Note 1.

3. Jill Serbousek, "More on ACDF with Dr. Kenneth Burkus" *InsideSpine* (June 26, 2007):2 http://www.insidespine.com/2007/06/26 (Accessed June 28, 2007).

4. Jill Serbousek, "Dr. Kenneth Burkus talks With Me about a Neck Surgery Procedure: Anterior Cervical Discectomy with Fusion" *InsideSpine* (June 7, 2007):1 http://www.insidespine.com/2007/06/07 (Accessed June 28, 2007).

5. Alan S. Hilibrand, Karthik Balasubramanian, Matthew Eichenbaum, John H. Thinnes, Scott Daffner, Scott Berta, Todd J. Albert, Alexander R. Vaccaro, and

Sorin Siegler, "The Effect of Anterior Cervical Fusion on Neck Motion" *Spine* 31 no. 15 (July 1, 2006): 2 http://gateway.tx.ovid.com/gw1/ovideweb.cgi (Access date unknown). [note: my copy of this article was obtained from the University of Arkansas for Medical Sciences Interlibrary Loan. The pages of my copy do not show the original page numbers so the citation within the chapter must be based on the page numbers from my ILL copy which run 1 through 9.]

6. Alan S. Hilibrand, Karthik Balasubramanian, Matthew Eichenbaum, John H. Thinnes, Scott Daffner, Scott Berta, Todd J. Albert, Alexander R. Vaccaro, and Sorin Siegler, "The Effect of Anterior Cervical Fusion on Neck Motion" *Spine* 31 no. 15 (July 1, 2006): 8 http://gateway.tx.ovid.com/gw1/ovideweb.cgi (Access date unknown). [note: my copy of this article was obtained from the University of Arkansas for Medical Sciences Interlibrary Loan. The pages of my copy do not show the original page numbers so the citation within the chapter must be based on the page numbers from my ILL copy which run 1 through 9.]

7. See Note 6.

8. Alan S. Hilibrand, Karthik Balasubramanian, Matthew Eichenbaum, John H. Thinnes, Scott Daffner, Scott Berta, Todd J. Albert, Alexander R. Vaccaro, and Sorin Siegler, "The Effect of Anterior Cervical Fusion on Neck Motion" *Spine* 31 no. 15 (July 1, 2006): 7 http://gateway.tx. ovid.com/gw1/ovideweb.cgi (Access date unknown). [note: my copy of this article was obtained from the University of Arkansas for Medical Sciences Interlibrary Loan. The pages of my copy do not show the original page numbers so the citation within the chapter must be based on the page numbers from my ILL copy which run 1 through 9.]

9. Alan Hilibrand, e-mail message to the author, July 20, 2007.

Chapter 74 Changes in Sensation After a Spinal Cord Injury

1. *Wikipedia*, s.v. "Proprioception," http://www.en.wikipedia.org/wiki/Proprioception (Accessed May 21, 2007).

2. *Wikipedia*, s.v. "Somatosensory system," http://www.en.wikipedia.org/wiki/Somatosensory _system (Accessed May 21, 2007).

3. Phillip J. Siddall and Joan McClelland. "Non-painful sensory phenomena after spinal cord injury" *J Neurol Neurosurg Psych* 66 (May 1999): 621.

Chapter 75 Claw Hand After a Spinal Cord Injury

1. *Wheeless' Textbook of Orthopedics*, s.v. "Intrinsic Weakness and Claw Hand," http://www.wheelessonline.com/ortho/intrinsic_weakness_and_claw_hand (Accessed June 28, 2007).

2. Eduardo A. Zancolli. "Claw-Hand Caused by Paralysis of the Intrinsic Muscles: A Simple Surgical Procedure for its Correction" *J Bone Joint Surg Am* 39 (1957): 1079.

Chapter 76 Dental Care After a Spinal Cord Injury

1. "New Study Confirms Periodontal Disease Linked to Heart Disease" American Academy of Periodontology (February 7, 2002): 1 http://www.perio.org/consumer/bacteria.htm (Accessed June 11, 2007).

2. "UB Researchers Identify Specific Oral Bacteria Most Likely to Increase Risk of Heart Attack" School of Dental Medicine State University of New York at Buffalo (March 12, 1999): 1 http://www.sdm.buffalo.edu/news/1990312_bacterial.html (Accessed June 1, 2007).

3. Paul Burtner, "Office Accessibility" in "Oral Health for Persons with Disabilities Traumatic Injury Spinal Cord Injury" Department of Pediatric Dentistry College of Dentistry University of Florida (undated): 1 http://www.dental.ufl.edu/Faculty/Pburtner/Disabilities/English/trauma2.htm (Accessed June 1, 2007).

4. Paul Burtner, "Coordination of Care" in "Oral Health for Persons with Disabilities Traumatic Injury Spinal Cord Injury" Department of Pediatric Dentistry College of Dentistry University of Florida (undated): 1 http://www.dental.ufl.edu/Faculty/Pburtner/Disabilities/English/trauma2.htm (Accessed June 1, 2007).

5. Paul Burtner, "Traumatic Injuries Spinal Cord Injury in "Oral Health for Persons with Disabilities Traumatic Injury Spinal Cord Injury" Department of Pedi-

atric Dentistry College of Dentistry University of Florida (undated): 1 http://www.dental.ufl.edu/Faculty/Pburtner/Disabilities/English/trauma2.htm (Accessed June 1, 2007).

6. See Note 5.

7. See Note 4.

Chapter 77 Eye Care After a Spinal Cord Injury

1. "Focus on Independence Gives Sight to Quadriplegics" The Spinal Cord Injury Zone.com (June 22, 2006): 1-2 http://www.thescizone.com/news/articles/717/1/Focus-on-Independence-Gives-Sight-to-Quadriplegics/Page-1.html (Accessed May 13, 2007).

2. "Focus on Independence Program Offers Vision Correction Surgery to Quadriplegic Patients" The National Spinal Cord Injury Association (January 12, 2006): 1-2 http://www.spinalcord.org/news.php?dep=1&page=6&list=1015.

Chapter 78 Exercise After a Spinal Cord Injury

1. Phil Klebine, "Physical Activity After SCI" *PN* (December 2006): 16.

2. See Note 1.

Chapter 79 Prescription Medication After a Spinal Cord Injury

1. Laurance Johnston, *Alternative Medicine and Spinal Cord Injury:Beyond the Banks of the Mainstream* (New York: Demos Publishing Company, 2006), 13-25, 44.

2. Laurance Johnston, *Alternative Medicine and Spinal Cord Injury: Beyond the Banks of the Mainstream* (New York: Demos Publishing Company, 2006), 25-31.

3. Laurance Johnston, *Alternative Medicine and Spinal Cord Injury: Beyond the Banks of the Mainstream* (New York: Demos Publishing Company, 2006), 28.

4. Laurance Johnston, *Alternative Medicine and Spinal Cord Injury:Beyond the Banks of the Mainstream* (New York: Demos Publishing Company, 2006), 177-8.

5. Laurance Johnston, *Alternative Medicine and Spinal Cord Injury:Beyond the Banks of the Mainstream* (New York: Demos Publishing Company, 2006), 39-40.

6. Laurance Johnston, *Alternative Medicine and Spinal Cord Injury:Beyond the Banks of the Mainstream* (New York: Demos Publishing Company, 2006), 40-43.

7. Laurance Johnston, *Alternative Medicine and Spinal Cord Injury:Beyond the Banks of the Mainstream* (New York: Demos Publishing Company, 2006), 83-88.

8. Laurance Johnston, *Alternative Medicine and Spinal Cord Injury:Beyond the Banks of the Mainstream* (New York: Demos Publishing Company, 2006), 60-67.

9. Laurance Johnston, *Alternative Medicine and Spinal Cord Injury:Beyond the Banks of the Mainstream* (New York: Demos Publishing Company, 2006), 105-11.

10. Laurance Johnston, *Alternative Medicine and Spinal Cord Injury:Beyond the Banks of the Mainstream* (New York: Demos Publishing Company, 2006), 113-28.

11. Laurance Johnston, *Alternative Medicine and Spinal Cord Injury:Beyond the Banks of the Mainstream* (New York: Demos Publishing Company, 2006), 129-63.

Chapter 80 Caregivers

1. "Introduction to Caregiving" Caring Connections (undated): 1 http://www.caringinfo.org/i4a/pages/Index.cfm?pageid=3437 (Accessed May 21, 2007).

2. Linda Lindsey, "Caregivers for SCI" SCI InfoSheet #17 Department of Physical Medicine & Rehabilitation University of Alabama, Birmingham (September 1998): 1 http://www.spinalcord.uab.edu/show/asp?/durki=22479 (Accessed May 21, 2007).

Chapter 81 Clothing After a Spinal Cord Injury

1. Everlyn S. Johnson, "Clothing for Special Needs: Clothing for the Disabled" *MSUcares* (November 27, 2002): 1 http://msucares.com/pubs/infosheets/is1559.htm (Accessed May 12, 2007).

2. Everlyn S. Johnson, "Clothing for Special Needs: Clothing for the Disabled" *MSUcares* (November 27, 2002): 2-3 http://msucares.com/pubs/infosheets/is1559.htm (Accessed May 12, 2007).

3. Everlyn S. Johnson, "Clothing for Special Needs: Clothing for the Disabled" *MSUcares* (November 27, 2002): 3 http://msucares.com/pubs/infosheets/is1559.htm (Accessed May 12, 2007).

4. Shana Sager, "Smart" Clothing Helps Disabled Wearers Move" *The Daily Northwestern* (January 5, 2007): 1-2 http://media.dailynorthwestern.com/media/storage/paper853/news/2007/01/05/Campus/smart.Clothing.Helps.Disabled.Wearers.Move-2600649.htm (Accessed May 12, 2007).

Chapter 82 Going Back to School After a Spinal Cord Injury

1. "Campus Beat" *Careers & the disABLED* (Fall 2006): 20.

2. "College Bound" *PN* (February 2007): 40.

3. Belinda M. Armstrong, "Finding an accessible college campus" *SpeciaLiving* (Fall 2006): 83, 86.

Chapter 83 Employment After a Spinal Cord Injury

1. Cynthia Salzman, "From Injury to Employment" *PN* (November 2006): 42.

2. See Note 1

3. Urban Miyares, "Starting a Business" *PN* (April 2006): 14-15.

4. See Note 3.

Chapter 84 Service Animals

1. "Service Animal Information" U.S. Department of Justice (July 26, 1996): 1-4 http://www.usdoj.gov/crt/ada/animal.htm (Accessed May 21, 2007).

2. See Note 1.

3. See Note 1.

4. Helping Hands (2005): 1 http://www.helpinghandsmonkeys.org (Accessed May 21, 2007).

Chapter 85 Pets as Therapy After a Spinal Cord Injury

1. Jill A. Kraus, "Stress in Pet Owners and Non-Pet Owners" Delta Society.org (undated): 5, 10 http://www.deltasociety.org/download/Jill%20Kraus StressOwnersNonPetOwners.pdf (Accessed May 3, 2007).

2. Jill A. Kraus, "Stress in Pet Owners and Non-Pet Owners" Delta Society.org (undated): 12-13 http://www.deltasociety.org/download/Jill%20Kraus StressOwnersNonPetOwners.pdf (Accessed May 3, 2007).

3. Jill A. Kraus, "Stress in Pet Owners and Non-Pet Owners" Delta Society.org (undated): 12 http://www.deltasociety.org/download/Jill%20Kraus StressOwnersNonPetOwners.pdf (Accessed May 3, 2007).

4. Jeanie Lerche Davis, "Hypertension/High Blood Pressure Health Center 5 Ways Pets Can Improve Your Health" *WebMD®* (2004): 1-2 http://www.webmd.com/hypertension-high-blood-pressure/features/health-benefits-of-pets (Accessed June 3, 2007).

5. "Healthy Reasons to Have a Pet" Delta Society.org (2005): 1 http://www.deltasociety.org/AnimalsHealthGeneralReasons.htm (Accessed June 3, 2007).

6. See Note 5.

7. Karen Allen, "Coping with Life Changes & Transitions: The Role of Pet [*sic*]" (1995): 2 http://www.deltasociety.org/AnimalsHealthGeneralReasons.htm (Accessed June 3, 2007).

8. Jennifer Foss, "Pet-i-cure: The Health Benefits of Owning Pets" Buzzle.com (February 18, 2002): 1-2 http://www.Buzzle.com/editorials/2-18-2002-11780.asp (Accessed June 3, 2007).

9. Jeanie Lerche Davis, "Hypertension/High Blood Pressure Health Center. 5 Ways Pets Can Improve Your Health" *WebMD®* (2004): 1 http://www.webmd.com/hypertension-high-blood-pressure/features/health-benefits-of-pets (Accessed June 3, 2007).

10. Chris Woolston, "Pets: Prescription for Senior Health" (March 23, 2006): 1 http://healthresources.caremark.com/topic/stresspets (Accessed June 3, 2007)

Chapter 86 Sports as Motivation After a Spinal Cord Injury

1. "History" Wheelchair Sports, USA.com (2007): 1 http://www.wsusa.org/about.htm (Accessed May 3, 2007).

2. "Advertisement 27th National Veterans Wheelchair Games" *PN* (March 2007): 47.

3. "Paralympic Sports" U.S. Paralympics Official Site (2005): 1-2 http://www.usolympicteam.com/paralympics/teams.html (Accessed July 6, 2007).

4. *Wikipedia*, s.v. "Boccia," http://en.wikipedia.org/wiki/Boccia (Accessed July 6, 2007).

5. *Wikipedia*, s.v. "Curling," http://en.wikipedia.org/wiki/Curling (Accessed July 6, 2007).

6. *Wikipedia*, s.v. "Goalball," http://en.wikipedia.org/wiki/Goalball (Accessed July 6, 2007).

7. "Advertisement National Paralyzed Veterans of America Bass Tournament" *PN* (February 2007): 50.

8. "Advertisement 11th Annual PVA National Trapshoot Circuit" *PN* (March 2007): 63.

9. "Extreme Wheelchair Sports" Apparelyzed.com (2005): 1-5 http://www.apparelyzed.com/support/sport/xtreme_wheelchair_sports_html (Accessed May 3, 2007).

10. Dave Baskin (Manager, National Rifle Association Disabled Shooting Services), phone conversation with the author, date unknown.

Chapter 87 Driving and Transportation After a Spinal Cord Injury

1. James Inkster, "Vehicle Modification Guide (Part I)" *PN* (August 2006): 66.

2. See Note 1.

3. See Note 1.

4. Glen W. Zumwalt, letter to the editor" *PN* (November 2006): 11-12.

5. See Note 1.

6. See Note 1.

7. James Inkster. "Vehicle Modification Guide (Part I)" *PN* (August 2006): 66-67.

8. Bob Nunn. "Adapted Vehicles: High Costs & Dangers" *PN* (June 2007): 14-15

Chapter 88 Travel and Accessibility After a Spinal Cord Injury

Chapter 89 Parking After a Spinal Cord Injury

1. "Disability-Parking Crackdowns" *New Mobility* (January 2006): 1 http://www.newmobility.com/review_article.cfm?id=1101 (Accessed May 15, 2007).

2. "United Spinal Sues for Parking in D.C." *New Mobility* (September 2006): 1 http://www. newmobility com/review_article.cfm?id=1197 (Accessed May 15, 2007).

Chapter 90 Selecting a Wheelchair After a Spinal Cord Injury

1. Lynn R. Halverson and Katherine A. Belknap, "Informed Consumer's Guide to Wheelchair Selection" Abledata.com (May 1994): 4 http://www.abledata.com/abledata_docs/icg_whel.htm (Accessed June 9, 2007).

2. "How to Select Wheelchairs or Wheeled Chairs?" UCan Health.com (2004): 1-2 http://www.uncanhealth.com/all_wheelchairs.htm (Accessed June 9, 2007).

3. "Sports Wheelchair Store" SpinLife.com (undated) 1-2 http://www.spinlife.com/category.cfm?categoryID=8 (Accessed June 9, 2007).

4. "A Sporty Solution" *PN* (May 2007): 82.

5. Gary Karp, "Choosing A Wheelchair" SpinLife.com (undated): 1-2 http://www.spinlife.com/spintips/details/k/Choosing-A-Wheelchair/a/329/c/3 (Accessed June 9, 2007).

6. Lynn R. Halverson and Katherine A. Belknap, "Fact Sheet on Manual Wheelchairs" Abledata.com (July 1994): 1-3 http://www.abledata.com/able/abledata_docs/manwhch.htm (Accessed June 9, 2007).

7. Kendra Betz, "Pushing a Wheelchair: Simple Task—or Accomplished Skill?" *PN* (March 2007): 30-35.

8. "Selecting a Power Chair" Stuart L. Portner website (April 8, 2004): 2 http://www.geocities.com/stuportner/files/power.htm (Accessed June 9, 2007).

9. "Choosing a Power Mobility-base, Power Wheelchair, or Scooter" University of Iowa Health Care (undated): 1-2 http://www.medicine.uiowa.edu/cdd/multiple/wc/wc_power.asp (Accessed June 9, 2007).

10. "Power Wheelchairs for PALS" ALS Society of Alberta (2006): 1-2 http://www.alsab.ca/equipment/powerchairs.aspx (Accessed June 9, 2007).

11. Carmen P. DiGiovine, "Power Wheelchair Batteries" SpinLife.com (2007): 1-5 http://www. spinlife.com/spintips/details/k/Power-Wheelchair-Batteries/a/121/c/3 (Accessed June 9, 2007).

12. Bradford C. Peterson, "Pardon the Cliché, but … a closer look" *PN* (September 2006): 74-75.

13. "Power Wheelchairs for PALS" ALS Society of Alberta (2006): 2 http://www.alsab.ca/equipment/powerchairs.aspx (Accessed June 9, 2007).

14. "Choosing a Power Mobility-base, Power Wheelchair, or Scooter" University of Iowa Health Care (undated): 2 http://www.medicine.uiowa.edu/cdd/multiple/wc/wc_power.asp (Accessed June 9, 2007).

15. See Note 3.

16. Richard C. Senelick and Karla Dougherty, *The Spinal Cord Injury Handbook* (Birmingham: HealthSouth Press, 1998), 49.

Chapter 91 Accessible Living, Home Modifications and Universal Design

1. Rosemarie Rossetti, "Accessible Homes: Building a Healthy Home" United Spinal.org (September 1, 2003): 2 http://www.unitedspinal.org/publications/action/2006/09/01/accessible-home-building-a-healthy-home/(Accessed September 28, 2006).

2. Susan Mack, "Increasing Housing Options Through Universal Design" *SpeciaLiving* (Winter 2005): 36.

Chapter 92 Equipment You May Need After a Spinal Cord Injury

1. Margaret C. Hammond and Stephen C. Burns, *Yes, You Can! A Guide to Self-Care for Persons with Spinal Cord Injury Third Edition* (Washington, D.C.: Paralyzed Veterans of America, 2000), 211-6.

Chapter 93 Self-Defense After a Spinal Cord Injury

1. *Wikipedia*, s.v. "Self-defense" http://en.wikipedia.org/wiki/Self-defense (Accessed July 2, 2007).

2. Richard P. Diamond, "How Can People with Disabilities Remain Both Mobile and Safe?" All About Multiple Sclerosis (January 2002): 1 http://www.mult-sclerosis.org/news/Jan2002/SelfDefenceForDisabled [*sic*] (Accessed June 8, 2007).

3. Randy LaHaie, "Self-Defense Articles The Nuts & Bolts of Awareness Learning to Detect Trouble" (2002): 1-8 http://www.protectivestrategies.com/awareness/html (Accessed June 8, 2007).

Chapter 94 In Case of Emergency

1. *Preparing Your Pets for Emergencies Makes Sense. Get Ready Now.* (Washington, D.C.: U.S. Department of Homeland Security, undated), 1.

2. *Preparing Your Pets for Emergencies Makes Sense. Get Ready Now.* (Washington, D.C.: U.S. Department of Homeland Security, undated), 2.

Chapter 95 Spinal Cord Syndromes as an Invisible Disability

1. "Nice to know I'm not alone with Brown Sequard" The National Spinal Cord Injury Association Discussion Forum (November 6, 2006): 1 http://www.spinalcord.org/forum/viewtopic.php/?t=416&highlight=brown+sequard (Accessed January 23, 2007).

2. Invisible Disabilities Advocate (November 23, 2003): 1-15 http://www.myida.org/disabled.htm (Accessed May 5, 2007).

3. David Moisan, "The Invisible Disabilities Page" (November 23, 2003): 1-2 http://mysite.verizon.net/vze20h45/invisible_disability.html (Accessed May 5, 2007).

4. *Wikipedia*, s.v. "Invisible disability," http://en.wikipedia.org/wiki/Invisible_disability (Accessed May 6, 2007).

Chapter 96 Disability Rights and Discrimination

1. "Disability Discrimination" Americans with Disabilities Act Equal Employment Opportunity Commission (May 17, 2007): 1 http://www.eeoc.gov/types/ada.html (Accessed June 19, 2007).

2. "Disabled People" Direct.gov (May 28, 2007): 1 http://www.direct.gov.uk/en/DisabledPeople/RightsAndObligations/DisabilityDiscriminationAct (Accessed April 26, 2007).

3. European Network on Independent Living. Independent Living Institute (December 15, 1999): 1-3 http://www.independentliving.org/docs2/index.html (Accessed April 26, 2007).

4. "Disability Rights" Australian Human Rights & Equal Opportunity Commission (June 8, 2007): 1 http://www.hreoc.gov.au/disability_rights/index.html (Accessed June 19, 2007).

5. National Disability Rights Network (undated): 1 http://www.ndrn.org (Accessed April 26, 2007).

6. National Council for Support of Disability Issues (2007): 1 http://www.ncsd.org (Accessed April 26, 2007).

Chapter 97 "My Introduction to Disabled People"

Chapter 98 Sexuality After a Spinal Cord Injury

1. Marca L. Sipski, "Sexuality and Spinal Cord Injury: where we are and where we are going" *American Rehabilitation* (Spring 1997): 1 http://www.ed.gov/pubs/AmericanRehab/spring97/sp9707.html (Accessed May 9, 2007).

2. K.D. Anderson, J.F. Borisoff, R.D. Johnson, S.A. Stiens, and S.L. Elliott, "The impact of spinal cord injury on sexual function: concerns of the general population" *Spinal Cord* (October 10, 2006): 2.

3. Miriam Kaufman, Cory Silverberg, and Fran Odette, *The Ultimate Guide to Sex and Disability* (San Francisco: Cleis Press, 2003), 1-12.

Chapter 99 Sex After a Spinal Cord Injury—Men

1. Marca L. Sipski, "Sexuality and Spinal Cord Injury: where we are and where we are going" *American Rehabilitation* (Spring 1997): 1 http://www.ed.gov/pubs/AmericanRehab/spring97/sp9707.html (Accessed May 9, 2007).

2. Phil Klebine and Linda Lindsey, "Sexual Function for Men with Spinal Cord Injury" Spinal Cord Injury InfoSheet #3 University of Alabama, Birmingham (May 2007): 1-6 http://www.spinalcord.uab.edu/show.asp?durki=22405 (Accessed June 6, 2007).

3. K.D. Anderson, J.F. Borisoff, R.D. Johnson, S.A. Stiens, and S.L. Elliott, "Long-term effects of spinal cord injury on sexual function in men: implications for neuroplasticity" *Spinal Cord* (October 10, 2006): 2.

4. Stanley Ducharme, "Testosterone & SCI." *PN* (May 2007): 33-34.

5. K.D. Anderson, J.F. Borisoff, R.D. Johnson, S.A. Stiens, and S.L. Elliott. "Long-term effects of spinal cord injury on sexual function in men: implications for neuroplasticity" *Spinal Cord* (October 10, 2006): 8.

Chapter 100 Sex After a Spinal Cord Injury—Women

1. Marca L. Sipski, "Sexuality and Spinal Cord Injury: where we are and where we are going" *American Rehabilitation* (Spring 1997): 1 http://www.ed.gov/pubs/AmericanRehab/spring97/sp9707.html (Accessed May 9, 2007).

2. Phil Klebine, Linda Lindsey, and Patricia Rivera, "Sexuality for Women with Spinal Cord Injury" University of Alabama, Birmingham (April 2004): 3 http://www.spinalcord.uab.edu/show.asp?durki=51275 (Accessed June 7, 2007).

3. K.D. Anderson, J.F. Borisoff, R.D. Johnson, S.A. Stiens, and S.L. Elliott, "Spinal cord injuries influences psychogenic as well as physical components of female sexual ability" *Spinal Cord* (October 10, 2006): 4.

4. K.D. Anderson, J.F. Borisoff, R.D. Johnson, S.A. Stiens, and S.L. Elliott, "Spinal cord injuries influences psychogenic as well as physical components of female sexual ability" *Spinal Cord* (October 10, 2006): 6.

5. K.D. Anderson, J.F. Borisoff, R.D. Johnson, S.A. Stiens, and S.L. Elliott, "Spinal cord injuries influences psychogenic as well as physical components of female sexual ability" *Spinal Cord* (October 10, 2006): 8.

6. Amie B. Jackson and Linda Lindsey, "Women's Health and Sexual Function after a Spinal Cord Injury" University of Alabama, Birmingham (2000): 2 http://www.spinalcord.uab.edu/show.asp?durki=32375 (Accessed July 11, 2007) Taken from Research Review, Fall 2000. Published by the UAB-RRTC on Secondary Conditions of SCI, Birmingham, AL. ©2000 Board of Trustees, University of Alabama.

7. See Note 6.

8. "Frequently Asked Questions About Human Papilloma Virus (HPV) Vaccines" Cancer Reference Information. American Cancer Society (January 18, 2007): 1-5 http://www.cancer.org/docroot/CRI/content/CRI_2_6x_FAQ_HPV_Vaccines.asp (Accessed June 19, 2007).

Chapter 101 "How Do I Find a Family Doctor Who Is Familiar with Spinal Cord Injuries After I'm Recovered?"

1. Gale G. Whiteneck, Susan W. Charlifue, Kenneth A. Gerhart, Daniel P. Lammertse, Scott Manley, Robert R. Menter, and Kathie R. Seedroff, *Aging With Spinal Cord Injury* (New York: Demos Publishing Company, 1993), 229.

2. "The World Factbook—United States" Central Intelligence Agency (June 19, 2007): 3 http://www.cia.gov/library/publications/the-world-factbook/print/us.html (Accessed June 29, 2007).

3. "Facts and Figures at a Glance Spinal Cord Injury" Spinalcord [*sic*] Injury Information Network University of Alabama, Birmingham (June 2006): 1 http://www.spinalcord.uab.edu/show.asp?durki=21446 (Accessed May 2, 2007).

4. Gale G. Whiteneck, Susan W. Charlifue, Kenneth A. Gerhart, Daniel P. Lammertse, Scott Manley, Robert R. Menter, and Kathie R. Seedroff, *Aging With Spinal Cord Injury* (New York: Demos Publishing Company, 1993), 276.

5. See Note 4.

6. Gale G. Whiteneck, Susan W. Charlifue, Kenneth A. Gerhart, Daniel P. Lammertse, Scott Manley, Robert R. Menter, and Kathie R. Seedroff, *Aging With Spinal Cord Injury* (New York: Demos Publishing Company, 1993), 297.

7. Gale G. Whiteneck, Susan W. Charlifue, Kenneth A. Gerhart, Daniel P. Lammertse, Scott Manley, Robert R. Menter, and Kathie R. Seedroff, *Aging With Spinal Cord Injury* (New York: Demos Publishing Company, 1993), 273.

8. Gale G. Whiteneck, Susan W. Charlifue, Kenneth A. Gerhart, Daniel P. Lammertse, Scott Manley, Robert R. Menter, and Kathie R. Seedroff, *Aging With Spinal Cord Injury* (New York: Demos Publishing Company, 1993), 305.

9. Gale G. Whiteneck, Susan W. Charlifue, Kenneth A. Gerhart, Daniel P. Lammertse, Scott Manley, Robert R. Menter, and Kathie R. Seedroff, *Aging With Spinal Cord Injury* (New York: Demos Publishing Company, 1993), 305-6.

Chapter 102 "Should I Go To a Chiropractor After a Spinal Cord Injury?"

1. "Incomplete c5 injury/spastic walking" The National Spinal Cord Injury Association Discussion Forum (January 24, 2005): 1 http://www.spinalcord.org/forum/viewtopic.php?t=256 (Accessed May 24, 2007).

2. Chung, O.M., "MRI confirmed cervical cord injury caused by spinal manipulation in a Chinese patient" *Spinal Cord* 40 no. 4 (April 2002): 197 http://www.nature.com/sc/journal/v40/n4/full/3101274a.html (Accessed May 24, 2007).

3. "Chiropractors" *Occupational Outlook Handbook, 2006-07Edition.* U.S. Department of Labor. Bureau of Labor Statistics (2006): 1 http://www.bls.gov/oco/print/ocos071.htm (Accessed May 24, 2007).

4. See Note 2.

5. Allan Rubin, "Does Medicare Cover Chiropractic Care?" therubins.com (undated): 1 http://www.therubins.com/geninfo/chiroprac.htm (Accessed June 28, 2007).

6. *Wikipedia,* s.v. "Subluxation," http://en.wikipedia/wiki/Subluxation (Accessed June 28, 2007).

7. See Note 5.

8. Gail A. Jensen, Robert D. Mootz, Paul G. Shekelle, and Daniel C. Cherkin, "Chiropractic in the United States: Training, Practice, and Research" (July 13, 1999): 8 http://www.Ncschiropractic.com/ahpr/part6.htm (Accessed June 28, 2007).

9. Gail A. Jensen, Robert D. Mootz, Paul G. Shekelle, and Daniel C. Cherkin. "Chiropractic in the United States: Training, Practice, and Research" (July 13, 1999): 2 http://www.ncschiropractic.com/ahpr/part6.htm (Accessed June 28, 2007).

Chapter 103 "Should I Go To a Massage Therapist After a Spinal Cord Injury?"

1. Ruth Werner, "Working with Clients Who Have Spinal Cord Injuries" *MassageToday* 02 no. 5 (May 2002): 3 http://www.massagetoday.com/mpacms/mt/article.php?id=10465 (Accessed June 28, 2007).

2. Ruth Werner, "Working with Clients Who Have Spinal Cord Injuries" *MassageToday* 02 no. 5 (May 2002): 4 http://www.massagetoday.com/mpacms/mt/article.php?id=10465 (Accessed June 28, 2007).

3. See Note 2.

4. See Note 2.

5. John McKinzie, "Experts: Spinal Cord Injury" AllExperts.com (2006): 1 http://en.allexperts.com/q/Spinal-Cord-Injury-2097/indexExp_39306.htm (Accessed July 20, 2007).

6. Laurel Chesky. "Therapists fight Medicare exclusion" *Massage* no. 119 (2005): 1 http://www.massagemag.com/ExtraEdit/119Therapists.php (Accessed June 28, 2007).

7. Stephen Nohlgren. "Yes, Medicaid pays for this" *St. Petersburg Times Online* (October 2, 2006): 1 http://www.sptimes.com/2006/10/02/Tampabay/Yes__Medicaid_pays_fo.shtm (Accessed June 28, 2007).

Chapter 104 "Should I Participate in a Clinical Trial After a Spinal Cord Injury?"

1. "Experimental treatments for spinal cord injury: what you should know if you are considering participation in a clinical trial. A guide for people with spinal cord injury, their families, friends & caregivers" International Campaign for Cures of spinal cord injury Paralysis (February 2007): 7 http://www.campaign-forcure.org (Access date unknown).

2. "Experimental treatments for spinal cord injury: what you should know if you are considering participation in a clinical trial. A guide for people with spinal cord injury, their families, friends & caregivers" International Campaign for Cures of spinal cord injury Paralysis (February 2007): 8 http://www.campaign-forcure.org (Access date unknown).

3. See Note 2.

4. *Wikipedia*, s.v. "Informed Consent," http://en.wikipedia.org/wiki/Informed_consent (Accessed July 19, 2007).

5. See Note 4.

6. See Note 2.

7. "Experimental treatments for spinal cord injury: what you should know if you are considering participation in a clinical trial. A guide for people with spinal cord injury, their families, friends & caregivers" International Campaign for Cures of spinal cord injury Paralysis (February 2007): 9 http://www.campaign-forcure.org (Access date unknown).

8. See Note 7.

9. "Experimental treatments for spinal cord injury: what you should know if you are considering participation in a clinical trial. A guide for people with spinal cord injury, their families, friends & caregivers" International Campaign for

Cures of spinal cord injury Paralysis (February 2007): 39 http://www.campaignforcure.org (Access date unknown).

10. See Note 7.

Chapter 105 "Final Thoughts"

Chapter 106 "A Word of Warning"

Bibliography

"A Sporty Solution" *PN* (May 2007): 82.

"Active State Medical Marijuana Programs" The National Organization for the Reform of Marijuana Laws (December 1, 2004): 1-10 http://www.norml.org/index.cfm?GroupID=3391 (Accessed July 5, 2007).

"Advertisement 11th Annual PVA National Trapshoot Circuit" *PN* (March 2007): 63.

"Advertisement 27th National Veterans Wheelchair Games" *PN* (March 2007): 47.

"Advertisement National Paralyzed Veterans of America Bass Tournament" *PN* (February 2007): 50.

Allen, Gemmy. "Communicating" Modern Management BMGT-1301 (1998): 1-5 http://www.telecollege.dcccd.edu/mgmt1374/book_contents/3organizing/commun/communic.htm+communication+process&hl=en&ct=clnk&cd=1&gl=us (Accessed May 27, 2007).

Allen, Karen. "Coping with Life Changes & Transitions: The Role of Pet [*sic*]" Delta Society.org (1995): 1-3 http://www.deltasociety.org/AnimalsHealthGeneralReasons.htm (Accessed June 3, 2007).

"Alpha Blockers" DrugDigest.org (undated): 1 http://www.drugdigest.org/DD/HC/HCDrugClass/0,4055,5-550246,00.html (Accessed May 8, 2007).

"Amitriptyline" MedlinePlus (April 1, 2005): 1-4 http://www.nlm.nih.gov/medlineplus/druginfo/memaster/a682388.html (Accessed May 24, 2007).

"Anatomy of the Urinary System" Ohio State University Medical Center (2007): 1-2 http://medicalcenter.osu.edu/patientcare/healthinformation/otherhealthtopics/Urology/AnatomyoftheUrinarySystem5114/index.cfm (Accessed May 8, 2007).

Anderson, K.D., J.F. Borisoff, R.D. Johnson, S.A. Stiens, and S.L. Elliott. "Long-term effects of spinal cord injury on sexual function in men: implications for neuroplasticity" *Spinal Cord* (October 10, 2006): 1-11.

Anderson, K.D., J.F. Borisoff, R.D. Johnson, S.A. Stiens, and S.L. Elliott. "Spinal cord injuries influences psychogenic as well as physical components of female sexual ability" *Spinal Cord* (October 10, 2006): 1-11.

Anderson, K.D., J.F. Borisoff, R.D. Johnson, S.A. Stiens, and S.L. Elliott. "The impact of spinal cord injury on sexual function: concerns of the general population" *Spinal Cord* (October 10, 2006): 1-10.

Anonymous. "Spinal cord injury without radiographic abnormality (SCIWORA) in the adult: A case presentation and literature review." *J Neurol Sciences Turkey* 21 (2004): 1-6 http://med.ege.edu.tr/~norolbil/2004/NBD31604.htm (Accessed February 11, 2005).

"Anterior Cord Syndrome" Apparelyzed.com (2005): 1 http://www.apparelyzed.com/spinal-cord-injury/anterior-cord-syndrome.html (Accessed July 15, 2007).

"Anterior Cord Syndrome" *Wheeless' Textbook of Orthopedics Online* (undated): 1 http://www.wheelessonline.com/ortho/anterior_cord_syndrome (Accessed July 15, 2007).

"Arachnoiditis Information & Support" Circle of Friends with Arachnoiditis (COFWA) (September 15, 2006): 1-3 http://www.cofwa.org (Accessed June 19, 2007).

"Arizona Grand Canyon State" 50states.com (2007): 1-4 http://www.50states.com/arizona.html (Accessed August 2, 2005).

Armstrong, Belinda M. "Finding an accessible college campus" *SpeciaLiving* (Fall 2006): 83.

"Autonomic Dysreflexia" The National Spinal Cord Injury Association (NSCIA) (2006): 1-3 http://www.spinalcord.org/html/factsheets/aut_dysreflexia.php (Accessed April 30, 2007).

Avitzur, Orly. "Avoid Insult to Brain Injury" *Neurology Now* (March/April 2007): 44-45.

Bangalore, Lakshmi. "Rebuilding Circuits" *PN* (February 2007): 25-29.

Barker, Lenette. letter to the editor *New Mobility* (September 2005): 6.

Barrett, Julia. "Dizziness" Health A to Z.com (August 14, 2006): 1-3 http://www.healthatoz.com/healthatoz/atoz/common/standard/transform.jsp?requestURI=/heathatoz/Atoz/ency/dizziness.jsp (Accessed May 24, 2007).

Barton, Vickeri. "Nutrition Guidelines for Individuals with SCI" SCI Forum Reports (from a lecture given June 13, 2006): 1-7 Northwest Regional Spinal Cord Injury System (NWRSCIS) http://depts.washington.edu/rehab/sci/nutrition.html (Accessed June 3, 2007).

Beeson, Michael S. and Scott T. Wilber. "Brown-Sequard Syndrome" *emedicine* (February 1, 2007): 1-6 http://www.emedicine.com/emerg/topic70.htm (Accessed July 15, 2007).

"Before You Ride" ATV Safety Institute (undated):1 http://www.atvsafety.org/asi.cfm?spl=2&action=display&pagename=Before%20You%20Ride (Accessed May 28, 2007).

Berg, David. "Introduction to Central Pain" PainOnline.org (2001): 1-4 http://www.painonline.org/intro.htm (Accessed May 9, 2007).

Betz, Kendra. "Pushing a Wheelchair: Simple Task—or Accomplished Skill?" *PN* (March 2007): 30-35.

Bhatoe, HS. "Cervical spinal cord injury without radiographic abnormality in adults" *Neurol India* 48 no. 3 (2000): 243-8 http://www.neurologyindia.com/

article.asp?issn=0028-3886;year=2000;volume=48;issue=3;spage=243;epage=8;aulast=Bhatoe (Accessed February 11, 2005).

"Bladder Care and Management" SpinalInjury.net (undated): 1-4 http://www.spinalinjury.net/html/_bladder_care_and_management.html (Accessed May 8, 2007).

Bloom, Karen K. "Spasticity and Spinal Cord Injury" Spinal Cord Injury Association of Kentucky (February 13, 2004): 1-2 http://www.sciak.org/articles/5/1/Spasticity-and-Spinal-Cord-Injury (Accessed May 14, 2007).

Blumenfeld, Hal. "Finger Flexors" neuroexam.com (undated): 1 http://www.neuroexam.com/content/.php?p=33 (Accessed April 30, 2007).

Boden, Barry P., Robin Tachetti, and Fred O. Mueller. "Catastrophic Injuries in High School and College Baseball Players" *Am J Sports Med* 32 no. 5 (July 1, 2004): 1189-95.

Bosch, Albert, E. Shannon Stauffer, and Vernon L. Nickel. "Incomplete Traumatic Quadriplegia: A Ten Year Review" *JAMA* 216 no. 3 (April 19, 1971): 473-8.

"BOTOX® Cosmetic" University of Washington Medical Center (2007): 1-2 http://www.uwmedicine.org/PatientCare/MedicalSpecialties/SpecialtyServices/botox.htm (Accessed May 14, 2007).

Boyarsky, Igor and Gary Godorov. "C2 Fractures" *emedicine* (March 15, 2006): 1-9 http://www.emedicine.com/orthoped/topic597.htm (Accessed July 15, 2007).

"Brain & Spinal Cord Injury Program Facility Designation Standards" *The Florida Department of Health Facility Designation Standards* (April 18, 2005): 1-56 http://www.doh.state.fl.us/workforce/brainsc/Facilities/Facility Standards2005.pdf (Accessed July 4, 2007).

Brohi, Karim. "Indications for spinal immobilisation" trauma.org 7 no. 4 (April 2002): 1-4 http://www.trauma.org/archive/spine/cspine-stab.html (Accessed July 9, 2007).

"Brown Sequard" PeaceHealth.org (July 5, 2005): 1-3 http://www.peacehealth.org/kbase/nord/nord950.htm (Accessed July 15, 2007).

Buechner, Jay S., Mary C. Speare, and Janice Fontes. "Hospitalizations for Spinal Cord Injuries, 1994-1998" 2 no. 3 *Health by Numbers Web Edition* Office of Health Statistics Rhode Island Department of Health (March 2003): 1-2 http://www.health.state.ri.us/chic/statistics/Hbn2-3.pdf (Accessed July 13, 2007).

"Burners and Stingers" American Academy of Orthopaedic Surgeons (January 2006): 1-5 http://orthoinfo.aaos.org/fact/hr_report.cfm?Thread_ID=226&topcategory=Shoulder (Accessed July 10, 2007).

Burtner, Paul. "Coordination of Care" in "Oral Health for Persons with Disabilities Traumatic Injury Spinal Cord Injury" Department of Pediatric Dentistry College of Dentistry University of Florida (undated): 1 http://www.dental.ufl.edu/Faculty/Pburtner/Disabilities/English/trauma2.htm (Accessed June 1, 2007).

Burtner, Paul. "Office Accessibility and Accommodation" in "Oral Health for Persons with Disabilities Traumatic Injury Spinal Cord Injury" Department of Pediatric Dentistry College of Dentistry University of Florida (undated): 1-2 http://www.dental.ufl.edu/Faculty/Pburtner/Disabilities/English/trauma2.htm (Accessed June 1, 2007).

Burtner, Paul. "Traumatic Injuries Spinal Cord Injury" in "Oral Health for Persons with Disabilities Traumatic Injuries Spinal Cord Injury" Department of Pediatric Dentistry College of Dentistry University of Florida (undated): 1-2 http://www.dental.ufl.edu/Faculty/Pburtner/Disabilities/English/trauma2.htm (Accessed June 1, 2007).

Burton, C.V. "The Infamous 'Transitional Syndrome'" The Burton Report® (undated): 1-3 http://www.burtonreport.com/infspine/SurgstabilTransitionalSynd.htm (Accessed January 26, 2007).

Byzek, Josie, Tim Gilmer, and Roxanne Furlong. "Active Aging" *New Mobility* (May 2007): 34, 35+.

"Campus Beat" *Careers & the disABLED* (Fall 2006): 20.

Cantu, Robert C. "Stingers, transient quadriplegia, and cervical spinal stenosis: return to play criteria" *Medicine & Science in Sports & Exercise* 29 no. 7 (Supplement July 1997): 233-5.

"Cars," an episode of *Crash Test Human.*

Carswell, Lindsay. "Paralysis Push" *ScienCentralNews* (April 5, 2005): 1-2 http://www.sciencentral.com/articles/view.php3?article_id=21839251 (Accessed May 2, 2007).

"Census 2001 at a glance" *Statistics South Africa Census 2001* (undated): 1 http://www.statssa.gov.za/census01/html/default.asp (Accessed July 4, 2007).

"Central Cord Syndrome" American Association of Neurological Surgeons (2007): 1-3 http://www.neurosurgerytoday.org/what/patient_e/central_cord_syndrome (Accessed July 11, 2007).

"Central Cord Syndrome" The National Spinal Cord Injury Association Discussion Forum (February 3, 2005): 1-8 http://www.spinalcord.ord/forum/viewtopic.php/?t=261&highlight =central+cord+syndrome (Accessed January 30, 2007).

"Cervical Artificial Disc Preserves Neck Mobility An Interview with Richard Guyer, MD" Spineuniverse.com (August 18, 2006): 1-3 http://www.spineuniverse.com/displayarticle.php/article2522.html (Accessed January 26, 2007).

"Cervical Artificial Disc Preserves Neck Mobility: Part 2 An Interview with Richard Guyer, MD" Spineuniverse.com (August 16, 2006): 1-3 http://www.spineuniverse.com/displayarticle.php/article2525.html (Accessed January 26, 2007).

Chesky, Laurel. "Therapists fight Medicare exclusion" *Massage* no. 119 (2005): 1 http://www.massagemag.com/ExtraEdit/119Therapists.php (Accessed June 28, 2007).

"Chiropractors" *Occupational Outlook Handbook, 2006-07Edition.* U.S. Department of Labor Bureau of Labor Statistics (2006): 1 http://www.bls.gov/oco/print/ocos071.htm (Accessed May 24, 2007).

"Choosing a Power Mobility-base, Power Wheelchair, or Scooter" University of Iowa Health Care (undated) 1-3 http://www.medicine.uiowa.edu/cdd/multiple/wc/wc_power.asp (Accessed June 9, 2007).

"Chronic dizziness may have several psychiatric and neurologic causes" *Medical Research News* (February 20, 2007): 1-2 http://www.news-medical.net/print_article.asp?id=22022 (Accessed May 24, 2007).

Christian, W. Jay. "Traumatic Brain & Spinal Cord Injury Surveillance Project Fiscal Year 2003 Final Report" Kentucky Injury Prevention and Research Center University of Kentucky (July 1, 2003): 1-32 http://www.kiprc.uky.edu/projects/tbi/tbi_FY03.doc (Accessed July 13, 2007).

Chung, O.M. "MRI confirmed cervical cord injury caused by spinal manipulation in a Chinese patient" *Spinal Cord* 40 no. 4 (April 2002): 196-9 http://www.nature.com/sc/journal/v40/n4/full/3101274a.html (Accessed May 24, 2007).

"Closed head injury" Providence Health & Services Alaska (2007): 1 http://www.providence.org/alaska/tchap/glossary/C.htm (Accessed June 10, 2007).

Cody, Thomas and Veronica (Roni) Zieroff. "Autonomic Dysreflexia" Northeast Rehabilitation Health Network (September 7, 2005): 1-2 http://www.northeastrehab.com/Articles/dysreflexia.html (Accessed April 30, 2007).

Cohn, Loma. "Mother of son with Baclofen pump warns others: proceed with caution" (undated): 1-2 http://www.nbiadisorders.org/baclofenpumpcaution.htm (Accessed May 14, 2007).

Cole, Jonathan. *Still Lives Narratives of Spinal Cord Injury.* Cambridge, Massachusetts: MIT Press, 2004.

"College Bound" *PN* (February 2007): 38-41.

"Communicating with Your Doctor" Ohio State University Medical Center (2007): 1-2 http://medicalcenter.osu.edu/patientcare/findadoctor/choosing/communication (Accessed May 24, 2007).

"Complications" Mayo Clinic Rochester, Minnesota (August 22, 2005): 1-13 http://www.mayoclinic.com/health/spinal-cord-injury/DS00460/DSECTION=7 (Accessed May 29, 2007).

"Current Trends Trends [*sic*] in Traumatic Spinal Cord Injury—New York, 1982-1988," *Morbidity and Mortality Weekly Report* 40 no. 31 (August 9, 1991): 535-7, 543;

Centers for Disease Control and Prevention http://www.cdc.gov/mmwr/preview/mmwrhtml/00014953.html (Accessed August 2, 2005).

Darbey, Mary. "Urology Nurses Online: Interview with a Nurse Entrepreneur" *Digital Urol J* (November 1997): 1-8 http://www.duj.com/Asta.html (Accessed May 8, 2007).

Davis, Jeanie Lerche. "Hypertension/High Blood Pressure Health Center 5 Ways Pets Can Improve Your Health" *WebMD®* (2004): 1-2 http://www.wedmd.com/hypertension-high-blood-pressure/features/health-benefits-of-pets (Accessed June 3, 2007).

Dawodu, Segun T. and Nicholas Lorenzo. "Cauda Equina and Conus Medullaris Syndromes" (January 16, 2007): 1-20 http://www.emedicine.com/neuro/topic667.htm (Accessed July 15, 2007).

Deitrick, George, Joseph Charalel, William Bauman, and John Tuckman. "Reduced Arterial Circulation to the Legs in Spinal Cord Injury as a Cause of Skin Breakdown Lesions" *Angiology* 58 no. 2 (2007): 174-85.

Del Bigio, Marc R. and Garth E. Johnson. "Clinical Presentation of Spinal Cord Concussion" *Spine* 14 no. 1 (January 1989): 37-40.

"Department of Disabilities and Special Needs Annual Accountability Report Fiscal Year 1995-1996 Program-Head and Spinal Cord Injury" South Carolina

General Assembly (May 24, 2005): 1-12 http://www.scstatehouse.net/reports/16aar96.htm (Acccessed September 26, 2005).

"Depression After Spinal Cord Injury" Drugs.com (undated): 1-2 http://www.drugs.com/cg/depression-after-spinal-cord-injury.html (Accessed June 28, 2007)

"Depression and Spinal Cord Injury" Research: Spinal Cord Injury Update University of Washington Rehabilitation Medicine 10 no. 2 (Summer 2001): 1-3 http://depts.washington.edu/rehab/sci/updates/01sum_depression.html (Accessed May 9, 2007).

"Dermatology" University of Maryland Medical Center (2007): 1-2 http://www.umm.edu/dermatology~info/anatomy.htm (Accessed May 29, 2007).

"Device Liberates Quadriplegic From Ventilator" *ScienceDaily* (May 15, 2001): 1-3 http://www.sciencedaily.com/releases/2001/05/010515075604.htm (Accessed May 11, 2007).

DeVivo, Michael. "Prevention of Spinal Cord Injuries that Occur in Swimming Pools" *Pushin' On Newsletter* 15 no. 1 (Winter 1997): 1-3 http://www.spinalcord.uab.edu/show.asp?durki =21422 (Accessed May 28, 2007).

DeWitt, David. "Bone graft site pain and morbidity after spinal fusion" Spine-health.com (June 20, 2007): 1-3 http://www.spine-health.com/topics/surg/graft-pain/graftpain.html (Accessed July 7, 2007).

Diamond, Richard P. "How Can People with Disabilities Remain Both Mobile and Safe?" All About Multiple Sclerosis (January 2002): 1-2 http://www.mult-sclerosis.org/news/Jan2002/SelfDefenceForDisabled [*sic*] (Accessed June 8, 2007).

DiGiovine, Carmen P. "Power Wheelchair Batteries" SpinLife.com (2007): 1-5 http://www.spinlife.com/spintips/details/k/Power-Wheelchair-Batteries/a/121/c/3 (Accessed June 9, 2007).

"Disability Discrimination" *The Americans with Disabilities Act* (May 17, 2007): 1-2 http://www.eeoc.gov/types/ada.html (Accessed June 19, 2007).

"Disability Rights" Australian Human Rights & Equal Opportunity Commission (June 8, 2007): 1-3 http://www.hreoc.gov.au/disability_rights/index.html (Accessed June 19, 2007).

"Disability-Parking Crackdowns" New Mobility (January 2006): 1 http://www.newmobility.com/review_article.cfm?id=1101 (Accessed May 15, 2007).

"Disabled People" Direct.gov (May 28, 2007): 1-3 http://www.direct.gov.uk/en/DisabledPeople/RightsAndObligations/DisabilityDiscriminationAct (Accessed April 26, 2007).

"Drug Rehab & Treatment The Disease of Addiction" Casa Palmera Treatment Center (undated): 1 http://www.casapalmera.com/treatments/drug-rehab-treatment.php (Accessed July 9, 2007).

Dryden, Donna M., L. Duncan Saunders, Brian H. Rowe, Laura A. May, Niko Yiannakoulias, Lawrence W. Svenson, Donald P. Schopflocher, and Donald C. Voaklander. "Depression following Traumatic Spinal Cord Injury" *Neuroepidemiology* 25 no. 2 (2005): 55-61.

Ducharme, Stanley. "Testosterone & SCI" *PN* (May 2007): 33-34.

Eimer, Bruce. "Hypnosis and Pain Management" (undated): 1-2 http://www.hypnosisgroup.com/hypnosis/pain_mgmt.html (Accessed May 9, 2007).

Elias, Ilian, Michael A. Pahl, Adam C. Zoga, Maurice L. Goins, and Alexander R. Vaccaro. "Recurrent burner syndrome due to presumed cervical spine osteoblastoma in a collision sport athlete—a case report" *J Brachial Plexus and Periph Nerve Inj* (June 6, 2007): 1-6 http://www.jbppni.com/content/2/1/13 (Accessed July 10, 2007).

Elmore, Judith. "Are You in Pain?" *PN* (November 2005): 16-17.

European Network on Independent Living. Independent Living Institute (December 15, 1999): 1-3 http://www.independentliving.org/docs2/index.html (Accessed April 26, 2007).

"Experimental treatments for spinal cord injury: what you should know if you are considering participation in a clinical trial. A guide for people with spinal cord injury, their families, friends & caregivers" International Campaign for Cures of spinal cord injury Paralysis (February 2007): 1-39 http://www.campaign-forcure.org/(Accessed July 19, 2007).

"Extreme Wheelchair Sports" Apparelyzed.com (2005): 1-5 http://www.apparelyzed.com/support/sport/xtreme_wheelchair_sports_html (Accessed May 3, 2007).

"Evaluating spinal fusion surgery" Spine-health.com (2007): 1-2 http://www.spine-health.com/topics/surg/discorfusion/discorfusion02.html (Accessed January 26, 2007).

"Facts & Figures" Arizona Governor's Council on Spinal and Head Injuries (May 2003): 1 http://www.azheadspine.org/spinal_facts.htm (Accessed August 2, 2005).

"Facts & Prevention Strategies Head & Spinal Cord Injuries in Pennsylvania 1995" Injury Prevention Program Pennsylvania Department of Health (1998): 4 http://www.dsf.health.state.pa.us/health/cwp/view.asp?a=174&Q=197963 (Accessed September 12, 2007).

"Facts and Figures at a Glance Spinal Cord Injury" Spinalcord [*sic*] Injury Information Network University of Alabama, Birmingham (June 2006): 1-4 http://www.spinalcord.uab.edu/show.asp?durki=21446 (Accessed May 2, 2007).

"Factsheet #2: Spinal Cord Injury Statistics" National Spinal Cord Injury Association Resource Center (May 1996): 1-5 http://www.makoa.org/nscia/fact02.html (Accessed May 2, 2007).

"Fatigue" Craig Hospital (undated): 1-3 http://www.craighospital.org/SCI/METS/fatigue.asp (Accessed June 3, 2007).

"Fecal impaction" *MedlinePlus* (October 13, 2006): 1 http://www.nlm.nih.gov/medlineplus/print/ency/article000230.htm (Accessed July 15, 2007).

Fiffer, Steve. *Three Quarters, Two Dimes and A Nickel A Memoir of Becoming Whole*. New York: The Free Press, 1999.

"Finger Flexors" neuroexam.com (undated): 1 http://www.neuroexam.com/content.php?p=33 (Accessed April 30, 2007).

"Focus on Independence Gives Sight to Quadriplegics" The Spinal Cord Injury Zone.com (June 22, 2006): 1-2 http://www.thescizone.com/news/articles/717/1/Focus-on-Independence-Gives-Sight-to-Quadriplegics/Page-1.html (Accessed May 13, 2007).

"Focus on Independence Program Offers Vision Correction Surgery to Quadriplegic Patients" The National Spinal Cord Injury Association (January 12, 2006): 1-2 http://www.spinalcord.org/news.php?dep=1&page=6&list=1015 (Accessed May 13, 2007).

Foss, Jennifer. "Pet-i-cure: The Health Benefits of Owning Pets" Buzzle.com (February 18, 2002): 1-2 http://www.Buzzle.com/editorials/2-18-2002-11780.asp (Accessed June 3, 2007).

"Frequently Asked Questions About Human Papilloma Virus (HPV) Vaccines" Cancer Reference Information. American Cancer Society (January 18, 2007): 1-5 http://www.cancer.org/docroot/CRI/content/CRI_2_6x_FAQ_HPV_Vaccines.asp (June 19, 2007).

Furlong, Roxanne. "Pay It Forward" *New Mobility* (June 2007): 45-51.

"Genetics and Spina Bifida" Spina Bifida Association (2007): 1-2 http://www.sbaa.org/site/c.liKWL7PLLrF/b.2700269/k.5527/Genetics_and_Spina_Bifida.htm (Accessed June 23, 2007).

Goldstein, Lee. *So Far So Good!* Palm Coast, Florida: Paraplegia Press, 2005.

Green, Barth A., M. Alexander Gabrielsen, Wiley J. Hall, and James O'Heir. "Analysis of swimming pool accidents resulting in spinal cord injury" *Paraplegia* 18 no. 2 (April 1980): 94-100.

Groopman, Jerome. *The Anatomy of Hope*. New York: Random House, 2004.

Grove, Ryan, John Norwig, and Joseph Maroon. "Management of a Cerebral and Spinal Cord Concussion in a Professional Football Player" *Pro Football Athletic Trainer* 21 no. 1 (Summer 2003): 1, 3, 8.

Hain, Timothy C. "Benign Paroxysmal Positional Vertigo" Timothy C. Hain, MD (February 27, 2007): 1-13 http://www.dizziness-and-balance.com/disorders/bppv/bppv.html (Accessed May 24, 2007).

Hain, Timothy C. "Vestibular Testing" Timothy C. Hain, MD (November 4, 2004): 1-7 http://www.tchain.com/otoneurology/testing/engrot.html (Accessed May 24, 2007).

Halabi, Safwan. "Hangman's Fracture" MyPACS.net Radiology Teaching Files Case 1775820 MyPACS.net (June 22, 2005): 1-2 http://www.mypacs.net/cases/HANGMANS-FRACTURE-1775820.html (Accessed July 15, 2007).

Halverson, Lynn R. and Katherine A. Belknap. "Fact Sheet on Manual Wheelchairs" Abledata. com (July 1994): 1-3 http://www.abledata.com/able/abledata_docs/manwhch.htm (Accessed June 9, 2007).

Halverson, Lynn R. and Katherine A. Belknap. Abledata.com "Informed Consumer's Guide to Wheelchair Selection" (May 1994):1-6 http://www.abledata.com/abledata_docs/icg_whel.htm (Accessed June 9, 2007).

Hammond, Margaret C. and Stephen C. Burns. *Yes, You Can! A Guide to Self-Care for Persons with Spinal Cord Injury Third Edition.* Washington, D.C.: Paralyzed Veterans of America, 2000.

Hanigan, William C. and Chris Sloffer. "Nelson's Wound: Treatment of Spinal Cord Injury in the 19th and Early 20th Century Military Conflicts" *Neurosurg Focus* 16 (March 2004): 1-12 http://www.medscape.com (Accessed January 31, 2007).

Harrison, Paul. *The first 48 hours.* Oldbrook, Milton Keynes U.K: Spinal Injuries Association, 2000.

Haupt, Jennifer. "Exercise Rx for Nerve Pain" *Neurology Now* (March/April 2007): 32-35.

"Hawaii health status indicators and baseline data (1990)" Hawaii State Department of Health (undated): 1 http://www.hawaii.gov/health/healthy-lifestyles/healthy_hawaii/opd-h2ex.htm (Accessed September 23, 2005).

"Hangman Fracture of the Cervical Spine" SpineUniverse.com (undated): 1 http://www.spineuniverse.com/Ip/ejournal/ag_030400danek_hangman.html (Accessed July 14, 2007).

"Heads Up, Don't Duck! A Player & Coaches Guide to Help Decrease the Risk of Spinal Cord Injuries in Hockey" Michigan Amateur Hockey Association (November 30, 2006): 1-3 http://www.maha.org/coaches/headsup/(Accessed May 3, 2007).

"Health Snapshot Spinal Cord Injury and SCI personal assistant services in Missouri (1995-2000)" Missouri Department of Health and Senior Services and contained in the Missouri Department of Health and Senior Services Missouri Information for Community Assessment database (April 2004): 1-2 http://www.muhealth-org/~momscis/snaps/sciinmoa.htm (Accessed February 7, 2006).

"Healthy People 2010 Chapter 15 Section 15-2 Injury and Violence Prevention" Safetypolicy. org (August 19, 2001): 1-2 http://www.safetypolicy.org/hp2010/15-2.htm (Accessed May 28, 2007).

"Healthy Reasons to Have a Pet" (2005): 1-2 http://www.deltasociety.org/AnimalsHealthGeneralReasons.htm (Accessed June 3, 2007).

"Heart and Circulatory System" KidsHealth® (February 2004): 1-5 http://www.kidshealth.org/parent/general/body_basics/heart.html (Accessed May 29, 2007).

Helping Hands (2005): 1 http://www.helpinghandsmonkeys.org (Accessed May 21, 2007).

Hendey, Gregory W., Allan B. Wolfson, William R. Mower, and Jerome R. Hoffman. "SCIWORA—It's Not Just Child's Play Analysis of the NEXUS Data." *Acad Emer Med* 9 no. 5 (2002): 1.

Hilibrand, Alan S., Karthik Balasubramanian, Matthew Eichenbaum, John H. Thinnes, Scott Daffner, Scott Berta, Todd J. Albert, Alexander R. Vaccaro, and Sorin Siegler. "The Effect of Anterior Cervical Fusion on Neck Motion" *Spine* 31 no. 15 (July 1, 2006): 1688-92 http://gateway.tx.ovid.com/gw1/ovideweb.cgi (Access date unknown). [note: my copy of this article was obtained from the University of Arkansas for Medical Sciences Interlibrary Loan. The pages of my copy do not show the original page numbers so the citation within the chapter must be based on the page numbers from my ILL copy which run 1 through 9.]

"History" Wheelchair Sports, USA (2007): 1-2 http://www.wsusa.org/about.htm (Accessed May 3, 2007).

"Hoffmann's reflex (Johann Hoffmann)" Whonamedit.com (undated): 1 http://www.whonamedit.com/synd.cfm/1560.html (Accessed April 30, 2007).

Hollicky, Richard. *Roll Models: People Who Live Successfully Following Spinal Cord Injury and How They Do It.* Victoria, British Columbia: Trafford Publishing, 2004.

Hollis, Ben. "A History of Spinal Cord Injury" (lecture, Arkansas Spinal Cord Commission monthly support group meeting, Sherwood, AR, February 16, 2006).

"Hollister—US: Continence Care FAQS" Hollister—Continence Care (undated): 1-3 http://www.hollister.com/us/continence (Accessed May 8, 2007).

"Hollister—US: Continence Care—Shadow Buddies" Hollister (2007): 1 http://www.hollister.com/us/continence/learning/shadow_buddies.html (Accessed May 8, 2007).

"Hospital Discharge Database Inpatient Interactive Query Results" Illinois Department of Public Health Health Statistics 2nd Quarter 1998, 3rd Quarter 1998, 4th Quarter 1998 (2004): 1-6 http://app.idph.state.il.us/hospitaldischarge/IPResults.asp (Accessed July 4, 2007).

"How to Help Your Doctor—Easy Steps To Improve Your Medical Care" MedicineNet.com (September 16, 2004): 1-9 http://www.MedicineNet.com/pdf/howtohelpyourdoctor.pdf (May 24, 2007).

"How to Select Wheelchairs or Wheeled Chairs?" uCan Health (2004): 1-2 http://www.uncanhealth.com/all_wheelchairs.htm (Accessed June 9, 2007).

Hudgins, Nancy and Kathleen Charter. "Neurosurgeon Named Head of TIRR's Mission Connect" *Texas Medical Center News* 24 no. 5 (March 15, 2002): 1-3 http://www.tmc.edu/(Accessed September 25, 2005).

"Illinois Estimated Population 2000-2004" Illinois Department of Public Health Health Statistics (undated): 1-3 http://www.idph.state.il.us/health/estpop2000_2009.htm (Accessed July 4, 2007).

"Incomplete C1 Quad" The National Spinal Cord Injury Association Discussion Forum (August 18, 2005): 1-5 http://www.spinalcord.ord/forum/viewtopic.php/?t=416&highlight =brown+sequard (Accessed January 23, 2007).

"Incomplete c5 injury/spastic walking" The National Spinal Cord Injury Association Discussion Forum (January 24, 2005): 1-7 http://www.spinalcord.org/forum/viewtopic.php?t=256 (Accessed May 24, 2007).

"Injury Complications" Paraplegic-Online.com (February 2, 2007): 1-6 http://www.paraplegic-online.com/einjuricomplic01.html (Accessed August 2, 2007).

"Injury Research and Prevention Program Summary" (undated): 1 http://www.oph.dhh.louisiana.gov/injuryprevention/page5316.htm (access date unknown).

Inkster, James. "Vehicle Modification Guide (Part I)" *PN* (August 2006): 66-67.

"Intrathecal Baclofen Pump System" Cleveland Clinic (2005): 1 http://www.clevelandclinic.org/health/health-info/docs/0300/0369.asp? (Accessed May 14, 2007).

"Intrinsic Weakness and Clay Hand" *Wheeless' Textbook of Orthopedics Online* (undated): 1 http://www.wheelessonline.com/ortho/intrinsic_weakness_and_claw_hand (Accessed June 28, 2007).

"Introduction to Caregiving" Caring Connections (undated): 1 http://www.caringinfo.org/i4a/pages/Index.cfm?pageid=3437 (Accessed May 21, 2007).

Invisible Disabilities Advocate (November 23, 2003): 1-15 http://www.myida.org/disabled.htm (Accessed May 5, 2007).

Jackson, Amie B. and Linda Lindsey. "Women's Health and Sexual Function after a Spinal Cord Injury" University of Alabama, Birmingham (2000): 2 http://www.spinalcord.uab.edu/show.asp?durki=32375 (Accessed July 11, 2007) Taken from Research Review, Fall 2000. Published by the UAB-RRTC on Secondary Conditions of SCI, Birmingham, AL. ©2000 Board of Trustees, University of Alabama.

Jacobson, Kurt E. "Stingers and Burners," *Hughston Health Alert* Hughston Sports Medicine Foundation (December 2, 2001): 1-3 http://www.hughston.com/hha/a_12_2_1.htm (Accessed May 3, 2007).

Jaworski, Theresa and J. Scott Richards. "Family Adjustment to Spinal Cord Injury" Spain Rehabilitation Center. Department of Rehabilitation Medicine University of Alabama, Birmingham. (1998): 1-12 http://images.main.uab.edu/spinalcord/pdffiles/FamilyAdjustment.pdf (Accessed July 10, 2007).

Jensen, Gail A., Robert D. Mootz, Paul G. Shekelle, and Daniel C. Cherkin. "Chiropractic in the United States: Training, Practice, and Research" (July 13, 1999): 1-11 http://www.ncschiropractic.com/ahpr/part6.htm (Accessed June 28, 2007).

Johnson, Everlyn S. "Clothing for Special Needs: Clothing for the Disabled" *MSUcares* Mississippi State University Extension Service (November 27, 2002): 1-4 http://msucares.com/pubs/infosheets/is1559.htm (Accessed May 12, 2007).

Johnson, Glen. "Common Indicators of a Head Injury" *Traumatic Brain Injury Survival Guide* (1998): 1-3 http://www.tbiguide.com/indicators.html (Accessed May 1, 2007).

Johnson, Glen. "How The Brain Is Hurt" *Traumatic Brain Injury Survival Guide* (1998): 1-3 (http://www.tbiguide.com/howbrainhurt.html (Accessed May 1, 2007).

Johnston, Laurance. *Alternative Medicine and Spinal Cord Injury: Beyond the Banks of the Mainstream*. New York: Demos Publishing Company, 2006.

Johnston, S. Laurance. "Methyl prednisolone Revisited" *PN* (December 2006): 35-36.

Kantor, Daniel. "Spasticity" *MedlinePlus* U.S. National Library of Medicine and the National Institutes of Health (March 5, 2007): 1-3 http://www.nlm.nih.gov/medlineplus/ency/article/003297.htm (Accessed May 14, 2007).

Karp, Gary. "Choosing A Wheelchair" SpinLife.com (undated): 1-2 http://www.spinlife.com/spintips/details/k/Choosing-a-Wheelchair/a/329/c/3 (Accessed June 9, 2007).

Kaufman, Miriam, Cory Silverberg, and Fran Odette. *The Ultimate Guide to Sex and Disability*. San Francisco: Cleis Press, 2003.

Kelly, Janis. "Late Recovery After Major Spinal Cord Injury—Is It Possible? The Christopher Reeve 'N of One' Study" *Neurology Reviews* 10 no. 11 (November 2002): 1-6 http://www.neurologyreviews.com/nov02/nr_nov02_superman.html (Accessed July 1, 2007).

Kishi, Y, R.G. Robinson, and A.W. Forrester. "Comparison between acute and delayed onset major depression after spinal cord injury" *J. Nerv Ment Dis* 183 no. 5 (May 1995): 286-92.

Klebine, Phil. "Physical Activity After SCI" *PN* (December 2006): 16.

Klebine, Phil and Daniel Lammertse. "Summary Transcript from Aging with Spinal Cord Injury Teleconference for Consumers & Families" Aging with SCI. Department of Physical Medicine & Rehabilitation University of Alabama, Birmingham (October 26, 1999): 1-6 http://www.spinalcord.uab.edu/show.asp?durki=25829 (Accessed January 7, 2006).

Klebine, Phil and Linda Lindsey. "Pain After Spinal Cord Injury" University of Alabama, Birmingham (May 2001): 1-6 http://wwwspinalcord.uab.edu/show.asp?durki=41119 (Accessed May 9, 2007).

Klebine, Phil and Linda Lindsey. "Sexual Function for Men with Spinal Cord Injury" Spinal Cord Injury InfoSheet #3 University of Alabama, Birmingham (May 2007): 1-6 http://www.spinalcord.uab.edu/show.asp?durki=22405 (Accessed June 6, 2007).

Klebine, Phil, Linda Lindsey, and Patricia Rivera. "Sexuality for Women with Spinal Cord Injury" (April 2004): 1-7 University of Alabama Birmingham. http://www.spinalcord.uab.edu/show.asp?durki=51275 (Accessed June 7, 2007).

Klebine, Phil and Linda Lindsey. "Understanding and Managing Respiratory Complications after SCI" Spinal Cord Injury—InfoSheet #19 University of Alabama, Birmingham (September 2001): 1-8 http://www.spinalcord.uab.edu/show.asp?durki=44544 (Accessed May 29, 2007).

"Know Your Anesthesiologist" American Society of Anesthesiologists (1999): 1-3 http://www.asahq.org/patient/Education/know.htm (Accessed May 24, 2007).

Koyanagi, Izumi, Yoshinobu Iwasaki, Kazutoshi Hida, Minoru Akino, Hiroyuki Imamura, Hiroshi Abe. "Acute cervical cord injury without fracture or dislocation of the spinal column" *J Neurosurg Online* 93 no. 1 (July 2000 Suppl): 1-7 online 15-20 printed http://www.thejns-net.org/spine/issues/v93n1/pdf/s0930015.pdf (Accessed February 6, 2007).

Kraus, Jill A. "Stress in Pet Owners and Non-Pet Owners" Delta Society.org (undated): 1-31 http://www.deltasociety.org/download/Jill%20KrausStress OwnersNonPetOwners.pdf (Accessed May 3, 2007).

Kübler-Ross, Elisabeth and David Kessler. "An excerpt from *On Grief and Grieving*" Davidkessler.org (January 2007): 1-3 http://www.davidkessler.org (Accessed May 10, 2007).

LaHaie, Randy. "Self-Defense Articles The Nuts & Bolts of Awareness Learning to Detect Trouble" (2002): 1-8 http://www.protectivestrategies.com/awareness/html (Accessed June 8, 2007).

Lawrence, David W., Gregory W. Stewart, Dena M. Christy, Lynn I. Gibbs, and Marcy Ouellete. "High School Football-Related Cervical Spinal Cord Injuries in Louisiana: The Athlete's Perspective." (1996): 1-9 http://www.injuryprevention.org/states/la/football/football.htm (Accessed May 2, 2007).

"Leg Blood Clot Symptoms" *eMedicineHealth* (September 12, 2005): 1 http://www.emedicinehealth.com/blood_clot_in_the_legs/page3_em.htm#Leg%20Blood%20Clot%20Symptoms (Accessed May 29, 2007).

Letonoff, Eric J., Troy R.K. Williams, and Kanwaldeep S. Sidhu. "Hysterical paralysis: a report of three cases and a review of the literature" *Spine* 27 no. 15 (October 2002): E441-5.

"Life Expectancy Hits Record High" Center for Disease Control. National Center for Health Statistics (February 28, 2005): 1-3 http://www.cdc.gov/nchs/pressroom/05facts/lifeexpectancy.htm (Accessed June 2, 2007).

Lindsey, Linda. "Caregivers for SCI" Spinal Cord Injury InfoSheet #17 Department of Physical Medicine & Rehabilitation University of Alabama, Birmingham (September 1998): 1-7 http://www.spinalcord.uab.edu/show/asp?durki=22479 (Accessed May 21, 2007).

Lindsey, Linda and Suzan Lewey. "Bowel Management" Spinal Cord Injury InfoSheet #9 Department of Physical Medicine & Rehabilitation University of Alabama, Birmingham (September 1999): 1-4 http://www.spinalcord.uab.edu/show.asp?durki=21482 (Accessed April 30, 2007).

"Living with Brown Sequard Syndrome" The National Spinal Cord Injury Association Discussion Forum (February 8, 2006): 1-4 http://www.spinalcord.ord/forum/viewtopic.php/?t=416&highlight=brown+sequard (Accessed January 23, 2007).

"Low Back Artificial Disc Device Approved! PRODISC-L® Total Disc Replacement" Spineuniverse.com (August 16, 2006): 1-3 http://www.spineuniverse.com/displayarticle.php/article1987.html (Accessed January 26, 2007).

Mack, Douglass John. *The Walking Quadriplegic Defeating Paralysis*. Philadelphia: Xlibris Corporation, 2005.

Mack, Susan. "Increasing Housing Options Through Universal Design." *SpeciaLiving* (Winter 2005): 36.

"Mad Dogs and Servicemen," an episode of *M*A*S*H.*

Maroon, J.C. "'Burning Hands' in football spinal cord injuries" *JAMA* 238 no. 19 (November 7, 1977): 2049-51.

Marzo, Donna. "Why Not Me? Dealing with Survivor Guilt in the Aftermath of a Disaster" *SelfhelpMagazine* (September 24, 2001): 1-2 http://www.selfhelpmagazine.com/articles/trauma/guilt.html (Accessed May 11, 2007).

McCaffrey, Patrick. "Traumatic Brain Injury: Recovery and Remediation" The Neuroscience on the Web Series CMSD 636 Neuropathies of Language and Cognition, Unit 12. California State University, Chico (2001): 1-5 http://www.scuchico.edu/~pmccaffrey/syllabi/SPPA336/336unit12.html (Accessed May 1, 2007).

McCluer, Shirley. "Predicting Outcome (Prognosis) in Spinal Cord Injury—Fact Sheet #12" Spinalcord [*sic*] Injury Information Network (June 2003): 1-3 http://www.spinalcord.uab.edu/show.asp?durki=21502 (Accessed July 1, 2007).

McColl, M.A. "A house of cards: women, aging and spinal cord injury" *Spinal Cord* 40 no. 8 (August 2007): 371-3 http://www.nature.com/sc/journal/v40/n8/full/31013321.html (Accessed May 9, 2007).

McHenry, Kenneth. "Controlling Central Pain: What science can't do, doesn't know and won't learn unless you speak up" *New Mobility* (March 1998): 1-12 http://www.newmobility.com/review_article.cfm?id=85 (Accessed May 9, 2007).

McKinley, William, Susan V. Garstang, and Houman Danesh. "Cardiovascular Concerns in Spinal Cord Injury." *emedicine* (December 12, 2006): 1-13 http://www.emedicine.com/pmr/topic20.htm (Accessed May 29, 2007).

McKinzie, John. "Experts: Spinal Cord Injury" AllExperts.com (2006): 1-2 http://en.allexperts.com/q/Spinal-Cord-Injury-2097/indexExp_39306.htm (Accessed July 20, 2007).

"Mental Health: Ganser Syndrome" *WebMD®* (July 1, 2005): 1-2 http://www.webmd.com/mental-health/ganser-syndrome (Accessed July 10, 2007).

Merriam, W.F., T.K. Taylor, S.J. Ruff, and M.J. McPhail. "A reappraisal of acute traumatic central cord syndrome" *J Bone Joint Surg Br* 68 no. 5 (November 1986): 708-13.

Minns, Robert A. and Anthony Busuttil. "Letter Patterns of Presentation of the shaken baby syndrome Four types of inflicted brain injury predominate" *BMJ* 328 (2004): 766 http://www.bjm.com/cgi/content/full/328/7442/766 (Accessed July 15, 2007).

Miracle Mist Plus. http://www.healthylifeandtimes.com (Accessed May 29, 2007).

Miyares, Urban. "Starting a Business" *PN* (April 2006) 14-15.

Moisan, David. "The Invisible Disabilities Page" (November 23, 2003): 1-2 http://mysite.verizon.net/vze20h45/invisible_disability.html (Accessed May 5, 2007).

Morrow, Thomas. "Spinal Disc Technology Seeks To Replace Body's Engineering Marvel" *Managed Care* (June 2005): 1-3 http://www.managedcaremag.com/archives/0506/0506.biotech.html (Accessed January 26, 2007).

National Council for Support of Disability Issues (2007): 1-3 http://www.ncsd.org (Accessed April 26, 2007).

National Disability Rights Network (undated): 1-3 http://www.ndrn.org (Accessed April 26, 2007).

"National Institute of Neurological Disorders and Stroke Arachnoiditis Information Page" National Institute of Neurological Disorders and Stroke (August 4, 2006): 1 http://www.ninds.nih.gov/disorders/arachnoiditis/arachnoiditis.htm (Accessed January 24, 2007).

"NCAA® Guideline 2n 'Burners' (Brachial Plexus Injuries)" (2003): 1 http://www.ncaa.org/library/sports_sciences/sports_med_handbook/2003-04/2n.pdf (Accessed July 10, 2007).

"Nevada's Injury Data Surveillance Project" Bureau of Family Health Services Nevada State Health Division Department of Human Resources (October 2002): 1-90 http://health2k.state.nv.us/BFHS/injury/NevadaInjuryReportFinal.pdf (Accessed July 13, 2007).

"New Study Confirms Periodontal Disease Linked to Heart Disease" American Academy of Periodontology (February 7, 2002): 1-2 http://www.perio.org/consumer/bacteria.htm (Accessed June 11, 2007).

Newey, Martyn L., Pradeep K. Sen, and Robert D. Fraser. "The long-term outcome after central cord syndrome A study of the Natural History" *J Bone Joint Surg Br* 82-B no. 6 (Aug 2000): 851-5.

"Nice to know I'm not alone with Brown Sequard" The National Spinal Cord Injury Association Discussion Forum (November 6, 2006): 1-3 http://www.spinalcord.ord/forum/viewtopic.php/?t=416&highlight=brown+sequard (Accessed January 23, 2007).

"NINDS Arachnoiditis Information Page" National Institute of Neurological Disorders and Stroke (August 4, 2006): 1-2 http://www.ninds.nih.gov/disorders/arachnoiditis/arachnoiditis.html (Accessed June 19, 2007).

Nohlgren, Stephen. "Yes, Medicaid pays for this" *St. Petersburg Times Online* (October 2, 2006): 1-4 http://www.sptimes.com/2006/10/02/Tampabay/Yes__Medicaid_pays_fo.shtm (Accessed June 28, 2007).

Nordlie, Tom. "UF researchers find possible treatment window for spasticity in study of rats with spinal cord injury" *University of Florida News* (November 27, 2002): 1-3 http://news.ufl.edu/2002/1127/spasticity/(Accessed May 14, 2007).

"NRA Gun Safety Rules" The National Rifle Association (2007): 1-3 http://www.nrahq.org/education/guide.asp (Accessed May 28, 2007).

"Number of hospitalized spinal cord injuries by year of injury and survival status, Oklahoma, 1988-1994" OSDH surveillance data (fatal and nonfatal injuries) *Oklahoma Injury Facts* (undated): 1 http://www.health.state.ok.us/program/injury/okfacts/fig78.html (Accessed September 25, 2005).

Nunn, Bob. "Adapted Vehicles: High Costs & Dangers" *PN* (June 2007) 14-15.

Nydam, Katie B. "SCI Pain: What Makes It Worse" *Pain Research Newsletter* Brigham and Women's Hospital (Fall 2006): 1-4.

O'Hare, Pat and Karyl M. Hall. "Preventing Spinal Cord Injuries Through Safety Education Programs" *American Rehabilitation* (Spring 1997): 1-4 http://www.ed.gov/pubs/AmericanRehab/spring97/sp9705.html (Accessed August 2, 2005).

O'Higgins, Holly Laux. "spinal cord injury in wisconsin 2000" (December 2002): 1-48 http://dhfs.wisconsin.gov/disabilities/physical/SCI_00.pdf (Accessed July 13, 2007).

"Oklahoma Injury Facts" Oklahoma Injury Prevention Service (September 2003): 1-88 http://www.health.state.ok.us/PROGRAM/INJURY/(Accessed February 25, 2005).

"Other Complications of Spinal Cord Injury: Autonomic Dysreflexia (Hyperreflexia) Symptoms and Causes" The Louis Calder Memorial Library of the University of Miami/Jackson Memorial Medical Center (1998): 1 http://calder.med/miami/edu/pointis/automatic.html (Accessed April 30, 2007).

"Paralympic Sports" U.S. Paralympics Official Site (2005): 1-2 http://www.usolympicteam.com/paralympics/teams.html (Accessed July 6, 2007).

Peterson, Bradford C. "Pardon the Cliché, but … a closer look" *PN* (September 2006): 74-75.

"Physical Therapy Corner: Burner Syndrome" Nicholas Institute of Sports Medicine and Athletic Trauma (2007): 1-3 http://www.nismat.org/ptcor/burners (Accessed July 10, 1007).

Pointer, Jim. "The Case of the Mysterious Motorist" Alameda County EMS (undated): 1-35 http://www.acgov.org/ems/Presentations/25_The_Case_of_The_mysterious_motorist.ppt (Accessed May 22, 2007).

"Population by State" FactMonster (2007): 1-3 http://www.factmonster.com/ipka/A0004986.html (Accessed July 4, 2007).

"Population by State" Infoplease.com (2007): 1-2 http://www.infoplease.com/ipa/A0004986.html (Accessed July 4, 2007).

"Power Wheelchairs for PALS" ALS Society of Alberta (2006): 1-3 http://www.alsab.ca/equipment/powerchairs.aspx (Accessed June 9, 2007).

Preparing Your Pets for Emergencies Makes Sense. Get Ready Now. Washington, D.C.: U.S. Department of Homeland Security, undated, 1-4.

"Pressure Sore Stages" Spinal Injury.net (2004): 1-3 http://www.spinal-injury.net/pressure-sore-stages-sci.htm (Accessed June 17, 2007).

"Pressure Sores" familydoctor.org (December 2006): 1-5 http://www.familydoctor.org/online/fandocen/home/seniors/endoflife (Accessed May 24, 2007).

"Pressure Ulcer" *Medline Plus* (October 17, 2005): 1-3 http://www.nlm.nih.gov/medlineplus/ency/article007071.htm (Accessed May 24, 2007).

"Preventing Spinal Cord Injury" The Foundation for Spinal Cord Injury Prevention, Care & Cure (1999): 1-3 http://www.fscip.org/prevention.htm (Accessed May 28, 2007).

"Psychologist" *Medical Terminology & Drug Database* St. Jude Children's Research Hospital Memphis, Tennessee (2007): 1 http://www.stjude.org/glossary (Accessed June 10, 2007).

"Quality of Life: What's Important" Craig Hospital (undated): 1-4 http://www.craighospital.org/SCI/METS/quality.asp (Accessed June 1, 2007).

Reeve, Christopher. *Nothing is Impossible: Reflections on a New Life*. New York: Random House, 2002.

Regan, Audrey S. "Maryland State Board of Spinal Cord Injury Research 2003 Research Grant Competition Announcement" Maryland Department of Health & Mental Hygiene (March 1, 2004): 1-4 http://www.fha.state.md.us/oipha/html/spinal.html (Accessed February 7, 2006).

Rich, Valerie and Elizabeth McCaslin. "Central Cord Syndrome in a High School Wrestler: A Case Report" *J Athletic Training* 41 no. 3 (2006): 341-44 http://www.pubmedcentral.nih.gov/articlerender.fcgi?artid=1569555 (Accessed July 11, 2007). [note: my copy of this article was obtained on the Internet. The pages of my copy do not show the original page numbers so the citation within the chapter must be based on the page numbers from my copy which run 1 through 7.]

Richards, J. Scott and Laura Kezar. "Pain following SCI" *Pushin' On Newsletter* 14 no. 2 (Summer 1996): 1-6 http://www.spinalcord.uab.edu/show.asp?durki=21428 (Accessed May 9, 2007).

Richards, J. Scott and John D. Putzke. "Pain Management following Spinal Cord Injury" Spinal Cord Injury InfoSheet #10 (May 2001): 1-4 Department of Physical Medicine & Rehabilitation University of Alabama, Birmingham (Accessed May 9, 2007).

Ron, Maria. "Explaining the unexplained: understanding hysteria" *Brain* 124 no. 6 (June 2001): 1065-6 http://brain.oxfordjournals.org/cgi/content/full/124/6/1065 (Accessed July 10, 2007).

Rossetti, Rosemarie. "Accessible Homes: Building a Healthy Home" (September 1, 2006): 2 http://www.unitedspinal.org/publications/action/2006/09/01/accessible-home-building-a-healthy-home/(Accessed September 28, 2006).

Roy-Byrne, P. "The Neuroanatomy of Hysterical Paralysis" *J Watch Psych* (July 26, 2001): 1 http://psychiatry.jwatch.org/cgi/content/full/2001/26/7 (Accessed July 10, 2007).

Rubin, Allan. "Does Medicare Cover Chiropractic Care?" (undated): 1 http://www.therubins. com/geninfo/chiroprac.htm (Accessed June 28, 2007).

Ruge, J.R. and others [not listed]. "Spinal Cord Injury Without Radiographic Abnormality (SCIWORA) Recommendations" SpineUniverse.com (May 14, 2001): 1-15 http://www. spineuniverse.com/pdf/traumaguide/13.pdf (Accessed July 1, 2007).

Sager, Shana. "'Smart' Clothing Helps Wearers Move" *The Daily Northwestern* (January 5, 2007): 1-2 http://media.www.dailynorthwestern.com/media/storage/paper853/news/2007/01/05/Campus/smart.Clothing.Helps.Disabled.Wearers.Move-2600649.html (Accessed May 12, 2007).

Salzman, Cynthia. "From Injury to Employment" *PN* (November 2006): 42.

Salzman, Cynthia. "Ways to Prevent Pain" *PN* (March 2007): 39-41.

Sanan, Abhay and Setti S. Rengachary. "The History of Spinal Biomechanics" *Neurosurgery* 39 (1996): 1-17 http://www.c3.hu/~mavideg/ns/Sananetal.html (Accessed July 15, 2007).

Sanford, Catherine P., Katrina R. Baggett, and J. Michael Bowling. "Hospitalizations from Injuries: A Report on the Completeness of External-Cause-of-Injury Coding in the State's Hospital Discharge Data North Carolina 1997-1999" *NCPH SCHS Studies* no. 128 (December 2001): 1-10 http://www.schs.state.nc.us/SCHS/(Accessed July 4, 2007).

Schiff, Jeffrey S., Brian Moore, and Jeff Louie. "Pediatric Trauma—Unique Considerations in Evaluating and Treating Children" *Minnesota Medicine* Minnesota Medical Association 88 (January 2005): 1-11.

Schneider, Daniel and Brian R. Szetela. "Ganser Syndrome" *emedicine* (August 30, 2006): 1-6 http://www.emedicine.com/med/topic840.htm (Accessed July 10, 2007).

Schneider, R.C., Glenn Cherry, and Henry Pantek. "The Syndrome of Acute Central Cervical Spinal Cord Injury with Special Reference to the Mechanisms Involved in Hyperextension Injuries of Cervical Spine" *J Neurosurg* 11 (July 26, 1954): 546-77.

Schreiber, Donald. "Spinal Cord Injuries" *emedicine* (August 8, 2006): 1-14 http://www.emedicine.com/emerg/topic553.htm (Accessed January 31, 2007).

"Section 3: Being A Hunter Chapter 6: Hunter Safety" The Ohio Department of Natural Resources (2005): 34-44 http://www.dnr.state.oh.us/wildlife/PDF/chapter6.pdf (Accessed May 28, 2007).

"Selecting a Power Chair" Stuart L. Portner website (April 8, 2004): 1-8 http://www.geocities.com/stuportner/files/power.htm (Accessed June 9, 2007).

Senelick, Richard C. and Karla Dougherty. *beyond [sic] please and thank you: The Disability Awareness Handbook for Families, Co-Workers, and Friends.* Birmingham: HealthSouth Press, 2001.

Senelick, Richard C. and Karla Dougherty. *The Spinal Cord Injury Handbook.* Birmingham: HealthSouth Press, 1998.

Serbousek, Jill. "Dr. Kenneth Burkus talks With Me about a Neck Surgery Procedure: Anterior Cervical Discectomy with Fusion" *InsideSpine* (June 7, 2007):1-3 http://www.insidespine.com/2007/06/07 (Accessed June 28, 2007).

Serbousek, Jill. "More on ACDF with Dr. Kenneth Burkus" *InsideSpine* (June 26, 2007):1-6 http://www.insidespine.com/2007/06/26 (Accessed June 28, 2007).

"Service Animal Information" U.S. Department of Justice (July 26, 1996): 1-4 http://www.usdoj.gov/crt/ada/animal.htm (Accessed May 21, 2007).

Siddall, Phillip J. "Non-painful sensory phenoma after spinal cord injury" *J Neurol Neurosurg Psychiatry* 66 (May 1999): 617-22.

Sipski, Marca L. "Sexuality and Spinal Cord Injury: where we are and where we are going" *American Rehabilitation* (Spring 1997): 1-4 http://www.ed.gov/pubs/AmericanRehab/spring97/sp9707.html (Accessed May 9, 2007).

Smith, Sarah. "The Tale Of The Horse's Tail: Cauda Equina Syndrome" Cauda Equina Syndrome Support Group (August 2000): 1-10 http://www.caudaequina.org/definition.html (Accessed January 24, 2007).

"South Carolina" U.S. Census Bureau State & County Quick Facts U.S. Census Bureau (May 7, 2007): 1-2 http://quickfacts.census.gov/qfd/states/45000.html (Accessed July 13, 2007).

"Spasticity" Sci-Info-Pages.com (March 5, 2007): 1-2 http://www.sci-info-pages.com/other _issues.html (Accessed May 14, 2007).

"Spasticity and Spinal Cord Injury" SCI Forum Reports. Northwest Regional Spinal Cord Injury System (NWRSCSI) (January 14, 2003): 1-4 http://depts.washington.edu/rehab/sci/spasticity.html (Accessed May 14, 2007).

"Spinal Cord Injury Bladder Management" Sci-Info-Pages.com (undated): 1-6 http://www.sci-info-pages.com/bladder.html (Accessed May 8, 2007).

"Spinal Cord Injury" American Association of Neurological Surgeons (November 2005): 1-9 http://www.neurosurgerytoday.org/what/patient_e/spinal.asp (Accessed May 2, 2007).

"Spinal Cord Injury" Mayo Clinic Rochester, Minnesota (August 22, 2005): 1-14 http://www.mayoclinic.com/health/spinal-cord-injury/D00460/DSECTION=3 (Accessed May 2, 2007).

"Spinal Cord Injury" U*X*L Complete Health Resource: Sick! 4 (2007): 1-6 http://www.faqs.org/health/Sick-V4/Spinal-Cord-Injury.html (Accessed April 18, 2007).

"Spinal Cord Injury—Early Days" multikulti.org.uk (undated): 1-4 http://www.multikulti.org.uk/en/health/spinal-cord-injury-early-days/(Accessed April 18, 2007).

"Spinal Cord Injury Facts and Figures at a Glance—June 2006" University of Alabama, Birmingham (June 2006): 1-5 http://www.spinalcord.uab.edu/show.asp?durki=21446 (Accessed June 2, 2007).

"Spinal Cord Injury (SCI): Fact Sheet" National Center for Injury Prevention and Control Center for Disease Control (September 7, 2006): 1-3 http://www.cdc.gov/ncipc/factsheets/scifacts.htm (Accessed May 2, 2007).

"Spinal Cord Injury—Incidence and Prevalence—US and Europe" Google Answers.com (June 21, 2004): 1-6 http://answers.google.com/answers/threadview?id=364371 (Accessed July 4, 2007).

"Spinal Cord Injury (SCI): Prevention Tips" Center for Disease Control. National Center for Injury Prevention and Control (September 7, 2006): 1-5 http://www.cdc.gov/ncipc/factsheets/scipvention.htm (Accessed May 28, 2007).

"Spinal Cord Injury Skin Management" Sci-Info-Pages.com (June 25, 2006): 1-7 http://www.sci-info-pages.com/skin_man.html (Accessed May 29, 2007).

"Spinal Cord Injury Statistics Arkansas" Arkansas Spinal Cord Commission (June 2004): 1-5 http://www.spinalcord.ar.gov/General/stats.html (Accessed September 23, 2005).

"Spinal Cord Injury Statistical Information" Spinal Cord Injury Association of Illinois (undated): 1-3 http://www.sci-illinois.org/Pages/factsheets/literature/stats.htm (Accessed June 2, 2007).

"Spinal Cord Injury Treatment" The National Spinal Cord Injury Association Discussion Forum (April 30, 2004): 1-2 http://www.spinalcord.ord/forum/viewtopic.php/?t=416&highlight =brown+sequard (Accessed January 23, 2007).

"Spinal Cord Trauma" *WebMD InteliHealth®* (2007): 1-3 http://www.intelihealth.com/IH/ihtIH/WSIHW000/9339/28083.html (Accessed July 9, 2007).

"Sports Wheelchair Store" SpinLife.com (undated): 1-2 http://www.spinlife.com/category.cfm?categoryID=8 (Accessed June 9, 2007).

"ST-99-1 State Population Estimates and Demographic Components of Population Change: July 1, 1998 to July 1, 1999" U.S. Census Bureau (December 29, 1999): 1-3 http://www.census.gov/population/estimates/state/st-99-1.txt (Accessed July 4, 2007).

"ST-99-1 State Population Estimates: Annual Time Series, July 1, 1990 to July 1, 1999" U.S. Census Bureau (December 29, 1999): 1-4 http://www.census.gov/population/estimates/state/st-99-3.txt (Accessed July 13, 2007).
StadiumPal and StadiumGal (2006). http://www.stadiumpal.com/and http://www.stadiumgal.com/(Accessed May 8, 2007).

Stover, Samuel L. "Heterotopic Ossification" Spinal Cord Injury InfoSheet #12 University of Alabama, Birmingham (June 1997): 1-5 http://www.spinalcord.uab.edu/show.asp?durki=21485 (Accessed April 30, 2007).

Strauss, David J., Michael J. DeVivo, David R. Paculdo, and Robert M. Shavelle. "Trends in Life Expectancy After Spinal Cord Injury" *Arch Phys Med Rehab* (87) (August 2006): 1079-85.

Surkin, Joseph, Melissa Smith, Alan Penman, Mary Currier, H. Louis Harkey III, and Yue-Fang Chang. "Spinal Cord Injury Incidence in Mississippi: A Capture-Recapture Approach." *J Trauma-Injury Infection & Critical Care* 45 no. 3 (September 1998): 502-4.

Suzuki, Kensuke, Kotoo Megure, Mitsuyoshi Wada, Kei Nakai, and Tadao Nose. "Anterior Spinal Artery Syndrome Associated with Severe Stenosis of the Vertebral Artery" *AJNR Am N Neuroradiol* 19 (August 1998): 1353-5 http://www.ajnr.org/cgi/reprint/19/7/1353 (Accessed July 2, 2007).

Tator, Charles H. and Edward C. Benzel. "Clinical Manifestations of Acute Spinal Cord Injury" in *Contemporary Management of Spinal Cord Injury From Impact to Rehabilitation.* 2nd ed. American Association of Neurological Surgery (2000): 21-32.

"The Body Electric," an episode of *Discover Magazine.*

The Foundation for Spinal Cord Injury Prevention, Care & Cure (1999) 1-2 http://www.fscip.org (Accessed May 28, 2007).

"The World Factbook—United States" Central Intelligence Agency (June 19, 2007): 1-12 http://www.cia.gov/library/publications/the-world-factbook/print/us.html (Accessed June 29, 2007).

Thompson, Vincent. "Population Estimates for 2004: Indiana Barely Maintains Its Rank" *incontext* 6 no. 1 (January-February 2005): 1-4.

Torg, Joseph S., James T. Guille, and Suzanne Jaffe. "Injuries to the Cervical Spine in American Football Players" *J Bone Joint Surg Am* 84 (2002): 112-122.

Torg, J.S., R.J. Naranja Jr., H. Pavlov, B.J. Galinat, R. Warren, and R.A. Stine. "The relationship of developmental narrowing of the cervical spinal canal to reversible and irreversible injury of the cervical spinal cord in football players." *J Bone Jnt Surg Am* 80 no. 10 (Oct 1998): 1554-5.

"Trampoline Injuries" The Foundation for Spinal Cord Injury Prevention, Care & Cure (1999): 1-2 http://www.fscip.org/tramp.html (Accessed May 28, 2007).

"Types of Paralysis" Apparelyzed.com (2005): 2 http://www.aparelyzed.com/quadriplegia.htm (Accessed July 15, 2007).

"UB Researchers Identify Specific Oral Bacteria Most Likely to Increase Risk of Heart Attack" School of Dental Medicine State University of New York at Buffalo (March 12, 1999): 1-2 http://www.sdm.buffalo.edu/news/1990312_bacterial.html (Accessed June 1, 2007).

Ullrich, Phil, Marylou Guihan, and Frances M. Weaver. "Feature Article: Psychological Treatments for Pain and Depression After Spinal Cord Injury: Rationale and Challenges to Implementation." United Spinal Association (March 8, 2007): 1-11 http://www.unitedspinal.org/publications/process/2007/03/08/feature-article-psychological-treatments-for-pain-and-depression-after-spinal-cord-injury-rationale-and-challenges-to-implementation/(Accessed May 10, 2007).

"Uncontrollable Trauma, PTSD and Alcohol Addiction" eNotAlone.com (2006): 1-4 http://www.enotalone.com/article/11325.html (Accessed July 9, 2007).

"Understanding Damage in Human Injury" *The Miami Project E-News* (January 2006): 1-2.

"United Spinal Sues for Parking in D.C." *New Mobility* (September 2006): 1 http://www.newmobility.com/review_article.cfm?id=1197 (Accessed May 15, 2007).

"United States Prescribing Information Lyrica" Pfizer (June 2007): 1-44 http://www.pfizer.com/pfizer/download/uspi_lyrica.pdf (Accessed July 19, 2007).

Vanek, Zeba F. and John H. Menkes. "Spasticity" *eMedicin*e (May 23, 2005): 1-17 http://www.emedicine.com/neuro/topic706.htm (Accessed May 14, 2007).

"Verified Trauma Centers" American College of Surgeons (May 10, 2007): 1-8 http://www.facs.org/trauma/verified.html (Accessed June 19, 2007).

Wald, David A. "Spinal Cord Injuries" AHC Media freecme.com (undated): 1-14 http://www.thrombosis-consult.com/articles/Textbook/42_spinalcordinjuries (Accessed February 11, 2005).

Walsh, Mary Claire. "Arachnoiditis" SpineUniverse.com (September 20, 2006): 1-3 http://www.spineuniverse.com/displayarticle.php/article180.html (Accessed January 24, 2007).

Warren, Sam, Martha Moore, and Mark S. Johnson. "Traumatic head and spinal cord injuries in Alaska (1991-1993)" *Alaska Med* 37 no. 1 (Jan-Mar 1995): 11-19.

Werner, Ruth. "Working with Clients Who Have Spinal Cord Injuries" *Massage-Today* 02 no. 5 (May 2002): 1-4 http://www.massagetoday.com/mpacms/mt/article.php?id=10465 (Accessed June 28, 2007).

"What are the symptoms of an acute spinal cord injury?" Ohio State University Medical Center (2007): 1-6 http://medicalcenter.osu.edu/patientcare/healthcare_services/nervous_system/acutespinal/(Accessed July 6, 2007).

"What is a Neuropsychologist?" *A Neuropsychology Homepage* (1997): 1-2 http://www.tbidoc.com/Appel2.html (Accessed June 10, 2007).

"What is Posttraumatic Stress Disorder (PTSD)?" National Center for Posttraumatic Stress Disorder (2007): 1-3 http://www.ncptsd.va.gov/ncmain/information/what_is.jsp (Accessed May 2, 2007).

Whiteneck, Gale G., Susan W. Charlifue, Kenneth A. Gerhart, Daniel P. Lammertse, Scott Manley, Robert R. Menter, and Kathie R. Seedroff. *Aging With Spinal Cord Injury.* New York: Demos Publishing Company, 1993.

Widerström-Noga, Eva G. and Dennis C. Turk. "Exacerbation of Chronic Pain following Spinal Cord Injury" *J Neurotrauma* 21 no. 10 (Oct 2004): 1384-95.

Wilder, Esther Isabelle. *Wheeling and Dealing: Living with Spinal Cord Injury.* Nashville: Vanderbilt University Press, 2006.

"Winter Season Prompts Concern on Snowmobile Safety" United Spinal Association (January 16, 2007): 1 http://www.unitedspinal.org/2007/01/16/339/#more-339/ (Accessed January 19, 2007).

"Women and Asthma" Women's Health Zone.net (2004): 1 http://www.womenshealthzone.net/zone.net/lung-conditions/asthma/women (Accessed June 3, 2007).

Wood, Jeffrey, Michael O'Brien, Thomas Lowe, Paul Alongi, James Eule, and Robert Vraney. "Transition Zone Syndrome: latrogenic Instability or Natural History?" SpineUniverse.com (January 11, 2003): 1-3 http://www.spineuniverse.com/displayarticle.php/article581.htm (Accessed January 26, 2007).

Wood-Dauphinée, S., G. Exner, and the SCI Consensus Group. "Quality of life in patients with spinal cord injury—basic issues, assessment, and recommendations" (Quality of Life after Multiple Trauma Conference Wermelskirchen, Germany September 29-October 2, 1999): 135-49.

Woodruff, Bradley A. and Roy C. Baron. "A Description of Nonfatal Spinal Cord Injury Using a Hospital-Based Registry" *Am J Prev Medicine* 10 no. 1 (1994): 11.

Woolston, Chris. "Pets: Prescription for Senior Health" (March 23, 2006): 1-2 http://healthresources.caremark.com/topic/stresspets (Accessed June 3, 2007).

Young, Wise. "Spinal Cord Injury Levels & Classification." Sci-Info-Pages.com (June 25, 2006): 1-10 http://www.sci-info-pages.com/levels.html (Accessed January 29, 2007).

Zancolli, Eduardo A. "Claw-Hand Caused by Paralysis of the Intrinsic Muscles: A Simple Surgical Procedure for its Correction" *J Bone Joint Surg Am* 39 (1957): 1076-80.

Zimmer, Lynn and John Morgan. "Marijuana myths facts" Drugpolicy.org (1997): 1-4 http://www.drugpolicy.org/marijuana/factsmyths/index.cfm? (Accessed July 5, 2007).

Zuber, William F., Max R. Gaspar, and Philip D. Rothschild. "The Anterior Spinal Artery Syndrome—A Complication of Abdominal Aortic Surgery" *Ann Surg* 172 no. 5 (November 1970): 909-15 http://www. pubmedcentral.nih.gov/picrender.fcgi?artid=1397362&blobtype=pdf (Accessed July 2, 2007).

Zumwalt, Glen W. letter to the editor *PN* (November 2006): 11-12.

Zwimpfer, Thomas J. and Mark Bernstein. "Spinal Cord Concussion" *J Neurosurg* 72 no. 6 (June 1990): 894-900.

Resources

Note: This is a basic list. It is not intended to be inclusive of every resource in every area. Information listed is included based on my research. I have received no compensation in any form for including or excluding any resource listed. Not all resources will be appropriate for every individual.

*=highly recommended

General

Ableware (catalog)
Independent Living from Maddak, Inc.
6 Industrial Rd
Pequannock, NJ 07440-1993 USA
(973) 628-7600
Fax (973) 305-0841
http://www.maddak.com
custservice@maddak.com

ABLEDATA (information on assistive products)
http://www.abledata.com

An Introduction to Spinal Cord Injury Understanding The Changes 4th edition (free download)
Paralyzed Veterans of America
http://www.pva.org

Crutches and Crutch Accessories
Thomas Fetterman, Inc.
1680 Hillside Road
Southampton, PA 18966 USA
Toll-free 1-888-582-5544
http://www.fetterman-crutches.com/

Disability Product Postcards
P.O. Box 200
Horsham, PA 19044-0220 USA
http://www.disabilitypostcards.com

Disabled Living Foundation (DLF) (UK)
http://www.dlf.org.uk/

e-Bility (list of websites)
http://www.ebility.com

Funding organizations
ftp:/trace.wisc.edu/PUB/TEXT/FUNDING/

Hobbies
http://www.gardenforever.com/index.htm
http://www.gotofreegames.com
http://www.cut-the-knot.org
http://www.puzzledepot.org
http://terrystickels.com8

Human Services Information: Dial 211

Learning About Spinal Cord Injury (free download)
http://www.spinalcord.uab.edu

On The Move: A Financial Guide for People with Spinal Cord Injuries (2002)
The PVA Distribution Center
Toll-free 1-888-860-7244

Pathways to Health: You Do Have a Choice (for cost)
http://www.craighospital.org

Resource Directory and Health Issues
http://www.sci-info-pages.com/orgs_inter.html

Social Security information: http://www.ssa.gov/

Spinal Cord Injury Recovery Center
http://www.sci-recovery.org

Spinal Cord Injury Resources by State
http://www.sci-info-pages.com/state-resources.htm

The Spinal Cord Injury Information Network (free)
http://www.spinalcord.uab.edu

The Status of SCI Research
PVA Publications/Reprints
2111 E. Highland Ave, Suite 180
Phoeniz, AZ 85016 USA
(602) 224-0500 ex. 19
http://www.pn-magazine.com

WRAP (Wellness and Risk Assessment Profile) (free)
Craig Hospital Research Department
3425 South Clarkson St
Englewood, CO 80110 USA
(303) 789-8202
http://www.craighospital.org/scripts/wrap/enter.asp
HealthResources@craighospital.org

Organizations

American Spinal Injury Association (ASIA)
2020 Peachtree Road, NW
Atlanta, GA 30309-1402 USA
(404) 355-1826
Fax (404) 355-1826
http://www.asia-spinalinjury.org

(educates members, healthcare professionals, patients and their families about spinal cord injuries, and other services)

Christopher and Dana Reeve Foundation
636 Morris Turnpike, Suite 3A
Short Hills, NJ 07078 USA
Toll-free 1-800-225-0292
http://www.christopherreeve.org

Institut pour la Recherche sur la Moelle épinière et l'Encéphale
33 0 1 44 05 15 43
http://www.irme.org/

International Campaign for Cures of spinal cord injury Paralysis (ICCP)
http://www.campaignforcure.org

Japan Spinal Cord Foundation
81 42 366 5153
http://www.jscf.org
jscf@jscf.org

List of Organizations
http://www.sci-info-pages.com/orgs.html

Miami Project to Cure Paralysis
P.O. Box 016960
R-48
Miami, FL 33101-6960 USA
(305) 243-6001
Fax (305) 243-6017
Toll-free 1-800-STANDUP
http://www.themiamiproject.org
mpinfo@miamiproject.med.miami.edu

Mobility International USA
P.O. Box 10767
Eugene, OR 97440 USA

(541) 343-1284
http://www.miusa.org

National Association for Continence
http://www.nafc.org/

National Institute of Neurological Disorders and Stroke (NINDS)
31 Center Drive, 8A07
Bethesda, MD 20892-2540
(301) 496-5751
Fax (301) 402-2186
Toll-free 1-800-352-9424
http://www.ninds.nih.gov/
braininfo@ninds.nih.gov/

National Rehabilitation Information Center
4200 Forbes Blvd Suite 202
Lanham, MD 20706 USA
(301) 459-5900
(301) 459-5984 (V/TTY)
Toll-free 1-800-346-2742
http://www.naric.com/
naricinfo@heitechservices.com

National Spinal Cord Injury Association (NSCIA)
5701 Democracy
Suite 300-9
Bethesda, MD 20817 USA
(301) 214-4006
Fax (301) 881-9817
Toll-free National Office 1-800-962-9629
Resource Center (301) 588-6959
http://www.spinalcord.org
info@spinalcord.org

Neil Sache Foundation (Australia)
141 Ifould Street
Adelaide, South Australia, 5000

61 8 8227 1777
Fax 61 8 8232 4311
http://www.nsf.org.au/

Neuropathy Association
(212) 692-0662
http://www.neuropathy.org

Neuropathy Action Foundation
88 Townsend Street, #225
San Francisco, CA 94107 USA
(415) 512-7262
Toll-free 1-877-512-7262
http://www.neuropathyaction.org
info@neuropathyaction.org

Open Doors Organization
2551 N. Clark St Suite 301
Chicago, IL 606014 USA
(773) 388-8839
Fax (413) 460-5995

Paralyzed Veterans of America
801 Eighteenth Street, NW
Washington, D.C. 2006-3517
Toll-free 1-800-424-8200
TTY 1-800-795-3427
http://www.pva.org
Toll-free publication distribution center 1-888-860-7244
(You do not have to be a veteran to purchase publications or subscribe to *PN*)

Rick Hansen Man in Motion Foundation (Canada)
1 (604) 876-6800
http://www.rickhansen.com

Spina Bifida Association
http://www.sbaa.org

Spinal Cord Injury Information Network
http://www.spinalcord.uab.edu

Spinal Cord Injury Network International Hotline
3911 Princeton Drive
Santa Rosa, CA 95405-7013 USA
(707) 577-8796
Fax (707) 577-0605
Toll-free 1-800-548-2673
http://www.spinalcordinjury.org
library@spinalcordinjury.org

Spinal Cord Society
19051 County Highway 1
Fergus Falls, MN 56537
(218) 739-5252 or (218) 739-5261
Fax (218) 739-5262
http://members.aol.com/scsweb

Spinal Cure Australia
61 2 9660 1040
http://www.spinalcure.org.au

Spinal Injuries Association
SIA House
2 Trueman Place
Oldbrook Milton Keynes MK6 2HH
UK
0845 678 6633
Fax 0845 070 6911
Toll-free 0800 980 0501 Open 9.30am to 4.30pm (closed 1pm to 2pm) Mon to Fri
sia@spinal.co.uk
Typetalk number is *0800 95 95 98*
Our Language Line number for people who prefer to speak in another language is *0800 980 0501*
http://www.spinal.co.uk/

Spinal Research (UK)
44 1483 898 786
http://www.spinal-research.org/

The Foundation for Spinal Cord Injury Prevention, Care & Cure
19223 Roscommon
Harper Woods, MI 48225 USA
Toll-free 1-800-342-0330
Fax (313) 245-0812
http://www.fscip.org
info@fscip.org

The Morton Cure Paralysis Foundation
P.O. Box 580396
Minneapolis, MN 55458-0396 USA
(612) 904-1420
http://www.mcpf.org
info@mcpf.org

The Travis Roy Foundation
111 Huntington Ave
Prudential Center, 19th Floor
Boston, MA 02199-7613 USA
http://www.travisroyfoundation.org
(offers grants for home modification, vehicle modifications, wheelchair maintenance)

ThinkFirst National Injury Prevention Foundation
5550 Meadowbrook Drive, Suite 110
Rolling Meadows, IL 60008
(847) 290-8600
Fax (847) 290-9005
http://www.thinkfirst.org
thinkfirst@thinkfirst.org

United Spinal Association
75-20 Astoria Blvd
Jackson Heights, NY 11370-1177 USA

Toll-free 1-800-404-2898
http://www.unitedspinal.org
info@unitedspinal.org

Usersfirst Alliance
http://www.usersfirst.org

Wheelin' Sportsmen NWTF
Toll-free 1-800-THE-NWTF
http://www.wheelinsportsmen.org

Wings For Life Foundation (Austria)
43 0 662 65824206
http://www.wingsforlife.com

Magazines

Ability
PO Box 10878
Costa Mesa, CA 92627 USA
http://www.abilitymagazine.com

Action
United Spinal Association
75-20 Astoria Blvd
Jackson Heights, NY 11370-1177 USA
Toll-free 1-800-404-2898
http://www.unitedspinal.org
info@unitedspinal.org

Audacity Magazine (online)
http://audacitymagazine.com

Careers & the disABLED
http://www.eop.com to susbscribe

Challenge (sports for the disabled)
http://www.dsusa.org/challenge.html

Forward
Spinal Injuries Association
SIA House
2 Trueman Place
Oldbrook Milton Keynes MK6 2HH
UK
0845 678 6633
Fax 0845 070 6911
Toll-free 0800 980 0501 Open 9.30am to 4.30pm (closed 1pm to 2pm) Mon to Fri
sia@spinal.co.uk
Typetalk number is *0800 95 95 98*
Our Language Line number for people who prefer to speak in another language is *0800 980 0501*
http://www.spinal.co.uk/

Neurology Now (free)
P.O. Box 1908
Lowell, MA 01853-9932 USA
Fax (978) 671-0460
http://www.neurologynow.com to subscribe

New Mobility
(publishes consumer guide once a year as part of subscription)
No Limits Communications
P.O. Box 220
Horsham, PA 19044 USA
http://www.newmobility.com

Palaestra (sports, physical education, and recreation for those with disabilities)
Challenge Publications, Ltd.
PO Box 508
Macomb, IL 61455
1-309-833-1902 (Phone/FAX)/Editorial
http://www.palaestra.com
challpub@macomb.com

Paralinks
http://www.paralinks.net

PN
Paralyzed Veterans of America
801 Eighteenth Street, NW
Washington, D.C. 2006-3517
Toll-free 1-800-424-8200
TTY 1-800-795-3427
http://www.pva.org

Reach Out Magazine
http://wwwreachoutmag.com

SCI Life
National Spinal Cord Injury Association
http://www.spinalcord.org/html/sci/

SpeciaLiving
P.O. Box 1000
Bloomington, IL 61702
(309) 661-9277
http://www.specialiving.com
gareeb@aol.com

Sports 'n Spokes
Paralyzed Veterans of America
2111 E. Highland Ave Suite 180
Phoenix, AZ 85016-9611 USA
http://www.pvamagazines.com/sns/

Today's Caregiver
http://www.caregiver.com to subscribe

Internet Communities

Apparelyzed
http://www.apparelyzed.com

CareCure Community
http://sci.rutgers.edu/

Dangerwood The Site to Survive Spinal Cord Injury and Paralysis
http://www.survivingparalysis.com/

DisabledOnline
http://www.disabledonline.com

MobileWomen
http://www.mobilewomen.org

NSCIA Forum
http://www.spinalcord.org/forum

Paraplegic-Online
http://www.paraplegic-online.com

Sci-Info-Pages
http://www.sci-info-pages.com/

Skip's List
http://www.SkipsList.org

SpinalNet
http://www.spinalnet.co.uk/

Spinal cord injury resource center
http://www.spinalinjury.net/

The Paralysis Community
http://spinal-cord-injury.clinicahealth.com/

Newsletters

Emerging Horizons—The Accessible Travel Newsletter
http://www.candy-charles.com/Horizons/index.html

Pushin' On (free)
University of Alabama at Birmingham
Department of PM&R
Spain Rehabilitation Center
619 19th St South-SRC 529
Birmingham, AL 35249 USA
(205) 934-3283
rtc@uab.edu

Spinal Column (free)
Alumni and Donors Shepherd Center Atlanta
2020 Peachtree Road, NW
Atlanta, GA 30309 USA
(404) 352-2020
http://www.shepherd.org

Spinal Cord Injury Update (free)
University of Washington
Department of Rehabilitation Medicine
Box 356490
Seattle, WA 98195 USA
(206) 543-3600
http://depts.washington.edu/rehab/sci
rehab@u.washington.edu

Support Groups

Arkansas Spinal Cord Commission Support Groups (various locations)
1501 North University Ave, Suite 470
Little Rock, AR 72207 USA
Toll-free 1-800-459-1517
Fax (501) 296-1787
http://www.spinalcord.ar.gov/

Spinal Cord Injury Support Group
1918 Birch Ave
Fayetteville, AR 72703 USA

(479) 443-5600
http://www.arsources.org/

Baton Rouge, LA USA
(225) 933-4961
HealthSouth Rehabilitation Hospital

National Spinal Cord Injury Association Chapters and Support Groups
http://www.spinalcord.org/chapters/

Spinal Cord Injury Resources by State including Support Groups
http://www.sci-info-pages.com/state-resources.html

Motivational Speakers

Glenn McIntyre*
McIntyre & Associates
753 Jewel Court
Camarillo, CA 93010 USA
(805) 988-6533
Fax (805) 988-6534
Voice Mail (805) 444-7025
http://www.glennmcintyre.com
glenn@glennmcintyre.com
(keynote speaker, trainer, and consultant)

Joe Rhea
Kansas City, MO USA
http://www.joerhea.com

Arkansas-Specific Resources

Arkansas Assistive Technology Alternative Financing Program
(Low interest loans for equipment purchase, vehicle purchase/mods, home mods)
Arkansas Rehabilitation Services
Attn: Alternative Financing Program
26 Corporate Hill Dr.
Little Rock, Arkansas 72205

(501) 686-2806
http://www.arkansas-ican.org/Alternate%20Financing.htm

Arkansas Disability Coalition
1123 S. University Avenue, Suite 225
Little Rock, AR 72204 USA
(501) 614-7020 (V/TDD)
Toll-free 1-800-223-1330 (V/TDD)
Fax (501) 614-9082
http://www.adcpti.org

Arkansas Governor's Commission on People with Disabilities
P.O. Box 3781
Little Rock, AR 72203 USA
1616 Brookwood Drive
Little Rock, AR 72202 USA
(501) 296-1637 (V/TDD)
(501) 413-1954 (Voice)
Toll-free 1-800-330-0632

Arkansas Rehabilitation Services
1616 Brookwood Dr
Little Rock, AR 72202 USA
(501) 296-1600 (V/TTY)
Toll-free 1-800-330-0632 (V/TTY)
http://www.arsinfo.org

Arkansas Spinal Cord Commission
1501 North University Ave, Suite 470
Little Rock, AR 72207 USA
Toll-free 1-800-459-1517
Fax (501) 296-1787
http://www.spinalcord.ar.gov/
Provides case management and limited financial assistance for spinal cord injury survivors

Disability Rights Center
1100 N. University, Suite 201

Little Rock, AR 72207 USA
(501) 296-1775 (V/TTY)
Toll-free 1-800-482-1174 (V/TTY)
Fax (501) 296-1779
http://www.arkdisabilityrights.org
panda@arkdisabilityrights.org

Disabled Sportsmen of Arkansas
1701 Airport Road
Jonesboro, AR 72401 USA

Employment Services Hotline
Toll-free 1-866-283-7900

Increasing Capabilities Access Network (ICAN)
Arkansas Rehabilitation Services
26 Corporate Hill Drive
Little Rock, AR 72205 USA
Toll-free 1-800-828-2799 (V/TDD)
(501) 666-8868

Mainstream (resource center for people with disabilities)
300 S. Rodney Parham, Suite 5
Little Rock, AR 72205 USA
(501) 280-0012
(501) 280-9262 TDD
Fax (501) 280-9267
http://www.mainstreamilrc.com
mainstreamlr@sbcglobal.net

Preface

Chapter 9 "Thoughts"

Chapter 10 Ways The Spinal Cord Can Be Injured

Chapter 11 The Neck Bone is Connected to the Hip Bone....?

Chapter 12 You Are Not Alone

Chapter 13 A Brief History of Spinal Cord Injury and Treatment

Chapter 14 Why You Need a Sense of Humor After a Spinal Cord Injury

Chapter 15 Know Your Surgeon and Anesthetist

Chapter 16 Surgery for Spinal Cord Injuries

Chapter 17 Communicating With Your Doctor

Chapter 18 The Importance of Peer Support After a Spinal Cord Injury

Chapter 19 Family and Friends Adjustment to a Spinal Cord Injury

Family Adjustment to Spinal Cord Injury (free download)
http://www.spinalcord.uab.edu

Chapter 20 Trauma Centers

Chapter 21 How an Incomplete Spinal Cord Injury is Diagnosed

Chapter 22 Hoffman's and Babinski's Signs

Chapter 23 What Does Paralysis After a Spinal Cord Injury Feel Like?

Chapter 24 An Introduction to Spinal Cord Injuries and Syndromes

Expected Outcomes: What You Should Know A Guide for People with C1-3 Spinal Cord Injury (2002) (booklet 20 pages) (free download)
http://www.pva.org/site/PageServer?pagename=pubs_generalpubs

Expected Outcomes: What You Should Know A Guide for People with C4 Spinal Cord Injury (2002) (booklet 20 pages) (free download)
http://www.pva.org/site/PageServer?pagename=pubs_generalpubs

Expected Outcomes: What You Should Know A Guide for People with C5 Spinal Cord Injury (2002) (booklet 20 pages) (free download)
http://www.pva.org/site/PageServer?pagename=pubs_generalpubs

Expected Outcomes: What You Should Know A Guide for People with C6 Spinal Cord Injury (2002) (booklet 20 pages) (free download)
http://www.pva.org/site/PageServer?pagename=pubs_generalpubs

Expected Outcomes: What You Should Know A Guide for People with C7-8 Spinal Cord Injury (2002) (booklet 20 pages) (free download)
http://www.pva.org/site/PageServer?pagename=pubs_generalpubs

Expected Outcomes: What You Should Know A Guide for People with T1-9 Spinal Cord Injury (2002) (booklet 20 pages) (free download)
http://www.pva.org/site/PageServer?pagename=pubs_generalpubs

Expected Outcomes: What You Should Know A Guide for People with T10-L1 Spinal Cord Injury (2002) (booklet 20 pages) (free download)
http://www.pva.org/site/PageServer?pagename=pubs_generalpubs

Expected Outcomes: What You Should Know A Guide for People with L2-S5 Spinal Cord Injury (2002) (booklet 20 pages) (free download)
http://www.pva.org/site/PageServer?pagename=pubs_generalpubs

Outcomes Following Traumatic Spinal Cord Injury: Clinical Practice Guidelines for Health-Care Professionals (1999) (booklet 31 pages) (free download)
http://www.pva.org/site/PageServer?pagename=pubs_generalpubs

Paralyzed Veterans of America
801 Eighteenth Street, NW
Washington, D.C. 2006-3517
Toll-free 1-800-424-8200
TTY 1-800-795-3427
http://www.pva.org
Toll-free publication distribution center 1-888-860-7244
http://www.scipg.org

Chapter 25 Anterior Cord Syndrome

Chapter 26 Brown-Sequard Syndrome

Chapter 27 Central Cord Syndrome

Chapter 28 Posterior Cord Syndrome

Chapter 29 Cauda Equina

Chapter 30 Arachnoiditis

Chapter 31 Conus Medullaris

Chapter 32 Cervicomedullary Syndrome

Chapter 33 Anterior Spinal Artery Syndrome

Chapter 34 Spinal Cord Concussion aka Spinal Cord Shock aka Spinal Shock

Chapter 35 SCIWORA (Spinal Cord Injury Without Radiographic Abnormality)

Chapter 36 SCIWORET (Spinal Cord Injury Without Radiographic Evidence of Trauma)

Chapter 37 Burning Hands Syndrome

Chapter 38 Bruising of the Spinal Cord (Contusio Cervicalis)

Chapter 39 The Hangman's Fracture

Chapter 40 Hysterical Paralysis

Chapter 41 Closed Head Injury aka Traumatic Brain Injury

List of doctors for brain trauma
http://www.bjscloset.org
http://www.geocities.com/bjscloset/2.html

(I used Dr. Dale Halfaker in Springfield, MO who is in the list)*

Chapter 42 Spina Bifida

Chapter 43 Prognosis After a Complete Spinal Cord Injury

Chapter 44 Prognosis After an Incomplete Spinal Cord Injury

Chapter 45 Prognosis After an Incomplete Central Cord Syndrome Spinal Cord Injury

Chapter 46 Rehabilitation After a Spinal Cord Injury

Chapter 47 Aging with a Spinal Cord Injury

Aging & SCI
PVA Publications/Reprints
2111 E. Highland Ave, Suite 180
Phoenix, AZ 85016 USA
(602) 224-0500 ex. 19
http://www.pn-magazine.com

Chapter 48 Life Expectancy After a Spinal Cord Injury

Chapter 49 Quality of Life After a Spinal Cord Injury

Chapter 50 The Importance of Hope After a Spinal Cord Injury

Meeting Life's Challenges
http://meetinglifeschallenges.com

Chapter 51 Religion and Faith After a Spinal Cord Injury

Chapter 52 Survivor Guilt I—"What Did I Do To Deserve This?"

Chapter 53 Survivor Guilt II—"I Did Something Stupid To Get Hurt"

Chapter 54 Survivor Guilt III—"My Actions Unintentionally Killed or Seriously Injured Another Person"

Chapter 55 Survivor Guilt IV—"Why Wasn't I Hurt Worse or as Badly as So-and-So?"

Chapter 56 Depression After a Spinal Cord Injury

Chapter 57 Addiction After a Spinal Cord Injury

Chapter 58 Spinal Cord Injury Statistics

Chapter 59 Spinal Cord Injury Prevention

Chapter 60 Sports as a Cause of Spinal Cord Injury

Chapter 61 Breathing Problems After a Spinal Cord Injury

Chapter 62 Blood Flow Problems After a Spinal Cord Injury

Chapter 63 Digestive System Problems After a Spinal Cord Injury

Colosan
American Lifestyle
http://www.aragonproducts.com/theproducts.cfm?master=7241
Health Springs
http://www.healthsprings.net/Colosan/colosan.htm
The Finchley Clinic
26 Wentworth Avenue
London N3 1YL
UK
44 0 208 349 4730
http://www.thefinchleyclinic.com/shop/colosan-p-6.html
Oxygen America
http://www.oxygenamerica.com/ProductDetails.aspx?ProductID=523
Health Savers
http://www.healthsavers.info/Colosan-MoreInfo.htm

Enzyme Magic
Concepts in Confidence
2500 Quantum Lakes Dr #214
Boynton Beach, FL 33426 USA
Toll-free 1-800-822-4050
http://www.conceptsinconfidence.com

Neurogenic Bowel Management in Adults with Spinal Cord Injury (booklet) (39 pages)
Paralyzed Veterans of America
801 Eighteenth Street, NW
Washington, D.C. 2006-3517
Toll-free 1-800-424-8200
TTY 1-800-795-3427
http://www.pva.org
Toll-free publication distribution center 1-888-860-7244
(You do not have to be a veteran to purchase publications or subscribe to *PN*)

The Magic Bullet (suppositories)
Concepts in Confidence
2500 Quantum Lakes Dr #214
Boynton Beach, FL 33426 USA
Toll-free 1-800-822-4050
http://www.conceptsinconfidence.com

Chapter 64 Autonomic Dysreflexia (Hyperreflexia): A Life-Threatening Condition After a Spinal Cord Injury

Chapter 65 Skin Problems After a Spinal Cord Injury

Chapter 66 Fatigue After a Spinal Cord Injury

Chapter 67 Nutrition After a Spinal Cord Injury

Alternative Medicine Primer for Spinal-cord Dysfunction
PVA Publications/Reprints
2111 E. Highland Ave, Suite 180
Phoenix, AZ 85016 USA

(602) 224-0500 ex. 19
http://www.pn-magazine.com

EATRIGHT Home-Based Weight Management Program for Individuals with Spinal Cord Impairments
Office of Research Services
University of Alabama at Birmingham
Department of Physical Medicine and Rehabilitation
(205) 934-3283
http:/www.spinalcord.uab.edu/
sciweb@uab.edu

Chapter 68 Pain After a Spinal Cord Injury

Nerve Pain Information
http://www.nervepaininformation.com
(will say it is for diabetic nerve pain or neuropathy)

Chapter 69 Kidney and Bladder Problems After a Spinal Cord Injury

Asta-Cath Female Self-Catheter Guide
http://www.brucemedical.com/ab10001.htm

Cran Magic+
Concepts in Confidence
2500 Quantum Lakes Dr #214
Boynton Beach, FL 33426 USA
Toll-free 1-800-822-4050
http://www.conceptsinconfidence.com

Female Urinary Directors (non-disposable)
My Sweet Pee
http://www.mysweetpee.com
Pee-Zee
http://pee-zees.tripod.com
Stadium Gal
http://www.stadiumgal.com
TravelMate

http://www.travelmateinfo.com
OnTheGo
http://www.womenstandtogo.com
Whiz
http://www.whizaway.com or http://www.jbol.co.uk
Freshette
http://www.freshette.com or http://www.rei.com
G-Funnel
http://www.biorelief.com/store/G-Funnel.html
Shewee
http://www.shewee.com

Female Urinary Directors (disposable)

EZ2P
Kiki Curry
2705 Rosedale
Dallas, TX 75205 USA
(214) 616-5454
http://www.ez2p.com
kiki@ez2p.com
P-Mate
http://www.pmate.com
http://www.pmateusa.com
http://www.pmate.co.uk/(UK & Ireland)
http://www.pmate.nl (Netherlands)

A good website for female urinary products is:
http://www.whenyougottago.com

Specialty Women's Clothing
P-Tights
http://www.ORGear.com
Cabela's QRS system
http://www.cabelas.com

Urinals
Compact Folding Urinal (Male)

http://fulloflife.com
(formerly sold by Rolli-Moden)

Female Urinals
Kant Wate Female Kit
http://www.kantwate.com
Compact Folding Urinal (Female)
http://fulloflife.com
(formerly sold by Rolli-Moden)
UrSec
http://www.gouget.com
Millie
http://www.valuemedicalsupplies.com/millie.htm
Feminal
http://www.brucemedical.com/femfemur.html

Urine Bottle Holder
Posey Urine Bottle Holder
Devine Medical Supplies
http://store.devinemedical.us/8270.html

Incontinence/Take Control
PVA Publications/Reprints
2111 E. Highland Ave, Suite 180
Phoenix, AZ 85016 USA
(602) 224-0500 ex. 19
http://www.pn-magazine.com

Mannose Magic
Concepts in Confidence
2500 Quantum Lakes Dr #214
Boynton Beach, FL 33426 USA
Toll-free 1-800-822-4050
http://www.conceptsinconfidence.com
U-Tract D-Mannose
Kordial Nutrients
Toll-free 1-877-567-3425

Solaray D-Mannose
The Vitamin Shoppe
Toll-free 1-866-293-2267
http://www.vitaminshoppe.com

Chapter 70 Spasticity After a Spinal Cord Injury

Exploring Spasticity
http://www.exploringspasticity.com/

Chapter 71 Chronic Dizziness After a Spinal Cord Injury

Chapter 72 Transitional Syndrome aka Adjacent Segment Disease

Chapter 73 Range of Motion After Neck Disc Fusion

Chapter 74 Changes in Sensation After a Spinal Cord Injury

Chapter 75 Claw Hand After a Spinal Cord Injury

Chapter 76 Dental Care After a Spinal Cord Injury

Chapter 77 Eye Care After a Spinal Cord Injury

Chapter 78 Exercise After a Spinal Cord Injury

Adaptive Cycle Resources
The SKIFORALL Foundation
1621 114th Ave, SE Suite 132
Bellevue, WA 98004-6905 USA
(425) 462-0978
http://www.skiforall.org
info@skiforall.org

Bowflex Versatrainer
(Search the Internet for a used set)

Ergys2
Therapeutic Alliances, Inc.
333 North Broad St
Fairborn, OH 45324 USA
(937) 879-0734
Fax (937) 879-5211
http://www.ERGYS.com
info@ERGYS.com

Exercise Program for Individuals with Spinal Cord Injuries: Paraplegia DVD
Christopher & Dana Reeve Paralysis Resource Center
http://www.ncpad.org/videos/fact_sheet.php?sheet=271

exerSCIzing
http://rrtc-sci.livejournal.com

Flexciser
Toll-free 1-888-353-9462

GameCycle
http://www.thegamecycle.com

Oxycycle
various websites on the Internet

Reck MOTOMed
Toll-free 1-866-738-6552

Recumbent Aqua Bike
Aquatics by Sprint
Toll-free 1-800-235-2156
http://www.sprintaquatics.com

RTI (electric stimulation peddler)
Toll-free 1-800-609-9166
http://www.restorative-therapies.com

Uppertone
GPK
535 Floyd Smith Dr
El Cajon, CA 92020 USA
(619) 593-7381
Fax (619) 593-7514
Toll-free 1-800-468-8679
http://www.gpk.com

VitaGlide
ReHa Medical
Toll-free 1-800-577-4424
http://www.grouprmt.com

Chapter 79 Prescription Medication After a Spinal Cord Injury

Alcohol, Drug and Prescription Medicine Use After SCI (pamphlet) (free)
Spinal Cord Injury Center
Froedtert Memorial Lutheran Hospital
9200 West Wisconsin Avenue
Milwaukee, WI 53226 USA
(414) 259-3657
http://www.mcw.edu/spinal/index.htm

Chapter 80 Caregivers

Caring Connections
http://www.caringinfo.org

National Family Caregivers Association (NFCA)
10400 Connecticut Ave, Suite 500
Kensington, MD 20895-3944 USA
http://www.thefamilycaregiver.com

Preventing Secondary Medical Complications: A Guide for Personal Assistants to People with Spinal Cord Injury (free download)
http://www.spinalcord.uab.edu

Taking Care of Yourself While Providing Care (for cost)
Richard Hollicky
http://www.craighospital.org

Chapter 81 Clothing After a Spinal Cord Injury

Fashion Game
PVA Publications/Reprints
2111 E. Highland Ave, Suite 180
Phoenix, AZ 85016 USA
(602) 224-0500 ex. 19
http://www.pn-magazine.com

Able2wear
Queenslie Business Centre,
Blairtummock Road,
Glasgow G33 4AN
0141-774-8000

AbleApparel
2121 Hillside Ave
New Hyde Park, NY 11040 USA
(516) 873-6552
http://www.ableapparel.com
sales@abbleapparel.com

Access Clothing
Sarah Harruthoonyan
(778) 229-4235
Canada
info@accessclothing.ca

Accessible Corporate Clothing
4 Countisbury Drive
Oakwood, Derby
Derbyshire, DE21 2PA (East Midlands)
01332831102
Fax 01332835201

Accessible Threads
http://www.accessiblethreads.com

Adaptations by Adrian
P.O. Box 7
San Marcos, CA 92079-0007 USA
Toll-free 1-877-6-ADRIAN
http://www.adaptationsbyadrian.com
adrians1@sbcglobal.net

Adaptive Clothing
P.O. Box 936
Exeter, NH 03833 USA
Toll-free 1-800-572-2224
http://www.adaptiveclothing.com
info@adaptiveclothing.com
Adaptive Clothing Showroom
Toll-free 1-877-2-SHOWROOM
Fax (845) 352-3919
adaptiveclothingshowroom@kewnet.com

Adaptive Designs Apparel
43 Oak St
Middleboro, MA 02346 USA

Adaptive Outlet.com
1701 E. Hennepin Ave
Minneapolis, MN 55414 USA
Toll-free 1-866-331-1122
http://www.adaptiveoutlet.com

Buck & Buck Designs
3111 27th Ave South
Seattle, WA 98144 USA
Toll-free 1-800-458-0600
http://www.buckandbuck.com

Clothing Solutions
1525 W. Alton Ave
Santa Ana, CA 92704 USA
Toll-free 1-800-336-2660
Fax 1-800-683-6510
http://www.clothingsolutions.com/
info@clothingsolutions.com

Comfort Clothing
P.O. Box 1396
Standish, ME 04084
Toll-free 1-888-640-0814
Fax (207) 642-7834
http://www.comfortclothing.com
info@comfortclothing.com

Crea Vie
Québec Canada
http://www.creavie.qc.ca
info@creavie.qu.ca

Creation Confort
6015, rue Louis-Hémon, angle Bellechusse
Montréal Québec H2G 2K5
Canada
(514) 728-6889
Toll-free 1-800-394-1513
Fax (514) 728-1807

Creations by Tu-RIGHTS
1097 Kohutek Rd
Victoria, TX 77904 USA
Toll-free 1-877-580-2540
Fax (361) 580-2540
turights@tisd.net

Creative Designs
Barbara Arnold

3704 Carlisle Court
Modesto, CA 95356 USA
(209) 523-3166
Toll-free 1-800-335-4852
http://www.robes4you.com
robes4you@aol.com

Creative Opportunities and Reality Expression
Oakville Ontario
Canada
(905) 339-2831
http://www.coare.com

Darlene's Silver Threads
P.O. Box 1853
Garibaldi Highlands, BC
Canada V0N 1T0
(604) 898-5677
Toll-free 1-877-988-5656
http://www.esCapesClothing.com

Dignity by Design
PMB 250
716 County Road 10 NE
Blaine, MN 55434-2389 USA
(612) 325-4889
http://www.dignitybydesign.com
info@dignitybydesign.com

Discovery Trekking Outfitters
919 Ironwood Rd
Campbell River, BC
Canada V9W 3E5
(250) 286-6577
Fax (250) 286-6576
http://www.discoverytrekking.ca

Easywear Australia
Suite 1/15 Howe Street
Osborne Park, WA 6017
Australia
(08) 9445 2333
Fax (08) 9445 2311
http://www.easywearaustralia.com.au/

Easy Access Clothing
PO Box 6521
26 Meadow DR
San Rafael, California 94903 USA
Toll-free 1-800-775-5536
http://www.easyaccessclothing.com

Easy Does It
P.O. Box 678
Marion, CT 06444-0678 USA
http://www.myeasydoesit.com
support@myeasydoesit.com

Ellipants
PO Box 16,
Ellesmere Port, CH66 2HA
0151 2005012
info@ellipants.co.uk

Epiphany Design
84 Carlton St, Ste 904
Toronto, ON M5B 2P4
Canada
(416) 410-2243
Toll-free 1-888-410-2223
http://www.epiphanydesign.ca
josephross@epiphanydesign.ca

EZYON
Endasa Corporation

Calgary, Alberta
Canada T2T 1E6
(403) 829-8133
Toll-free 1-866-3-ENDASA
http://www.ezyon.com
info@endasa.com
product@endasa.com

Fashion Apparel Magic
Ruth Clark
859 Battle St
Kamloops, British Columbia
Canada V2C 2M7
(250) 314-1849
http://www.fashionmagic.bc.ca
rjclark@fashionmagic.bc.ca

Fashion Freaks
http://www.independentliving.org/fashionfreaks
fashionfreaks@independentliving.org
sells clothing patterns for wheelchair users

Fashions for Special Needs
13A Albert St. W.
Thorold, Ontario
Canada L2V 2G1
(905) 227-1200
Toll-free 1-866-631-1200
Fax (905) 227-1205

Fledglings
Wenden Court, Station Approach,
Wendens Ambo
Saffron Walden CB11 4LB
0845 4581124

Forde's Functional Fashions
8020 East Dr, Suite #317

North Bay Village, FL 33141-4157 USA
(305) 754-4457
Toll-free 1-800-531-7705 or 1-877-754-4457
Fax (305) 757-5447
http://www.fordes.con
fashions@fordes.com

Golden Wear Clothing
Toll-free 1-888-551-9484
http://www.goldenwearclothing.com
info@goldenwearclothing.com

IndependentYou
434 Springfield Pike
Cincinnati, OH 45215 USA
http://www.independentyou.com

Innovative Plums
9906 Foster Ave
Cleveland, OH 44108-1034 USA
Toll-free 1-888-47-PLUMS
http://innovativeplums.com
customerservice@innovativeplums.com

Janska
P.O. Box 66
Colorado Springs, CO 80903 USA
Toll-free 1-866-452-6752
http://www.janska.com

Kutaways
Denise Julian (905) 668-3765
Jennifer Gallienne (905 666-5823
http://www.kutaways.com
Canada

LiftVestUSA
35 West 83 St

New York, NY 10024 USA
Toll-free 1-800-300-5671
Fax (212) 874-2499
http://www.liftvest.com
info@liftvest.com

MJ Designs
http://www.mjdesignsinc.com
contact@mjdesignsinc.com
Toll-free 1-800-722-2021

New Life Easy On Pants
http://members.aol.com/ezonpants.

Nice 'n Cozy
707 Greenwood Ave
Wilmette, IL 60091 USA
(847) 835-4275
Fax (847) 256-4720
http://www.nicencozy.com
info@nicencozy.com

Personal Touch Health Care Apparel
New York USA
(718) 375-1703
Toll-free 1-888-626-1703
http://www.nursinghomeapparel.com
info@adaptiveapparel.com

Pebbels
P.O. Box 5163
Alexandra Hills, Brisbane Queensland 4161
Australia

Professional Fit Clothing
831 North Lake St #1
Burbank, CA 91502 USA
(818) 563-1975

Fax (818) 563-1834
Toll-free 1-800-422-2348
http://www.professionalfit.com
sales@professionalfit.com or kurt@professionalfit.com

Rackety's Clothing
Hilwyn Farm, School Lane,
Longsdon, Stoke-on-Trent ST9 9QS
01538 381430
http://www.racketys.com
Revolution-Underwear
22 Springwell Drive, Countesthorpe, Leicester LE8 5SQ
UK
0116 2775316
http://www.revolution-underwear.co.uk/

Resident Shoppers Service
P.O. Box 4430
5946 Success Dr
Rome, NY 13442-4430 USA
Toll-free 1-800-537-3811
Fax 1-800-560-5575
http://wwwshoppersservice.com
shoppers@ntcnet.com

Sewfits
PMB #213
3005 S. Lamar Blvd Ste #D109
Austin, TX 78704 USA
Toll-free 1-888-SEWFITS
(512) 462-0783
http://www.sewfits.com
contact@sewfits.com

Sew Much Comfort
(sews clothing for injured American soldiers free of charge)
Distribution and fundraising questions
Ginger Doesedel

ginger@sewmuchcomfort.org
Money and fabric donations
Michelle Cuppy
michelle@sewmuchcomfort.org

Sheerlines International Healthcare Ltd
Unit 15, Gainsborough Trading Estate, Rufford Road, Stourbridge, West Midlands DY9 7ND
01384 379700 or 375600

Shop on the Net
82 Bartley Drive #3
North York, ON M4A 1C4
Canada
(416) 759-5755
Fax (416) 759-7706
http://www.shoponwheels.net
kbritto@shop-onthenet.com
maryfay@shop-onthenet.com

Silvert's Handicapped Clothing
Concord, ON
Canada
Toll-free 1-800-387-7088
http://www.silverts.com
customercare@silverts.com

Sizedwell Clothing
Unit 1A Lychgate Farm Industrial Estate
A127 Arterial Road, Rayleigh Weir, Essex SS6 7TZ
UK

Smartypants
5717 SE Ramona St
Portland, OR 97206 USA
(971) 219-5823
http://www.smartypantsworkshop.com

Special Care Clothing
1300 780 755
http://www.specialcareclothing.com.au/
info@specialcareclothing.com.au

Special Clothes, Inc
P.O. Box 333
E. Harwich, MA 02645 USA
(508) 430-2410 (phone, fax, TDD)
http://www.Special-Clothes.com
SPECIALCLO@aol.com

Specially For You
Carolynn Weinert
15621 309th Ave
Gettysburg, SD 57442 USA
(605) 765-9396
http://www.speciallyforyou.com

Spec-L
(209) 235-1981
Toll-free 1-800-445-1981
Fax (209) 235-0590
http://www.spec-l.com

Swartzie's Handicapped Custom Clothing
400 Elquist #2100-2
Battle Mountain, NV 98920 USA
Toll-free 1-800-685-4648
http://www.the-onramp.net/swartzie's/

Up Front Designwear
Feveralls Lodge, Roe End Lane, Markyate,
Herts AL3 8AG
01582 840797

USA Wheelchair Jeans
2600 Osuna RD, NE, #313

Albuquerque, NM 87109 USA
Toll-free 1-800-935-5170
http://www.USAJeans.net

Wardrobe Wagon
1-800-WWCARES
http://www.wardrobewagon.com
info@wardrobewagon.com

Wear-Ease
The Sarah Bra (made for women with upper body disability)
http://www.wearease.com

Wearable Clothing
Queenslie Business Centre
Blairtummock Road
Glasgow, G33 4AN
UK
0141 774 9000
Fax 0141 774 9064
enquiries@wearableclothing.com

YOUCAN TOOCAN
2223 S. Monaco Pkwy
Denver, CO 80222 USA
(303) 759-9525
Toll-free 1-888-663-9396
http://www.youcantoocan.com/

Chapter 74 Colleges and Universities: Returning to School After a Spinal Cord Injury

Contact the Higher Education agency in your state

Arizona State University
Disability Resource Center

Australian Government Department of Education, Science and Training
http://www.dest.gov.au/

Best U.S. Colleges and Universities for Wheelchair Accessibility (2005)
http://www.geocities.com/ketchum4/bestcollegesanduniversitiespg2.htm
(also has vocational rehabilitation information by state)

California Polytechnic State University (Cal Poly)
http://www.calpoly.edu/

Citrus College
Glendoa, California USA
(626) 914-8675
http://www.citruscollege.edu/
dsp&s@citruscollege.edu

Directorate-General for Education and Culture (Europe)
http://ec.europa.eu/dgs/education_culture/index_en.html
eac.info@ec.europa.eu

Disabled Scholarship Opportunities
http://www.scholarships-ar-us.org/disabilities.htm

Disabled Students Programs at College of Marin
Kentfield, CA USA
(415) 485-9406
www.marin.cc.ca.us/disabled/

Edinboro University of Pennsylvania
(814) 732-2761
http://www.edinboro.edu/

Education/Class Action
PVA Publications/Reprints
2111 E. Highland Ave, Suite 180
Phoenix, AZ 85016 USA
(602) 224-0500 ex. 19
http://www.pn-magazine.com

Foreign Languages
http://www.word2.word.com

Free courses
http://www.Suite101.com

Free education on the Internet
http://www.free-ed.net

HERO Higher Education & Research Opportunities in the United Kingdom
http://www.hero.ac.uk/uk/home/index.cfm

Higher Education Funding Council for England
http://www.hefce.ac.uk/

San Joaquin Delta College Disabled Student Services
Stockton, CA USA
(209) 954-5628

Southwest Minnesota State University
Marshall, Minnesota USA
(507) 537-7021
http://www.southwestmsu.edu/

Take It From Us: Strategies and Ideas About Going Back to School (pamphlet) (free)
Spinal Cord Injury Center
Froedtert Memorial Lutheran Hospital
9200 West Wisconsin Avenue
Milwaukee, WI 53226 USA
(414) 259-3657
http://www.mcw.edu/spinal/index.htm

The University of New South Wales
(wheelchair accessible colleges)
http://www.unsw.edu.au/

University of California at Berkeley
Disabled Students' Program
(510) 642-0518
TTY (510) 642-6376
http://dsp.berkeley.edu/sbin/dspACCESS.php?_page=home

University of Cambridge
Girton College-Wolfson Court
Clarkson Road, Cambridge, CB3 0EH
UK
01223 338 892
Fax 01223 311 566
http://www.girton.cam.ac.uk
warden@girton.cam.ac.uk
Access Issues
Mrs. Maureen Hackett, Warden
01223 338 891
Fax 01223 311 566
mh208@cam.ac.uk

University of Cambridge
Queens' College
Silver Street, Cambridge, CB3 9ET
UK
01223 335 511
Fax 01223 335 577
http://www.queens.cam.ac.uk
info@queens.cam.ac.uk
Access Issues
Junior Bursar
01223 335 520
Fax 01223 335 577
info@queens.cam.ac.uk

University of Illinois at Urbana-Champaign
Division of Rehabilitation-Education Services
(the author's undergraduate alma mater)
(217) 333-4603

University of Maine
(207) 581-2319
TDD (207) 581-2311
http://www.umaine.edu

University of Minnesota, Twin Cities
Disability Services
(612) 624-4037 (V/TTY)
http://www.umn.edu/

University of Washington
Disabilities, Opportunities, Interworking, and Technology (DO-IT) Program
http://www.u.washington.edu/
doit@u.washington.edu

University of Wisconsin-Madison
McBurney Disability Resource Center
(608) 263-2741
(608) 263-6393 TTY
http://www.uwis.edu/

University of Wisconsin-Whitewater
http://www.uwis.edu/

Chapter 75 Employment After a Spinal Cord Injury

Books and articles on self-employment
http://www.jan.wvu.edu/SBSES/BIBLIOGRAPHY.HTM

Employment Resources for the Disabled: the Riley Guide
http://www.rileyguide.com/abled.html

The Abilities Fund
(advances entrepreneurial opportunities for Americans with disabilities)
4177 Alyssa Court SW #1
Iowa City, IA 52240 USA
(319) 338-2521

Fax (319) 338-2528
Toll-free 1-866-720-3863
http://www.abilitiesfund.org
benbingle@abilitiesfund.org

Chapter 84 Service Animals

Canine Companions for Independence
http://www.caninecompanions.org

Dog AID (Dog Assistance In Disability)
25 Speechly Drive
Rugely, Staffordshire WS15 2PT
UK
http://www.dogaid.org.uk/
Jude McDermott 01547 510266
Midge Walster 01322 667058
Sandra Fraser 01743 891314

Hero Assistance Dogs (Florida)
http://www.heroassistancedogs.org

International Association of Assistance Dog Partners (IAADP)
http://www.iaadp.org

Service Animal Registry of America
http://www.affluent.net/sara/sara1.htm

Service Dogs (directory)
Cindy Moore
http://www.k9web.com/dog-faqs/service.html
Southwest Service Dogs
P.O. Box 158
Clarksville, AR 72830 USA
(479) 754-3682
http://www.southwestservicedogs.org

Susquehanna Service Dogs
http://www.keystonehumanservices.org/ssd/dogs.php

Top Dog (train your own service dog)
5049 E. Broadway Blvd Suite 102
Tucson, AZ 85711 USA
(520) 323-6677
http://www.topdogusa.org

Chapter 85 Pets After a Spinal Cord Injury

Chapter 86 Sports as Motivation After a Spinal Cord Injury

Disabled Sports USA
http://www.dsusa.org

Supracor Helmet
Supracor
Toll-free 1-800-787-7226
http://www.supracor.com

The National Sports Center for the Disabled
http://www.nscd.org/

Access to Recreation (catalog)
8 Sandra Court
Newbury Park, CA 91320-4302 USA
Toll-Free 1-800-634-4351
http://www.AccessTR.com

Don Krebs' Access to Recreation (catalog)
8 Sandra Court
Newbury Park, CA 91320-4302 USA
Toll-free 1-800-634-4351 (US and Canada)
International (805) 498-7535
Fax (805) 498-8186
http://www.accesstr.com

List of Websites
http://www.google.com/Top/Sports/Disabled
Sports Training and Athletic Competition (list of websites)
http://www.makoa.org/sports.htm

Chapter 87 Transportation After a Spinal Cord Injury

Behind the Wheel—Past and Present
PVA Publications/Reprints
2111 E. Highland Ave, Suite 180
Phoenix, AZ 85016 USA
(602) 224-0500 ex. 19
http://www.pn-magazine.com

Car Talk (radio show and Internet site)
http://www.cartalk.com/content/features/Special-Needs/mobility-links.html
Links to many websites related to adaptive equipment rebate programs, driver rehabilitation and more

National Mobility Equipment Dealers Association
A non-profit association that strives to increase independence for people with disabilities through the provision of safe adaptive transportation
11211 N. Nebraska Avenue
Suite A-5
Tampa, Florida 33612
Phone: (800) 833-0427
Fax: (813) 977-6402
www.nmeda.org

Wheelchairnet.org
Transportation Information
http://www.wheelchairnet.org/WCN_Living/transport.html

Chapter 88 Travel & Accessibility After a Spinal Cord Injury

ABLE to Travel Travel Agency (members of United Spinal Association)
Toll-free membership information 1-800-404-2898 ex. 222
membership@unitedspinal.org

Toll-free reservations 1-888-211-3635
http://www.abletotravel.org

Access Tours
Toll-free 1-800-929-4811
http://www.accesstours.org

Access Travel Center
http://www.accesstravelcenter.com

Access-Able Travel Source
http://www.access-able.com/

Accessible Cruise Planners
Steve
Toll-free 1-800-801-9002
http://www.Love2cruise.com

Accessible Cruises
Connie George Travel Associates
Toll-free 1-888-532-0989
http://www.WheelchairCruising.com

Accessible Journeys
Toll-free 1-800-846-4537
http://www.disabilitytravel.com/

Accessible Portugal
351 919 195 680
http://www.accessibleportugal.com
info@accessibleportugal.com

Amtrak Cascades Program
Discounts for Mobility Impaired Travelers (15%)
Toll-free 1-800-USA-RAIL
TTD/TTY 1-800-523-6590

Disability Travel and Recreation Resources
http://www.makoa.org/travel.html

Free Travel Information
Access-Able Travel Source
P.O. Box 1796
Wheat Ridge, CO 80034
(303) 232-2979
carol@access-able.com

Get Connected to accurate travel information
http://www.travelguides.org

Gimp On The Go
http://www.gimponthego.com/

Greyhound ADA Assist Line
Toll-free 1-800-752-4841 (48 hours in advance of travel)

Handicapped Travel Club (camping)
http://www.handicappedtravel.com

Resources for Disabled Travelers
http://www.disabilityinfo.gov

Society for Accessible Travel and Hospitality
(212) 447-7284
http://www.sath.org

Tent (Wheelchair Accessible)
BlueSky Designs
http://www.blueskydesigns.us/freedomtent.htm

Tips for Travelers With Disabilities
http://travel.state.gov/travel/tips/brochures/brochures_1228_html

Transitions Abroad
http://www.transitionsabroad.com/listings/travel/disability/

Chapter 89 Parking After a Spinal Cord Injury

Chapter 90 Selecting a Wheelchair After a Spinal Cord Injury

Absolute Power
PVA Publications/Reprints
2111 E. Highland Ave, Suite 180
Phoeniz, AZ 85016 USA
(602) 224-0500 ex. 19
http://www.pn-magazine.com

e-motion Push-Rim Power for manual wheelchairs
Frank Mobility Systems, Inc.
1003 International Drive
Oakdale, PA 15071-9226
Toll-free 1-888-426-8581
Fax (724) 695-3710
http://www.FrankMobility.com
Info@FrankMobility.com

Evaluating Wheelchair Cushions
PVA Publications/Reprints
2111 E. Highland Ave, Suite 180
Phoeniz, AZ 85016 USA
(602) 224-0500 ex. 19
http://www.pn-magazine.com

Magic Wheels 2-Gear Wheelchair Drive for Manual Wheelchairs
Magic Wheels Inc.
3837 13th Avenue West Suite #104
Seattle, WA 98119 USA
(206) 282-0760 (In Washington State)
Fax (206) 282-0765
Toll-free 1-866-MAGICWH (624-4294)
http://www.magicwheels.com
info@magicwheels.com

Maintaining Your Wheelchair
PVA Publications/Reprints
2111 E. Highland Ave, Suite 180
Phoeniz, AZ 85016 USA
(602) 224-0500 ex. 19
http://www.pn-magazine.com

Mobility-Advisor.com
http://www.mobility-advisor.com

USA TechGuide
United Spinal Association
http://www.usatechguide.org/index.php

Walking on Your Hands
PVA Publications/Reprints
2111 E. Highland Ave, Suite 180
Phoeniz, AZ 85016 USA
(602) 224-0500 ex. 19
http://www.pn-magazine.com

Whirlwind Wheelchair International (independent wheelchair-producing workshops in developing countries)
http://www.whirlwindwheelchair.org/

Chapter 91 Accessible Living, Home Modifications and Universal Design

Accessible Housing Packet #1
PVA Publications/Reprints
2111 E. Highland Ave, Suite 180
Phoeniz, AZ 85016 USA
(602) 224-0500 ex. 19
http://www.pn-magazine.com

Accessible Housing Packet #2
PVA Publications/Reprints
2111 E. Highland Ave, Suite 180
Phoeniz, AZ 85016 USA

(602) 224-0500 ex. 19
http://www.pn-magazine.com

Accessibility Services (architectural plan review)
United Spinal Association
Dominic Marinelli
Director, Accessibility Services
33 LeoCrest Court
West Seneca, NY 14224 USA
(716) 828-9139
Toll-free 1-866-249-2441
Fax (716) 828-9108
http://www.Accessibility-Services.com

ADAptations
http://www.adaptationsinc.com

Building an Accessible Home
B. Duerstock
http://www.vet.purdue.edu/cpr/bsd/building.html

Concord Elevator, Inc.
(905) 791-5555
Toll-free 1-800-661-5112
Fax (905) 791-2222
http://www.concordelevator.com
info@concordelevator.com

Easy Access for Easier Living
http://www.easterseals.com/easyaccess

Home Accessibility Resources
http://www.okrehab.org/guide/CH06/home-accessibility-resources.htm

Home Plans and list of Contractors, Architects and Interior Designers specializing in Universal Design, Home Modifications, or ADA Consulting
http://wwwuniversaldesignonline.com

Kitchen Design For The Wheelchair User
Kim A. Beasley and Thomas D. Davies, Jr.
http://www.pva.org/access/ackitch1.htm

Mobility Friendly Homes in the UK
http://www.mobilityfriendlyhomes.co.uk/

Silver Cross Home Elevator Guide (USA, Canada, England)
http:/www.silvercross-elevators.com

Simplicity Lift Ramp
Raase Lifts, Inc.
Toll-free 1-800-664-8030
http://www.raaseliftsinc.com
rraab@new.rr.com

The National Wheel-O-Vator Co., Inc.
Toll-free 1-800-551-9095
Fax (309) 923-5091
http://www.wheelovator.com
info@wheelovator.com

The Right Space
A Wheelchair Accessibility Guide for Single-Family Homes
http://www.trspace.com/

"The Visualizer" Device to check blueprint accessibility
2557 NE Robinson St
Bend, OR 97701 USA
Toll-free 1-877-887-2227
Fax (541) 389-7921
http://www.visualizerset.com
info@visualizerset.com

UDA Accessible Ideal Home Plans
http://www.uniteddesign.com/accessible_plans.html

Wheelchair Accessible Home Clearinghouse
http://www.waccess.org/

Chapter 92 Equipment You May Need After a Spinal Cord Injury

Chapter 93 Self-Defense After a Spinal Cord Injury

Accessible Safety (video/information packet)
Richard Diamond
Accessible Safety Tape and Information Packet
12 Sulak Lane, #31
Park Ridge, NJ 07656 USA
http://www.safetyshield.biz

California Personal Safety Programs for People with Special Needs
http://www.kidpower.org/Special-Needs.html

Chapter 94 In Case of Emergency

Chapter 95 Spinal Cord Syndromes as an Invisible Disability

Chapter 96 Disability Rights and Discrimination

Mainstream
http://mainstream-mag.com/

National Council for Support of Disability Issues
http://www.ncsd.org/

Chapter 97 My Introduction to Disabled People

Chapter 98 Sexuality After a Spinal Cord Injury

Sexuality and Spinal Cord Injury (booklet) (free)
Spinal Cord Injury Center
Froedtert Memorial Lutheran Hospital
9200 West Wisconsin Avenue
Milwaukee, WI 53226 USA

(414) 259-3657
http://www.mcw.edu/spinal/index.htm

Sexuality Reborn (video) (1992)
Kessler Medical Rehabilitation Research and Education Center
Kessler Institute for Rehabilitation
(9793) 243-6812
http://wwwkmrrec.org/nnjscis/consumer
info@kmrrec.org

Sex Advice for C5/6 (in French)
http://www.c5c6sex.com/scripts.index.php

Chapter 99 Sex After a Spinal Cord Injury—Men

A Guide and Resource Directory to Male Fertility Following Spinal Cord Injury/Dysfunction
Marie J. Amador, Charles M. Lynne, and Nancy L. Brackett
The Miami Project to Cure Paralysis (2000)
(303) 243-7108
http://www.scifertility.com free download

Sexy Cord
http://www.sexycord.com

Chapter 100 Sex After a Spinal Cord Injury—Women

Reproductive Health for Women with Spinal Cord Injury: Part I (video)(2003)
Reproductive Health for Women with Spinal Cord Injury: Part I (video)(2003)
Dr. Amie Jackson
Department of Physical Medicine and Rehabilitation (PM&R)
University of Alabama at Birmingham
(205) 934-3283
http://www.spinalcord.uab.edu
sciweb@uab.edu

Chapter 101 "How Do I Find a Family Doctor Who Is Familiar with Spinal Cord Injuries After I'm Recovered?"

Additional Reading and Movies

Note: This is a basic list. It is not intended to be inclusive of every resource in every area.
Information listed is included based on my research. I have received no compensation in any form for including or excluding any resource listed.

*=highly recommended

Books

General Guides to Spinal Cord Injury

Ida Bromley. *Tetraplegia and paraplegia 5th edition*. Foots Cray, Sidcup UK: Elsevier Science, 1998.

Adrian Cristian. *Living With Spinal Cord Injury: A Wellness Approach*. New York: Demos Medical Publishing, 2004.

Barry Corbet and others. *Spinal Network: The Total Wheelchair Resource Book*. Santa Monica, California: Nine Lives Press, 2002.

Bernadette Fallon. *so you're paralysed....* 2nd edition. Oldbrook Milton Keynes UK: Spinal Injuries Association, 1987.

Margaret C. Hammond and Stephen C. Burns. *Yes, You Can! A Guide to Self-Care for Persons with Spinal Cord Injury Third edition*. Washington, D.C.: Paralyzed Veterans Association, 2000.*

Paul Harrison. *Managing spinal injury—critical care The initial management of people with actual or suspected spinal injury in high dependency and intensive care units*. Oldbrook Milton Keynes UK: Spinal Injuries Association (date unknown).

Paul Harrison. *The first 48 hours The initial management of people with actual or suspected spinal cord injury from scene of accident to A&E department.* Oldbrook Milton Keynes UK: Spinal Injuries Association, 2000.

Dominic Joyeux. *Moving Forward 3 The guide to living with spinal cord injury.* Oldbrook Milton Keynes UK: Spinal Injuries Association, 2002.

Gary Karp. *Life on wheels—for the active wheelchair user.* Sebastopol, California: O'Reilly & Associates, 1999.

Sam Maddox. *Spinal network—the total resource for the wheelchair community 2nd edition.* Boulder, Colorado: Spinal Network, 1993.

Sam Maddox. *The Paralysis Resource Guide.* Short Hills, New Jersey: The Christopher Reeve Resource Center, 2003.

Sara Palmer, Kay Harris Kriegsman, Jeffrey B. Palmer. *Spinal Cord Injury A Guide For Living.* Baltimore: The Johns Hopkins University Press, 2000.

Richard C. Senelick and Karla Dougherty. *beyond please and thank you: The Disability Awareness Handbook for Families, Co-Workers, and Friends.* Birmingham: HealthSouth Press, 2001.

Richard C. Senelick and Karla Dougherty. *The Spinal Cord Injury Handbook.* Birmingham: HealthSouth Press, 1998.

Esther Isabelle Wilder. *Wheeling and Dealing Living with Spinal Cord Injury.* Nashville: Vanderbilt University Press, 2006.

Subject Specific Guides to Spinal Cord Injury.

Active! Sports, leisure and arts. Oldbrook Milton Keynes UK: Spinal Injuries Association (date unknown).

Peter Axelson, Jean Minkel, Anita Perr, and Denise Yamada. *The manual wheelchair training guide.* Minden, Nevada: PAX Press, 1998.

Peter Axelson, Jean Minkel, Anita Perr, and Denise Yamada. *The powered wheelchair training guide*. Minden, Nevada: PAX Press, 2002.

Rosemary Bakker. Elder Design: *Designing and Furnishing a Home for Your Later Years*. New York: Penguin Books, 1997.

Thomas D. Davies, Jr. and Carol Peredo Lopez. *Accessible Home Design*. Washington, D.C.: Paralyzed Veterans Association, 2006.

Thomas D. Davies, Jr. and Kim A. Beasley. *Home Design: Architectural Solutions for the Wheelchair Us*er. Washington, D.C.: Paralyzed Veterans Association, 1999.

Marcie Davis and Melissa Bunnell. *Working Like Dogs: The Service Dog Guidebook*. Crawford, Colorado: Alpine Publications, 2007.

Irma Dobkin and Mary Jo Peterson. *Gracious Spaces*. New York: McGraw-Hill Professional, 1991.

Stanley H. Ducharme and Kathleen M. Gill. *Sexuality After Spinal Cord Injury: Answers to Your Questions*. Baltimore: Paul H. Brookes Publishing Company, 1997.

Michael Farr and Daniel J. Ryan. *Quick Job Search for People with Disabilities*. St. Paul, Minnesota: JIST Publishing, 2007.

Jerome Groopman. *The Anatomy of Hope*. New York: Random House, 2004

Barbara Hansen. *The Strength Within*. Mahwah, New Jersey: HiddenSpring, 2000.

Candy B. Harrington. *101 Accessible Vacations*. New York: Demos Publishing, October 2007.

Candy B. Harrington. *Barrier-Free Travel: A Nuts and Bolts Guide for Wheelers and Slow Walkers 2nd edition*. New York: Demos Publishing, 2005.

Candy B. Harrington. *There is Room at the Inn: Inns and B&Bs for Wheelers and Slow Walkers*. New York: Demos Publishing, 2006.

Laurance Johnston. *Alternative Medicine and Spinal Cord Injury: Beyond the Banks of the Mainstream*. New York: Demos Publishing Company, 2006.

Gary Karp. *Disability & The Art of Kissing*. San Raphael, California: Life on Wheels Press, 2007.

Miriam Kaufman, Cory Silverberg, and Fran Odette. *The Ultimate Guide to Sex and Disability*. San Francisco: Cleis Press, 2003.

Andrea Kennedy and Craig Kennedy. *Access Anything: Colorad, Adventuring with Disabilities*. Steamboat Springs, Colorado: AccessAnything.net, 2007.

Andrea Kennedy and Craig Kennedy. *Access Anything: I Can Do That*! Steamboat Springs, Colorado: AccessAnything.net, 2007.

Ken Kroll and Erica Levy Klein. *Enabling Romance: A Guide to Love, Sex and Relationships for People With Disabilities*. Horsham, Pennsylvania: No Limits Communications, 2001.

Elisabeth Kübler-Ross and David Kessler. *On Grief and Grieving*. New York: HarperCollins, 2007.

Cynthia Leibrock and James Evan Terry. *Beautiful Universal Design: A Visual Guide*. Hoboken, New Jersey: John Wiley & Sons, 1999.

Cynthia Leibrock and Susan Behar. *Beautiful Barrier Free Design: A Visual Guide to Accessibility*. Hoboken, New Jersey: John Wiley & Sons, 1992.

Kate Lobley. *Sex Matters A guide to sexuality for spinal cord injured people*. Oldbrook Milton Keynes UK: Spinal Injuries Association, 2002.

Maria M. Meyer and Paula Derr. The Comfort of Home 3rd edition A Complete Guide for Caregivers. Berkeley, California: Transition Vendor (effective August 2007 Perseus Distribution), 2007.

Dorothy E. Northrop, Stephen Cooper, and Kimberly Calder. *Health Insurance Resources A Guide for People with Chronic Disease and Disability.* New York: Demos Publishing, 2007.

The Accessible Home: Updating Your Home for Changing Physical Needs. Chanhassen, Minnesota: Creative Publishing International, 2003.

Mark C. Weber. *Disability Harassment.* New York: New York University Press, 2007.

Gale G. Whiteneck, Susan W. Charlifue, Kenneth A. Gerhart, Daniel P. Lammertse, Scott Manley, Robert R. Menter, and Kathie R. Seedroff. *Aging With Spinal Cord Injury.* New York: Demos Publishing Company, 1993.

Margaret Wylde, Adrian Baron-Robbins, and Sam Clark. *Design Details for Health: Making the Most of Interior Design's Healing Potential.* New York: John Wiley & Sons, 1999.

Individual Stories of Spinal Cord Injury

Art E. Berg. *Finding Peace in Troubled Waters.* Salt Lake City, Utah: Deseret Book Company, 1998.

Scott Brown and Sam Carchidi. *Miracle in the Making: The Adam Taliaferro Story.* Chicago: Triumph Books, 2001.

Dennis Byrd and Michael D'Orso. *Rise & Walk: The Trial & Triumph of Dennis Byrd.* New York: HarperCollins Publishers, 1993.

Joni Earreckson and Joe Musser. *Joni.* Grand Rapids, Michigan: Zondervan Publishing House, 1976.

Brooke Ellison and Jean Ellison. *Miracles Happen.* New York: Hyperion, 2001.

Steve Fiffer. *Three Quarters, Two Dimes, and a Nickel A Memoir of Becoming Whole.* New York: The Free Press, 1999.

Richard Galli. *Rescuing Jeffrey: A True Story*. Chapel Hill, North Carolina: Algonquin Books, 2000.

Lee Goldstein. *So Far So Good!* Palm Coast, Florida: Paraplegia Press, 2005. (published only in manuscript form and CD-ROM)

Ron Heagy. *Never Give Up!: How Tragedy Taught Me That Life Is An Attitude.* Irvine, California: Harvest House Publishers, 2002.

Julie Hill. *Footprints in the Snow How Science Helped Turn Tragedy to Triumph.* London: MacMillan, 2000.

Eddie W. Hunt. *A Slide Through Time.* Sistersville, West Virginia: Prospect Press, 1998.

J. Michael Kanouff. *Letters from the Edge: A Travelogue through the Looking Glass of Paralysis.* Tamarc, Florida: Llumina Press, 2004.

Maxine Kumin. *Inside the Halo and Beyond: The Anatomy of a Recovery.* New York: W.W. Norton & Company, 2000.

Douglass John Mack. *The Walking Quadriplegic Defeating Paralysis.* Philadelphia: Xlibris Corporation, 2005.

Bruce McGhie. *Ascent: how one quadriplegic fought for a full life and soared.* New York: Ruder Finn Press, 2007.

Amy Montgomery. *Just An Accident.* Bloomington, Indiana: AuthorHouse, 2004.

Robert F. Murphy. *The Body Silent: The Different World of the Disabled.* New York: Henry Holt and Company, 1987.

Susan Parker. *Tumbling After: Pedaling Like Crazy After Life Goes Downhill.* New York: Crown, 2002.

Christopher Reeve. *Nothing is Impossible.* New York: Random House, 2002.

Christopher Reeve. *Still Me.* New York: Random House, 1998.

Dana Reeve. *Care Packages.* New York: Random House, 1999.

Peter Rennebohm. Be Not Afraid: Ben Peyton's Story. St. Cloud, Minnesota: North Star Press, 2004.

Travis Roy and E.M. Swift. *Eleven Seconds A Story of Tragedy, Courage & Triumph.* New York: Warner Books, 1998.

Matthew Sanford. *Waking A Memoir of Trauma and Transcendence.* Emmaus, Pennsylvania: Rodale Press, 2006.

Kevin Saunders. *There's Always A Way.* Waco, Texas: WRS Publishing, 1993.

Ronald C. Schultz. *Looking Upward: Facing and Reaching Beyond Spinal Cord Injury.* Baltimore: PublishAmerica, 2006.

Randy Snow. *Pushing Forward A Memoir of Motivation.* Dubuque, Iowa: Kendall-Hunt, 2001.

Tilman Spengler. *Spinal Discord: One Man's Wrenching Tale of Woe in Twenty-four Vertebral Segments.* New York: Metropolitan Books, 1997.

Kelvin Taylor. *What Now: A True Story About Overcoming Incredible Challenges.* Springville, Utah: Cedar Fort Publishing, 2003.

Stephen Thompson. *Genesis A Portrait of a Spinal Cord Injury.* Santa Fe: Sunstone Press, 2001.

Heidi Von Beltz. *My Soul Purpose: Living, Learning, and Healing.* New York: St. Martin's Paperbacks, 1998.

Mark Wellman and John Finn. *Climbing Back.* Waco, Texas: WRS Publishing, 1992.

Margie Williams. *Journey to Well Learning to Live After Spinal Cord Injury.* Newcastle, California: Altarfire Publishing, 1997.

Novelized Stories of Individual Spinal Cord Injury

Sherrance Henderson. *Sunshine Has Rain*. Baltimore: Imperious Publishing, 2004.

Kris Ann Piazza. *Impact*. Baltimore: PublishAmerica, 2002.

Collections of "My Story" of Spinal Cord Injury as Motivation for Recovery

Jonathan Cole. *Still Lives Narratives of Spinal Cord Injury*. Cambridge, Massachusetts: MIT Press, 2004. (United States)

David Grundy and Andrew Swain. *ABC of spinal cord injury*. Oxford UK: BMJ Books, 2002.

Richard Hollicky. *Roll Models: People Who Live Successfully Following Spinal Cord Injury and How They Do It*. Victoria, British Columbia: Trafford Publishing, 2004.

Gary Karp and Stanley D. Klein. *From There to Here Stories of Adjustment to Spinal Cord Inj*ury. Horsham, Pennsylvania: No Limits Communications, Inc., 2004. (United States)

Lydia Thomas and Kevin Mulhern. *Link to Life Spinal Cord Injury*. London: Bixtree Central, 1994. (United Kingdom)

Closed Head Injury

Michael Andary, Anthony Gamboa, Jr., Madhav Kulkami, Charles (Nick) Simpkins, John Stilson, Dr. Emanuel Tanay, and Donald Vogenthaler. *Closed Head Injury: A Common Complication of Vehicular Crashes*. Irving, Texas: Mothers Against Drunk Driving, 1995.

Richard C. Senelick and Cathy E. Ryan. *Living With Head Injury A Guide For Families*. Washington, D.C.: Rehab Hospital Services Press, 1991.

Movies

The Men. Stanley Kramer Productions, 1950.*

The Waterdance. No Frills Film Production, 1992.*

The Wings of Eagles. MGM, 1957.*

Appendix—Methodology

The methodology design used in the Spinal Cord Injury Statistics Chapter for estimating the incidence per 100,000 population for states where data is not tracked is courtesy of Phil Klebine, M.A., Assistant Director of Research Services, Department of Physical Medicine & Rehabilitation, University of Alabama, Birmingham.

The incidence of spinal cord injury in the United States is 40 cases per million or 4.0 cases per 100,000 population, as stated previously in this book. For each state for which data was not available, the most recent state population was obtained from the Internet. Assuming the incidence of spinal cord injury in each state was the same as the nationwide incidence, calculations were performed to estimate the state's incidence of spinal cord injury per 100,000 population.

Appendix—Disability Marketing

This is one subject I want to discuss briefly, although it is only indirectly related to the subject of the book. Therefore, I am including the discussion in an Appendix (I have an MBA in Marketing, and I simply could not let this topic go without mention). After all, if you have a spinal cord injury, you are now a member of a target market. Lucky you!

You may find yourself receiving materials in the mail from companies you did not know existed once you subscribe to any disability-related magazine, request product information from a disability-related product company (such as a wheelchair company), or any other source where your name and address can be purchased on a mailing list.

Marketing to the Disabled is a marketing activity that most companies have yet to discover. Disability comes in many forms. Some individuals are born disabled. Others acquire disability through accident, disease, or illness. Others do not become disabled until their elder years. It is a worldwide phenomenon, unconfined to a specific country or region of the world.

Most companies' familiarity with the disabled ends with attempts to accommodate the disabled related to the Americans with Disabilities Act or the equivalent in other countries. Some companies do not even have this level of familiarity.

I searched http://www.Amazon.com and http://www.Bookfinder.com and found one book on Marketing to the Disabled (Joel Reedy. *Marketing to Consumers with Disabilities.* Chicago: Probus Publishing Company, 1993).

I had a little more luck searching the Internet. I found one organization, The National Organization on Disability, with a section on Marketing to People with Disabilities. The organization and some of the resources it provides follow:

National Organization on Disability
910 Sixteenth Street, N.W. Suite 600
Washington, D.C. 20006
(202) 293-5960
Fax (202) 293-7999
TTY (202) 293-5968

http://www.nod.org
ability@nod.org

The website also includes publications and casting agencies for the disabled, a short course on Marketing to Customers with Disabilities for businesses, a section on website accessibility for the Disabled, guidelines for writing about the Disabled with sensitivity and using appropriate language, information on a Georgia website offering Disability sensitivity training, information from a 2004 Disability forum conference, and two articles, "Marketing the Disability Market: iCan!, But Can It?" and "What Marketers Should Know About People with Disabilities" among other resources.

I will admit I have mixed feelings on increasing the amount of marketing toward Disabled consumers. On the one hand, I want my needs as a Disabled consumer recognized. On the other hand, I'm not sure the world needs more Marketing.

One advantage I can see to the increased awareness on the part of companies toward consumers with Disabilities is perhaps those same companies will become more aware of the needs of their Disabled employees or will become less reluctant to hire the Disabled. Some corporate Diversity efforts also include the Disabled as a targeted group. Small companies are less likely to hire the Disabled because of the risk of insurance premiums skyrocketing.

Other Publications by Carolyn Boyles

Non-fiction

"Paralegal Management in the Rural Law Office," *The Paralegal* 4 no. 5(September/October 1988).
"Help Wanted: A Profile of Institutional Research 1970-1985" *Research in Higher Education* 28 no. 3 (May 1988).
Paul Langston and Carolyn Boyles, "The Search for a New Mission and New Admissions Standards: A Case Study" *College and University* 62 no. 3 (Spring 1987).

Fiction

"A 'SCI' of Relief" *Audacity Magazine* (online) (September 2007).
"A Time To Learn" *The Storyteller* (October/November/December 2007).
"The Great Winslow Train Robbery" *Echoes of the Ozarks Vol. III* Ozark Writers League (November 2007).

Contacting the Author

Carolyn Boyles
P.O. Box 94174
North Little Rock, AR 72190 USA
(AR is Arkansas)
www.carolynboyles.com
CBoyles@aol.com

If you would like to contact me relating to this book, my mailing address and e-mail address are above.

If the book helped you in any way, please post a positive comment on http://www.amazon.com about the book. Tell anybody you think might be benefitted by the book.

I am interested in freelance writing opportunities, fiction or non-fiction. I also do ghostwriting. If you have a proposal, please contact me.

Index

978-0-595-45864-
0-595-45864-5

14501989R00328

Made in the USA
Lexington, KY
02 April 2012